Endocrine Pathology

Editor

JUSTINE A. BARLETTA

SURGICAL PATHOLOGY CLINICS

www.surgpath.theclinics.com

Consulting Editor
JASON L. HORNICK

December 2019 • Volume 12 • Number 4

ELSEVIER

1600 John F. Kennedy Boulevard • Suite 1800 • Philadelphia, Pennsylvania, 19103-2899

http://www.theclinics.com

SURGICAL PATHOLOGY CLINICS Volume 12, Number 4
December 2019 ISSN 1875-9181, ISBN-13: 978-0-323-73307-6

Editor: Katerina Heidhausen
Developmental Editor: Donald Mumford

Surgical Pathology Clinics (ISSN 1875-9181) is published quarterly by Elsevier Inc., 360 Park Avenue South, New York, NY 10010. Months of issue are March, June, September, and December. Business and Editorial Office: Elsevier Inc., 1600 John F. Kennedy Blvd., Ste. 1800, Philadelphia, PA 19103-2899. Accounting and Circulation Offices: Elsevier Inc., 3251 Riverport Lane, Maryland Heights, MO 63043. Periodicals postage paid at New York, NY and at additional mailing offices. Subscription prices are $213.00 per year (US individuals), $279.00 per year (US institutions), $100.00 per year (US students/residents), $272.00 per year (Canadian individuals), $318.00 per year (Canadian Institutions), $263.00 per year (foreign individuals), $318.00 per year (foreign institutions), and $120.00 per year (international & Canadian students/residents). Foreign air speed delivery is included in all *Clinics*' subscription prices. All prices are subject to change without notice. **POSTMASTER:** Send address changes to *Surgical Pathology Clinics*, Elsevier, 3251 Riverport Lane, Maryland Heights, MO 63043. **Customer Service: 1-800-654-2452 (US). From outside the United States, call 1-314-447-8871. Fax: 1-314-447-8029. E-mail: JournalsCustomerServiceusa@elsevier.com (for print support)** and **JournalsOnlineSupport-usa@elsevier.com (for online support)**.

Reprints. For copies of 100 or more, of articles in this publication, please contact the Commercial Reprints Department, Elsevier Inc., 360 Park Avenue South, New York, NY 10010-1710. Tel. 212-633-3874; Fax: 212-633-3820; E-mail: reprints@elsevier.com.

Surgical Pathology Clinics of North America is covered in *MEDLINE/PubMed (Index Medicus)*.

Contributors

CONSULTING EDITOR

JASON L. HORNICK, MD, PhD
Director of Surgical Pathology and Immunohistochemistry, Brigham and Women's Hospital, Professor of Pathology, Harvard Medical School, Boston, Massachusetts, USA

EDITOR

JUSTINE A. BARLETTA, MD
Chief, Endocrine Pathology Service, Department of Pathology, Brigham and Women's Hospital, Associate Professor of Pathology, Harvard Medical School, Boston, Massachusetts, USA

AUTHORS

ADEBOWALE J. ADENIRAN, MD
Associate Professor of Pathology, Director of Cytopathology, Department of Pathology, Yale School of Medicine, New Haven, Connecticut, USA

TREVOR E. ANGELL, MD
Assistant Professor, Division of Endocrinology, Diabetes, and Metabolism, Keck School of Medicine of USC, University of Southern California, Los Angeles, California, USA

ANDREA BARBIERI, MD
Assistant Professor, Department of Pathology, Yale School of Medicine, Yale New Haven Hospital, New Haven, Connecticut, USA

JUSTINE A. BARLETTA, MD
Chief, Endocrine Pathology Service, Department of Pathology, Brigham and Women's Hospital, Associate Professor of Pathology, Harvard Medical School, Boston, Massachusetts, USA

JENNIFER CHAN, MD, MPH
Clinical Director, Program in Carcinoid and Neuroendocrine Tumors, Department of Medical Oncology, Dana-Farber Cancer Institute, Assistant Professor of Medicine, Harvard Medical School, Boston, Massachusetts, USA

NICOLE A. CIPRIANI, MD
Associate Professor, Department of Pathology, The University of Chicago, Chicago, Illinois, USA

WILLIAM C. FAQUIN, MD, PhD
Professor of Pathology, Harvard Medical School, Department of Pathology, Massachusetts General Hospital, Boston, Massachusetts, USA

JOANNA GIBSON, MD, PhD
Associate Professor, Department of Pathology, Yale School of Medicine, Yale New Haven Hospital, New Haven, Connecticut, USA

JULIE GUILMETTE, MD
Department of Pathology, Charles-Lemoyne Hospital, Sherbrooke University Affiliated Health Care Center, Greenfield Park, Quebec, Canada

MOHAMED RIZWAN HAROON AL RASHEED, MD
Department of Pathology, Memorial Sloan Kettering Cancer Center, New York, New York, USA

ETHAN JAMES HARRIS, BS
University of Illinois College of Medicine, Chicago, Illinois, USA

ANJELICA HODGSON, MD
Resident, Department of Laboratory Medicine and Pathobiology, University of Toronto, Toronto, Ontario, Canada

JULIAN HUANG, AB
Yale School of Medicine, New Haven, Connecticut, USA

YIN P. HUNG, MD, PhD
Assistant, Department of Pathology, Massachusetts General Hospital, Harvard Medical School, Boston, Massachusetts, USA

KERRY KILBRIDGE, MD
Brigham and Women's Hospital, Harvard Medical School, Department of Surgery, Lank Center for Genitourinary Oncology, Dana-Farber Cancer Institute, Boston, Massachusetts, USA

MELISSA G. LECHNER, MD, PhD
Division of Endocrinology, Diabetes, and Metabolism, David Geffen School of Medicine, University of California, Los Angeles, Los Angeles, California, USA

JOCHEN H. LORCH, MD, MS
Department of Medical Oncology, Dana-Farber Cancer Institute, Boston, Massachusetts, USA

OZGUR METE, MD
Consultant in Endocrine Pathology, Department of Pathology, University Health Network, Associate Professor, Department of Laboratory Medicine and Pathobiology, The University of Toronto, Toronto, Ontario, Canada

MATTHEW NEHS, MD
Brigham and Women's Hospital, Harvard Medical School, Department of Surgery, Dana-Farber Cancer Institute, Boston, Massachusetts, USA

SARA PAKBAZ, MD
Clinical Fellow, Department of Pathology, University Health Network, University of Toronto, Toronto, Ontario, Canada

NATALIE PATEL, MD
Fellow, Gastrointestinal and Pancreaticobiliary Pathology, Department of Pathology, Yale School of Medicine, Yale New Haven Hospital, New Haven, Connecticut, USA

KIMBERLY PEREZ, MD
Program in Carcinoid and Neuroendocrine Tumors, Department of Medical Oncology, Dana-Farber Cancer Institute, Assistant Professor of Medicine, Harvard Medical School, Boston, Massachusetts, USA

STEPHANIE SMOOKE PRAW, MD
Associate Professor, Division of Endocrinology, Diabetes, and Metabolism, David Geffen School of Medicine, University of California, Los Angeles, Los Angeles, California, USA

ESTHER DIANA ROSSI, MD, PhD, MIAC
Affiliated Professor of Anatomic Pathology, Division of Anatomic Pathology and Histology, Catholic University of Sacred Heart, Rome, Italy

PETER M. SADOW, MD, PhD
Director, Head and Neck Pathology Division, Massachusetts General Hospital, Associate Professor of Pathology, Harvard Medical School, Boston, Massachusetts, USA

ANAND VAIDYA, MD, MMSc
Division of Endocrinology, Diabetes and Hypertension, Department of Medicine, Center for Adrenal Disorders, Brigham and Women's Hospital, Harvard Medical School, Boston, Massachusetts, USA

KRISTINE S. WONG, MD
Department of Pathology, Brigham and Women's Hospital, Harvard Medical School, Boston, Massachusetts, USA

BIN XU, MD, PhD
Department of Pathology, Memorial Sloan Kettering Cancer Center, New York, New York, USA

Contents

Preface: Endocrine Pathology: Advances, Updates, and Diagnostic Pearls xi

Justine A. Barletta

Pitfalls in Thyroid Cytopathology 865

Esther Diana Rossi, Adebowale J. Adeniran, and William C. Faquin

Fine-needle aspiration (FNA) is among the first diagnostic tools used in the evaluation of thyroid nodules. It has the ability to triage patients with benign and malignant lesions, thus defining the optimum clinical and/or surgical management. The Bethesda System for Reporting Thyroid Cytopathology has found worldwide acceptance. Thyroid FNA offers high positive predictive value (97%–99%), with sensitivities and specificities of 65% to 99% and 72% to 100%, respectively. Nonetheless, many potential diagnostic pitfalls exist that can lead to false-positive and/or false-negative results. This article discusses several of the potential pitfalls in the cytologic evaluation of thyroid lesions.

Prognostic Parameters in Differentiated Thyroid Carcinomas 883

Nicole A. Cipriani

Differentiated thyroid carcinomas make up most thyroid malignancies. The AJCC staging system and the ATA risk prediction system are the best predictors of mortality and recurrence, respectively. Key factors to be identified and reported by pathologists are reviewed in this article and include: (1) aggressive histologic variants of papillary thyroid carcinoma (including tall cell, columnar cell, and hobnail variants); (2) presence of gross extrathyroidal extension (into skeletal muscle or adjacent organs); (3) angioinvasion (including number of foci); (4) number, anatomic level, and size of lymph node metastases; (4) extranodal extension; (5) genetics (especially BRAF V600E or TERT promoter mutation).

Thyroid Tumors You Don't Want to Miss 901

Kristine S. Wong and Justine A. Barletta

This article examines more uncommon thyroid entities, including anaplastic thyroid carcinoma, poorly differentiated thyroid carcinoma, rare papillary thyroid carcinoma variants, medullary thyroid carcinoma, non-invasive follicular thyroid neoplasm with papillary-like nuclear features (NIFTP), and multiple adenomatous nodules in the setting of Cowden syndrome. These entities were chosen based on their clinical significance and because they can be diagnostically challenging due to their morphologic diversity and overlap with other thyroid tumors. This article addresses the diagnostic features of each entity, focusing on how to avoid potential pitfalls and mimics while also highlighting the clinical implications of each diagnosis.

Molecular Alterations in Thyroid Carcinoma 921

Mohamed Rizwan Haroon Al Rasheed and Bin Xu

Thyroid carcinoma is the most common cancer in the endocrine system. Recent advances, using next-generation sequencing, have shed light on the molecular pathogenesis of thyroid cancer. Constitutional activation of the mitogen-activated protein kinase pathway through RAS mutation, BRAF mutation, and/or fusions involving receptor tyrosine kinase (eg, RET-PTC) plays a central role in tumorigenesis and opens doors to promising tyrosine kinase inhibitor therapy. Several molecular signatures, such as TERT promoter mutation and TP53 mutation, are associated with tumor progression. This article provides a concise and updated summary of the main genetic alterations in thyroid carcinoma.

Treatment of Differentiated Thyroid Carcinomas 931

Melissa G. Lechner, Stephanie Smooke Praw, and Trevor E. Angell

Differentiated thyroid cancer (DTC) is the most common thyroid cancer and is frequently encountered in clinical practice. The incidence of DTC has increased significantly over the past three decades. Surgical resection, radioactive iodine (RAI), and levothyroxine suppression therapy remain the primary modalities for DTC treatment. Active surveillance for low-risk thyroid cancer may be an alternative to immediate surgery for appropriately selected patients. Patient characteristics influence treatment selection and intensity. In the subset of patients with progressive distant metastatic disease not amenable to treatment with surgery or RAI, novel agents, including targeted therapies and immunotherapy, should be considered.

Treatment of Aggressive Thyroid Cancer 943

Julian Huang, Ethan James Harris, and Jochen H. Lorch

Although thyroid cancer generally has a good prognosis, there is a subset of patients for whom standard care (ie, treatment limited to surgery or surgery plus radioactive iodine) is either not appropriate because of the aggressive nature of their disease or not sufficient because of disease progression through standard treatment. Most of these tumors fall into 1 of 3 groups: radioactive iodine–refractory differentiated thyroid carcinoma, anaplastic thyroid carcinoma, or progressive medullary thyroid carcinoma. Major classes of treatments in clinical development for these aggressive thyroid tumors include tyrosine kinase inhibitors, mammalian target of rapamycin inhibitors, and mitogen-activated protein kinase kinase inhibitors.

A Guide to Pheochromocytomas and Paragangliomas 951

Julie Guilmette and Peter M. Sadow

Pheochromocytomas and extra-adrenal paragangliomas are rare neuroendocrine neoplasms with characteristic histologic and immunohistochemical features. These tumors can arise in several anatomic locations, necessitating that their diagnostic recognition extends beyond the realm of endocrine pathology. A practical and reproducible risk stratification system for these tumors is still in development. In this rapidly evolving era of molecular medicine, it is essential for pathologists to equip themselves with a framework for understanding the classification of paragangliomas and pheochromocytomas and be informed of how they might advise their colleagues with regard to prognostication and appropriate follow-up.

A Diagnostic Approach to Adrenocortical Tumors 967

Anjelica Hodgson, Sara Pakbaz, and Ozgur Mete

Adrenocortical tumors range from primary bilateral micronodular or macronodular forms of adrenocortical disease to conventional adrenocortical adenomas and carcinomas. Accurate classification of these neoplasms is critical given the varied pathogenesis, clinical behavior, and outcome of these different lesions. Confirmation of adrenocortical origin, diagnosing malignancy, providing relevant prognostic information in adrenocortical carcinoma, and correlation of laboratory results with clinicopathologic findings are among the important responsibilities of pathologists who evaluate these lesions. This article focuses on a practical approach to the evaluation of adrenocortical tumors with an emphasis on clinical and imaging findings, morphologic characteristics, and multifactorial diagnostic schemes and algorithms.

Treatment of Adrenocortical Carcinoma **997**

Anand Vaidya, Matthew Nehs, and Kerry Kilbridge

Adrenocortical carcinoma (ACC) is a rare malignancy with a poor prognosis. ACC is capable of secreting excess adrenocortical hormones, which can compound morbidity and compromise clinical outcomes. By the time most ACCs are diagnosed, there is usually locoregional or metastatic disease. Surgery is the most important treatment to offer possibility of cure or prolong survival. Several adjuvant therapies are used depending on grade and stage of the tumor and other patient-related factors. This review provides an overview of treatment approaches for ACC, highlighting evidence to support each treatment and acknowledging where more data and research are needed to improve care.

Parathyroid Pathology **1007**

Julie Guilmette and Peter M. Sadow

Proliferative pathologic lesions of parathyroid glands encompass a spectrum of entities ranging from benign hyperplastic processes to malignant neoplasia. This review article outlines the pathophysiologic classification of parathyroid disorders and describes histologic, immunohistochemical, and molecular features that can be assessed to render accurate diagnoses.

Neuroendocrine Tumors of the Gastrointestinal Tract and Pancreas **1021**

Natalie Patel, Andrea Barbieri, and Joanna Gibson

Neuroendocrine neoplasms (NENs) of the gastrointestinal tract and pancreas have undergone numerous nomenclature changes and classification updates as the understanding of the clinical, pathologic, and molecular features of these tumors has grown and evolved. This review will examine common features of gastrointestinal and pancreatic NENs as well as unique site-specific considerations, grading and classification protocols, prognostic parameters, and associations with hereditary syndromes.

Treatment of Gastroenteropancreatic Neuroendocrine Tumors **1045**

Kimberly Perez and Jennifer Chan

Neuroendocrine tumors (NETs) represent a group of biologically and clinically heterogeneous neoplasms arising from the diffuse neuroendocrine system. Although NETs may develop in almost any organ, they commonly arise in the gastrointestinal tract and pancreas and are referred to as gastroenteropancreatic (GEP)-NETs when they arise from these sites. In recent years, advances in understanding of the biology of NETs have resulted in an expansion in treatment options and improved survival for patients. This review focuses on treatment of GEP-NETS and highlights factors that govern the therapeutic approach.

Neuroendocrine Tumors of the Lung: Updates and Diagnostic Pitfalls **1055**

Yin P. Hung

Neuroendocrine tumors of the lung constitute approximately 20% of all primary lung tumors and include typical carcinoid, atypical carcinoid, small cell carcinoma, and large cell neuroendocrine carcinoma. Given their morphologic overlap with diverse mimics, neuroendocrine tumors of the lung can be diagnostically challenging. This review discusses the clinical, histologic, immunophenotypic, and molecular features of pulmonary neuroendocrine tumors, along with common diagnostic pitfalls and strategies for avoidance.

SURGICAL PATHOLOGY CLINICS

FORTHCOMING ISSUES

March 2020
Pulmonary Pathology
Kirk Jones, *Editor*

June 2020
Current Trends in Neuropathology
David M. Meredith, *Editor*

September 2020
Gastrointestinal Pathology
Paul S. Rodriguez, *Editor*

RECENT ISSUES

September 2019
Hematopathology
Mina Luqing Xu, *Editor*

June 2019
Gynecologic Pathology: Practical Issues and Updates
Brooke E. Howitt, *Editor*

March 2019
Soft Tissue Pathology
Elizabeth G. Demicco, *Editor*

SERIES OF RELATED INTEREST
Clinics in Laboratory Medicine

Preface
Endocrine Pathology: Advances, Updates, and Diagnostic Pearls

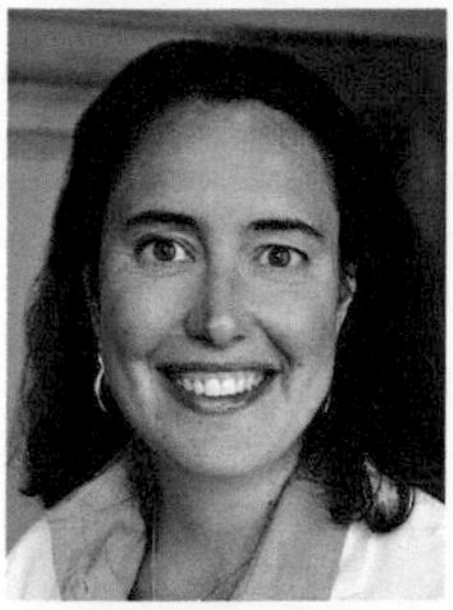

Justine A. Barletta, MD
Editor

It has been an exciting decade to practice endocrine pathology. Advances in our understanding of the molecular basis of thyroid tumors have changed the field. Recent iterations of molecular tests have further improved the triaging of patients with cytologically indeterminate nodules to surgery or surveillance. Insight into the molecular basis of thyroid tumors has also played a pivotal role in the reclassification of tumors, such as encapsulated follicular variant of papillary thyroid carcinoma, and is increasingly being used to refine risk stratification and inform treatment strategies. However, the advances in endocrine pathology are in no way limited to thyroid tumors. For example, virtually every year a new gene is found to be associated with the familial development of pheochromocytomas and paragangliomas. In addition, knowledge of the molecular underpinnings of pancreatic neuroendocrine neoplasms has impacted tumor classification.

This issue of *Surgical Pathology Clinics* is devoted to endocrine pathology. The issue is filled with articles outlining a practical approach to the diagnosis of an array of endocrine neoplasms. In addition, 4 articles written by experts in endocrinology, endocrine surgery, and oncology are meant to serve as a resource for pathologists to deepen their understanding of how patients with endocrine tumors are treated and how diagnostic parameters in our reports influence treatment decisions.

The first third of the issue is dedicated to thyroid pathology. Although the number of diagnostic entities in thyroid pathology is relatively small, diagnostic challenges arise due to pitfalls and controversies. The authors of the first article carefully review the many pitfalls in thyroid cytopathology (and how to avoid them). The next outstanding review not only provides an in-depth discussion of prognostic parameters for differentiated thyroid carcinoma but also tackles some of the controversies, including what constitutes vascular invasion. After that, uncommon (but clinically important) thyroid entities are reviewed, and the molecular basis of thyroid tumors is addressed. Two articles devoted to the treatment of thyroid tumors (differentiated thyroid tumors and aggressive thyroid carcinomas) complete the thyroid section. The next group of articles focuses on adrenal pathology. Drs Sadow and Guilmette (who deserve special mention because they contributed 2 articles to this issue!) inform the reader of the frequent familial basis and current state of risk stratification of pheochromocytomas and paragangliomas. The pathology of the adrenal cortex is examined in the following article, with an expert review of algorithms used to distinguish benign from malignant adrenal cortical tumors. This section ends with an article covering the basics of treatment of adrenal cortical carcinoma. Parathyroid pathology is next considered. From there, the issue turns to gastroenteropancreatic

Surgical Pathology 12 (2019) xi–xii
https://doi.org/10.1016/j.path.2019.08.013
1875-9181/19/© 2019 Published by Elsevier Inc.

(GEP) neuroendocrine tumors, with 2 outstanding reviews: the first provides a thorough overview of GEP neuroendocrine tumors at each site and updates the reader on tumor grading. The second article discusses treatment options for patients with these tumors. The issue concludes with a concise and practical guide to neuroendocrine tumors of the lung.

I would like to thank all of the authors who have contributed to this issue. I am grateful for the time they took from their exceedingly busy schedules to contribute thoughtful articles that are a true reflection of their expertise, insight, and passion for this field.

Justine A. Barletta, MD
Chief, Endocrine Pathology Service
Department of Pathology
Brigham and Women's Hospital
Associate Professor of Pathology
Harvard Medical School
75 Francis Street
Boston, MA 02115, USA

E-mail address:
jbarletta@bwh.harvard.edu

Pitfalls in Thyroid Cytopathology

Esther Diana Rossi, MD, PhD, MIAC[a], Adebowale J. Adeniran, MD[b], William C. Faquin, MD, PhD[c,*]

KEYWORDS

• Fine-needle aspiration • Cytology • Thyroid nodule • Thyroid cancer • False-positive diagnoses • False-negative diagnoses

ABSTRACT

Fine-needle aspiration (FNA) is among the first diagnostic tools used in the evaluation of thyroid nodules. It has the ability to triage patients with benign and malignant lesions, thus defining the optimum clinical and/or surgical management. The Bethesda System for Reporting Thyroid Cytopathology has found worldwide acceptance. Thyroid FNA offers high positive predictive value (97%–99%), with sensitivities and specificities of 65% to 99% and 72% to 100%, respectively. Nonetheless, many potential diagnostic pitfalls exist that can lead to false-positive and/or false-negative results. This article discusses several of the potential pitfalls in the cytologic evaluation of thyroid lesions.

OVERVIEW

Thyroid nodules are frequently detected in clinical practice, reflecting their prevalence in the general population and especially among women.[1,2] Fine-needle aspiration (FNA) is among the first and most valuable diagnostic tools for the presurgical discrimination of benign and malignant lesions. Although most thyroid nodules (90%–92%) are benign, the small subset of malignant nodules needs to be presurgically identified for optimal management.[3–6] The diagnostic value and accuracy of FNA in the evaluation of thyroid nodules has been well established in the literature.[1–8] Thyroid FNA has shown a high positive predictive value for identifying malignancy, ranging from 97% to 99% in the Bethesda System for Reporting Thyroid Cytopathology (TBSRTC) to 95% from the Royal College of Pathologists in the British thyroid system.[1,9] Using TBSRTC, Yang and colleagues[10] reported a sensitivity of 94% and specificity of 98.5% for malignancy, and sensitivity of 89.3% and specificity of 74% for identifying neoplastic disease.

Despite its overall success, FNA false-positive (FP) and/or false-negative (FN) results can occur for a variety of reasons, often caused by the quality of the aspirated material (**Table 1**). Yang and colleagues[10] found an overall 15.3% discrepancy rate between cytologic and histologic diagnoses, with FN results related mostly to issues of sample adequacy. Overall, approximately 3.2% of patients with a benign FNA result have been shown to be FNs. However, most studies only considered the FNA results of patients who proceeded to surgery.[10–21] FP results of thyroid FNA have a broad range of causes, but many are caused by tumors that can show a range of cytomorphologic appearances that overlap with other tumor subtypes. This overlap is seen in FNA of tumors such as medullary thyroid carcinoma (MTC), anaplastic thyroid carcinoma (ATC), and in certain variants of papillary

All the authors contributed equally to the article.
Conflicts of interest and funding: The authors have no conflicts of interest. This work did not receive any specific grant funding.
[a] Division of Anatomic Pathology and Histology, Catholic University of Sacred Heart, A. Gemelli Square, 1, Rome 20123, Italy; [b] Department of Pathology, Yale University School of Medicine, 333 Cedar Street, New Haven, CT 06510, USA; [c] Department of Pathology, WRN 219, Massachusetts General Hospital, 55 Fruit Street, Boston, MA 02114, USA
* Corresponding author.
E-mail address: wfaquin@partners.org

Surgical Pathology 12 (2019) 865–881
https://doi.org/10.1016/j.path.2019.08.001

Table 1
Examples of false-negative and false-positive thyroid fine-needle aspiration results

Diagnoses	FN	FP
ND	Few cells suggestive of benign condition	AUS/FLUS
Cystic lesions	Misinterpretation of cystic degeneration and squamous cells	Atypical cyst-lining cells, few cells with features suggestive for SFM or even PM
GD	None	PTC
LT	Scant diagnostic features of LT	Mostly PTC; lymphomas; FNHCT
Follicular-patterned lesions	Underestimate architectural and cellular features; intrathyroidal parathyroid adenoma; PTEN hamartoma	SFM/PM; PTC; FVPTC; FC
Hürthle cell neoplasm	HT; goiter, granular cell tumor; intrathyroidal parathyroid adenoma	PTC[a]; MTC; HTC
NIFTP	Follicular-patterned lesions	SFM or PM favoring PTC; MTC
PTC	HTT; LT; GD	MTC; PDC
FVPTC	AUS/FLUS or SFN/FN	NIFTP
NIFTP	AUS/FLUS; BL	SFM/PM
MTC	SFN/FN; FNHCT	PTC, HTC
PDC	SFN/FN; FNHCT	MTC; metastases; lymphoproliferative disorders
ATC	Few atypical cells classified as ND	PDC; MTC; metastases; lymphomas
Metastatic lesions	Few atypical cells classified as ND	PDC, MTC, ATC

Abbreviations: ATC, anaplastic thyroid carcinoma; AUS, atypia of undetermined significance; FC, follicular carcinoma; FLUS, follicular lesion of undetermined significance; FNHCT, follicular neoplasm, Hürthle cell type; FVPTC, follicular variant of PTC; GD, Graves disease; HT, Hashimoto thyroiditis; HTC, Hürthle cell carcinoma; LT, lymphocytic thyroiditis; MTC, medullary thyroid carcinoma; ND, nondiagnostic; NIFTP, noninvasive follicular neoplasm with papillarylike nuclear features; PDC, poorly differentiated carcinoma; PM, positive for malignancy; PTC, papillary thyroid carcinoma; PTEN, phosphatase and tensin homolog; SFM, suspicious for malignancy; SFN/FN, suspicious for follicular neoplasm/follicular neoplasm.

[a] Including oncocytic variant of PTC.

thyroid carcinoma (PTC). This article discusses several of the important diagnostic pitfalls for a range of diagnostic categories and tumor types that can be encountered in thyroid cytology and that can lead to both FN and FP thyroid FNA results.

NONDIAGNOSTIC THYROID FINE-NEEDLE ASPIRATIONS

Thyroid specimens that are inadequate for cytologic interpretation are classified as nondiagnostic (ND) in TBSRTC.[1] Different factors can contribute to an ND result, such as the inherent nature of the nodule (cystic vs solid vs fibrotic and calcified), as well as aspects of the FNA procedure and operator experience. In order to reduce the rate of ND results, the recommendation for these samples is to repeat the FNA under sonographic guidance targeting cellular areas of the nodule. Using this approach, several studies have documented a significant reduction (from 70% to 83%) in the ND rate.[14,22–25] TBSRTC reports a risk of malignancy (ROM) of 5% to 10% for ND samples.[1] PTC has been reported as the most frequent cause of an FN diagnosis in the ND category.[22–25] One important caveat in the evaluation of a thyroid FNA that might otherwise be interpreted as ND is that the presence of cytologic atypia should be reported as atypia of undetermined significance(AUS) or follicular lesion of undetermined significance (FLUS) even without the required minimal number of follicular cells.[1]

CYSTIC THYROID LESIONS

Cystic or predominantly cystic thyroid nodules are reported in approximately 15% to 25% of thyroid lesions and most are histologically benign.[22–26] The microscopic findings include foamy and hemosiderin-laden macrophages, scant colloid, and few follicular cells. On occasion, cyst-lining cells can show atypical nuclear features that can mimic PTC (**Fig. 1**). FNA of cystic thyroid nodules has been associated with both FN and FP results.

The ROM is generally low for thyroid nodules, with low suspicion ultrasonography pattern that is less than 2-3 cm in size.[26] The ROM, particularly for PTC, increases with larger and more complex cysts.[1] Jaragh and colleagues[27] analyzed 76 cyst fluid-only FNA cases, concluding that the only morphologic feature predictive of malignancy was the presence of follicular epithelium with atypical features. However, some atypical cells in benign cystic lesions can be derived from cyst-lining cells as epithelial repair.[28,29] Specific cytomorphologic features are associated with cyst-lining cells including (1) well-defined cellular borders, (2) dense granular cytoplasm, (3) enlarged nuclei with regular nuclear borders, and (4) occasional pale nuclei. A diagnosis of AUS/FLUS is considered more appropriate for these cases.[1]

In rare instances, squamous cells can be encountered in cystic thyroid FNAs, where they can be a diagnostic pitfall.[28–33] Their presence has been associated with a variety of different entities, including benign lymphoepithelial cysts, epidermoid cyst, thyroglossal duct remnants, and squamous metaplasia in long-standing Hashimoto thyroiditis (HT). Much less often, squamous cells reflect a malignant lesion such as PTC, ATC, primary or metastatic squamous carcinoma, mucoepidermoid carcinoma, or carcinoma with thymuslike differentiation. Gage and colleagues[28] analyzed a series of 15 thyroid lesions with a predominance of squamous cells, and suggested the presence of 3 main cytologic patterns: benign, mixed cellularity, and malignant. Most commonly, detection of abundant anucleated and bland squamous cells plus background lymphocytes was compatible with a benign lesion. In some cases, the squamous cells represented reactive squamous metaplasia in HT, whereas malignant lesions were usually easily recognized.[32]

GRAVES DISEASE

Graves disease (GD) is a common endocrine disorder that can pose diagnostic issues because of cellular changes overlapping with the nuclear features of PTC.[1,34,35]

GD is among the most frequent causes of hyperthyroidism, with a prevalence of palpable thyroid nodules 3-fold higher than in the general population, and FNA of these nodules can represent a significant diagnostic dilemma. Despite the low ROM (between 1.9% and 2.5%), the cytomorphologic changes in GD, especially after treatment, can be misinterpreted as PTC.[34,35] Cytologic features found in aspiration of GD include scattered follicular cell pleomorphism,

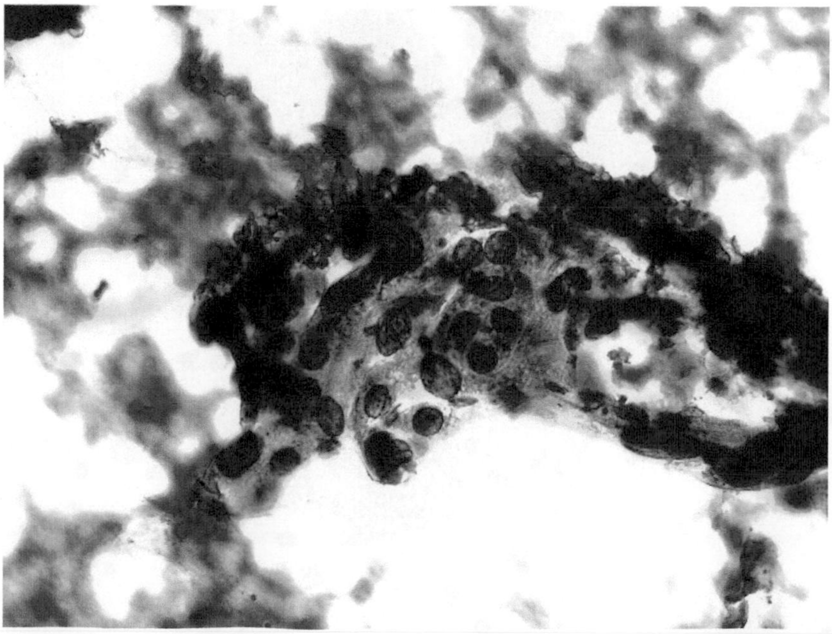

Fig. 1. FNA of cystic thyroid nodule. Rare groups of follicular cells with nuclear atypia are present. These atypical cyst-lining cells can mimic PTC (Papanicolaou stain, original magnification ×600).

fire-flare cells, Hürthle cell changes, and background lymphocytes. Because of the nonspecific nature of these findings, clinical correlation is essential to avoid an FP diagnosis. Treatment of GD with radioactive iodine is well known to cause significant follicular cell atypia, including nuclear and cellular enlargement, anisonucleosis, coarse chromatin, hyperchromasia, and cytoplasmic vacuolization. To avoid an FP diagnosis, it is helpful to note that these samples lack the fine powdery chromatin typically seen in PTC. In the attempt to differentiate GD from PTC, Anderson and colleagues[34] evaluated 11 cytomorphologic features in FNA cases of GD and PTC in GD. They concluded that only 4 of these features were predictive of PTC in GD, and all were based on nuclear characteristics, including oval nuclear shape, pale chromatin, and distinct eccentric nucleoli.[32]

INFLAMMATORY LESIONS

LYMPHOCYTIC THYROIDITIS

The term lymphocytic thyroiditis (LT) encompasses a variety of conditions ranging from chronic lymphocytic thyroiditis (HT) to subacute lymphocytic thyroiditis (postpartum and silent thyroiditis) and focal (silent) thyroiditis.[1] Other entities with LT include GD, nodular goiter, and immunoglobulin G4 thyroiditis.[1] HT represents both the most common form of autoimmune thyroiditis and the most common cause of hypothyroidism. It typically affects middle-aged women as a diffuse heterogeneous enlargement of the thyroid, but frequently the enlargement is localized as a pseudonodule (from 26% to 80% of cases) and raises suspicion of a neoplastic nodule.[36–39] HT is recognized as a multifaceted disease with an initial phase of hyperthyroidism followed by a chronic phase of hypothyroidism. In the initial phase of HT, there is antibody-mediated destruction of follicular structures with lymphocytic infiltration. The chronic phase shows the presence of atrophic follicles and fibrotic parenchyma. Depending on the stage of the disease, FNA specimens can result in a range of diagnostic pitfalls.[37–39] For instance, the prevalence of either the lymphoid or the oncocytic component may raise the possibility of lymphoma or a Hürthle cell neoplasm, respectively. The early phase of hyperthyroidism is characterized by a population of oncocytic cells arranged in flat sheets or as isolated cells. In some cases, the oncocytic cells show nuclear enlargement, grooves, and chromatin clearing, suggesting PTC (**Fig. 2**). FNA samples with a prominent population of lymphoid cells where lymphoma is a concern can be evaluated by flow cytometry.[38,39]

A recent study by Yi and colleagues[40] showed a higher prevalence of thyroiditis among patients with FP results than among those with PTC. Among 48 patients with FP results, thyroiditis was diagnosed in 54.2% (26 cases), whereas the rate of thyroiditis was only 9.4% in patients with

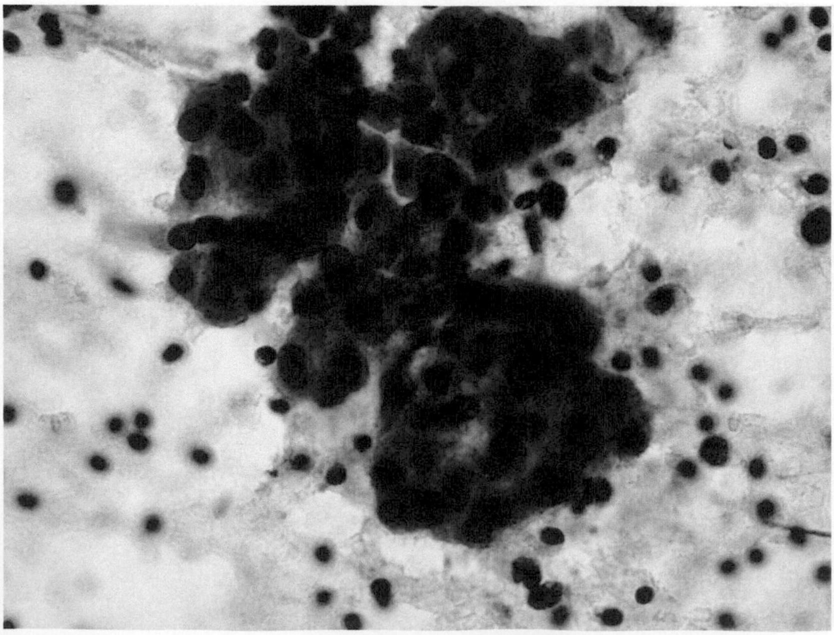

Fig. 2. FNA of chronic LT. The follicular cells are cohesive and have moderate amounts of oncocytic cytoplasm and mild nuclear atypia (Papanicolaou stain, original magnification ×600).

PTC. A key point is that, in the presence of a lymphocytic background, a definitive diagnosis of PTC should be made only when well-developed classic features of PTC are present.

A unique entity in patients with HT is the Warthin-like variant of PTC, which mimics the mixture of oncocytes and lymphocytes of HT[1] (**Fig. 3**). However, a careful evaluation of the cytologic features can resolve the dilemma. The Warthin-like variant of PTC has more pleomorphic and irregular nuclear membranes, nuclear pseudoinclusions, and less prominent nucleoli than the oncocytes of HT. In addition, the Warthin-like variant of PTC shows permeating lymphocytes and plasma cells.

GRANULOMATOUS THYROIDITIS

Granulomatous (de Quervain) thyroiditis (GT) is a self-limiting inflammatory process of the thyroid that is usually diagnosed clinically in patients with neck and ear pain and tenderness occurring a few weeks after a viral upper respiratory tract infection.[40–45] In rare cases, FNA is performed for nodular swelling that raises the possibility of a neoplastic condition. The cytologic features are variable and depend on the stage of disease. The initial stage shows neutrophils and eosinophils resembling an acute thyroiditis; the later stages show hypocellularity with giant cells, epithelioid cells, lymphocytes, macrophages, and scant degenerated follicular cells. In the involutional stage, there might only be giant cells and inflammatory cells. In the presence of granulomas, other entities, including sarcoidosis and infections, should be considered. Solano and colleagues[42] retrospectively analyzed 36 cases of GT to reassess the clinical and cytologic findings characteristic of GT: presence of follicular cells with intravacuolar granules and/or plump transformed follicular cells; epithelioid granulomas; multinucleated giant cells; an acute and chronic inflammatory background; absence of fire-flare cells, hypertrophic follicular cells, oncocytic cells, and transformed lymphocytes. Based on these findings, selected features of GT can mimic a variety of entities, such as hemorrhage and infarction in a nodular goiter, and final stages of HT.

INDETERMINATE FOLLICULAR-PATTERNED LESIONS

ATYPIA OF UNDETERMINED SIGNIFICANCE/ FOLLICULAR LESION OF UNDETERMINED SIGNIFICANCE AND FOLLICULAR NEOPLASM/ SUSPICIOUS FOR FOLLICULAR NEOPLASM

One of the most important challenges in thyroid cytology is represented by the so-called gray zone of indeterminate thyroid FNA lesions. Despite most thyroid lesions being correctly classified as either benign (70%–75%) or malignant (5%–10%), the remaining nodules (20%-25%) belong to indeterminate categories.[46–55]

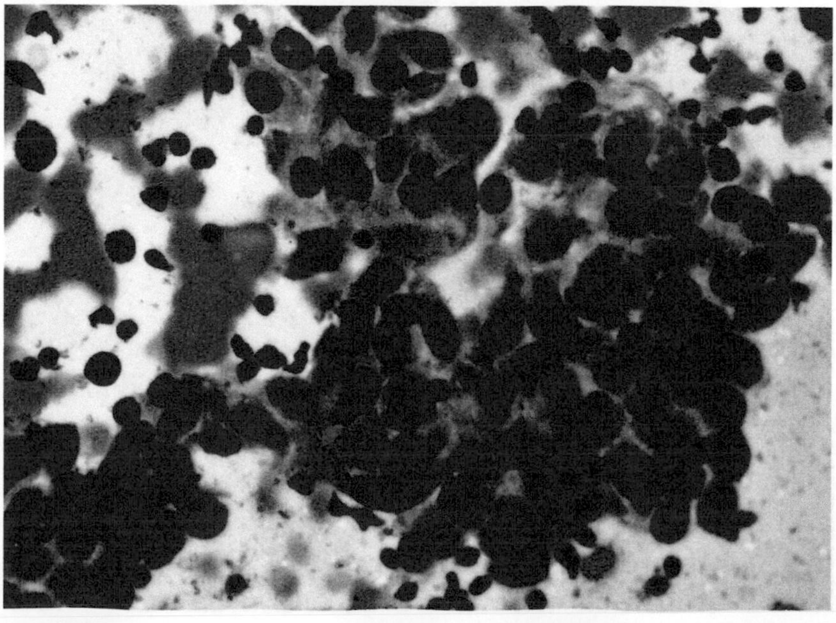

Fig. 3. FNA of Warthin-like variant of PTC. Cells have oncocytic features and nuclear atypia in a background of chronic inflammation (Diff-Quik stain, original magnification ×600).

The interpretation of follicular-patterned lesions is challenging and difficulties and limitations in discriminating whether these nodules are benign or malignant entities can result in unnecessary surgical resections (lobectomy or total thyroidectomy) and increased health care costs.[46,54–65]

The atypia in AUS/FLUS includes a range of nuclear and/or architectural changes.[1,66,67] Both nuclear and architectural patterns can result in diagnostic pitfalls even though most of these findings are caused by benign conditions such as hyperplastic-adenomatous nodules, toxic adenomas, and chronic LT. Two benign instances in which AUS/FLUS diagnosis can be avoided are the presence of few oncocytic cells and/or cyst-lining cells with mild atypia mixed with benign follicular cells, and the presence of papillary structures without any nuclear features of PTC.

Intrathyroidal parathyroid adenomas are often misclassified as suspicious for follicular neoplasm (SFN). Such aspirates can show a microfollicular pattern.[68–70] The ultrasonography detection of a posterior nodule, small hyperchromatic nuclei, scant cytoplasm, and crowded trabecular clusters without colloid can be a subtle clue for the diagnosis. The application of ancillary techniques in such instances, including immunostains for parathyroid hormone (PTH) and/or molecular analysis by Afirma or Thyroseqv 3, can recognize the expression profile supporting the diagnosis of a PTH lesion[11,17,71–77] (**Fig. 4**).

ONCOCYTIC/HÜRTHLE CELL NEOPLASM

Since the introduction of the term Hürthle cells to define thyroid follicular cells with abundant granular mitochondria-rich cytoplasm, their presence has been noticed in several conditions (**Fig. 5**),[78–83] including adenomatous/hyperplastic nodules, chronic lymphocytic (Hashimoto) thyroiditis, multinodular goiter, but also Hürthle cell adenoma and carcinoma.[80–82] A common diagnostic pitfall is misinterpreting the presence of a population of Hürthle cells in sheets admixed with background colloid with or without sheets of nononcocytic follicular cells[78–84] as Hurthle cell neoplasm (HCN). As a general guideline, the presence of a mixture of Hürthle and non-Hürthle cells especially is more consistent with a benign nodule.

Most chronic LT cases can be recognized because of the predominance of lymphocytes compared with Hürthle cells. In difficult and controversial cases, mostly when the lymphocytic component is scant, a clue to the correct interpretation is based on finding oncocytic cells organized in small clusters of 3 to 10 cells with large nuclei, with or without glassy chromatin and with nuclear features that may raise concern for PTC. A high threshold should be maintained when background lymphocytes are present.[84] However, in some cases the differential diagnosis between follicular neoplasm, Hürthle cell type (FNHCT) and the oncocytic variant of PTC is especially challenging and it may not be possible to distinguish between them. In some cases, the morphologic

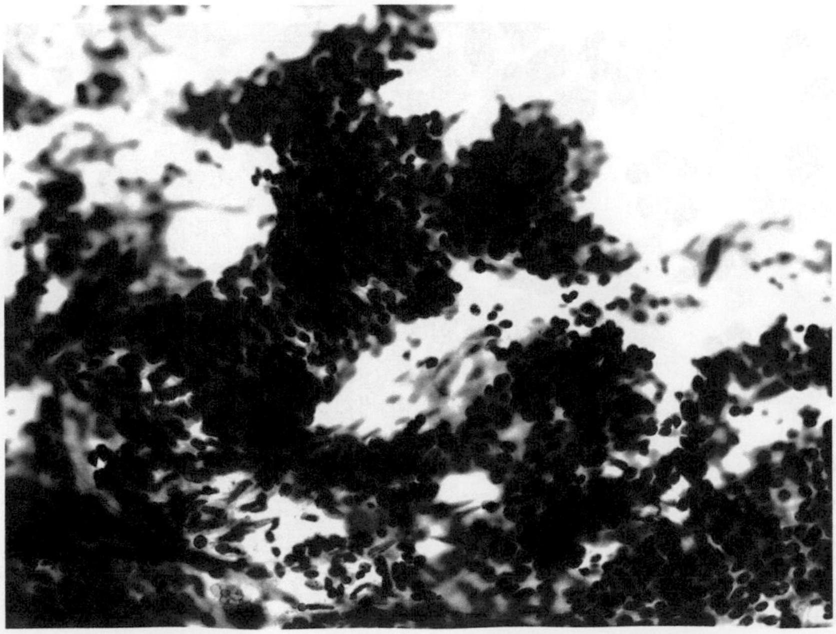

Fig. 4. FNA of parathyroid adenoma. Cells are cohesive and have small amounts of eosinophilic cytoplasm and uniform round dark nuclei. The microscopic features overlap with those of a follicular neoplasm (Papanicolaou stain, original magnification ×400).

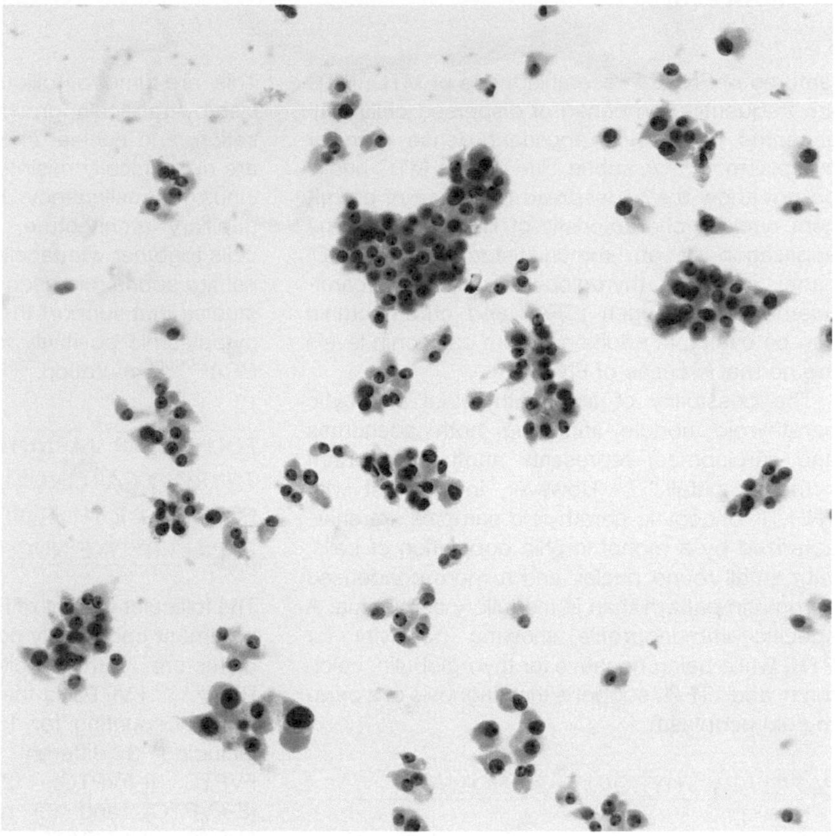

Fig. 5. FNA of Hürthle cell neoplasm. Hürthle cells in sheets, small clusters, and single cells. The dispersed cells often have eccentrically placed nuclei with prominent nucleoli, but the nuclei lack the salt-and-pepper chromatin of MTC (Papanicolaou stain, original magnification ×400).

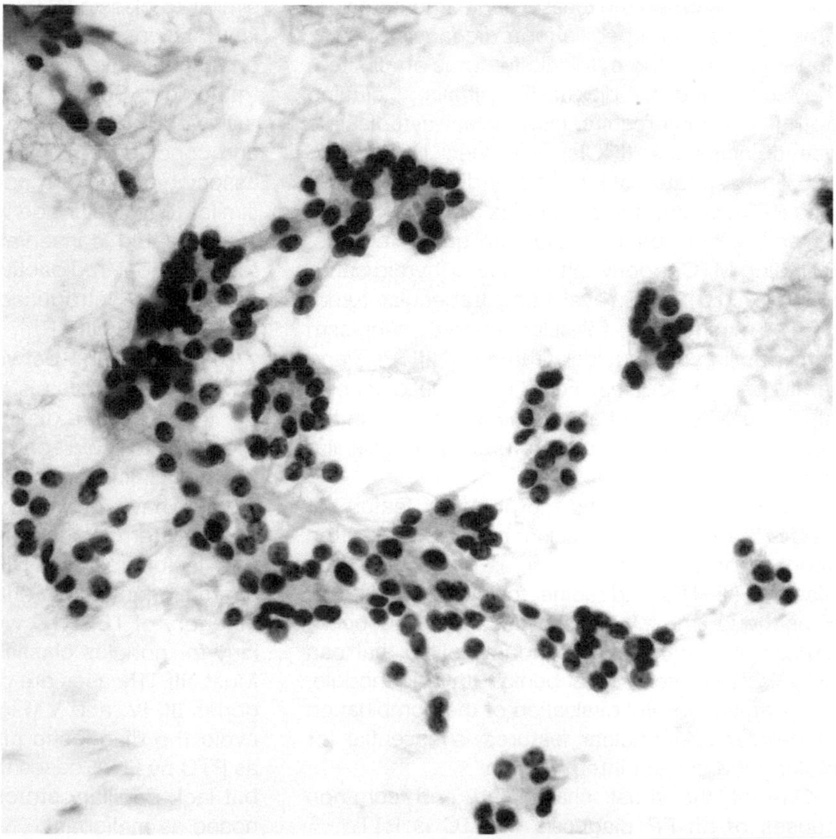

Fig. 6. FNA of NIFTP. Epithelial cells show a follicular architectural arrangement with rare grooves and elongation. The diagnosis on the original cytology was follicular neoplasm (Bethesda category IV) (Papanicolaou stain, original magnification ×600).

features of FNHCT resemble those of MTC. MTC are frequently composed of dispersed cells with eccentric nuclei and abundant dense granular cytoplasm.[79–87] A subtle clue is that MTC nuclei do not show the widespread presence of prominent nucleoli characteristic of Hürthle cells. The application of an immunohistochemistry (IHC) panel, including thyroglobulin, calcitonin, carcinoembryonic antigen (CEA), and chromogranin can be useful. In addition, serum calcitonin levels are normal in cases of FNHCT.

The possibility of an intrathyroidal oncocytic parathyroid nodule (including both adenomas and carcinomas) represents another important cytologic pitfall.[69,88] However, in contrast with FNHCT, oncocytic parathyroid samples are characterized by a monomorphic population of cells, with small round nuclei, and a more condensed chromatin pattern than in medullary carcinoma. A specific immunoprofile showing positivity for PTH, while being negative for thyroglobulin, calcitonin, and TTF-1, supports the diagnosis of a parathyroid neoplasm.

PAPILLARY THYROID CARCINOMA

PTC is the most common malignant tumor of the thyroid gland, with most having an indolent clinical course.[89–94] When the classic nuclear features are present, they are specific for a diagnosis of PTC; however, when the cytologic features are limited, they can lead to diagnostic pitfalls, including both FP and FN results. Intranuclear cytoplasmic pseudoinclusions (INCIs) are seen in 50% to 100% of aspirates of PTC, depending on the specific PTC variant; however, INCIs are also found in several other benign and malignant entities, including MTC, poorly differentiated thyroid carcinoma (PDTC), ATC, hyalinizing trabecular tumor (HTT), noninvasive follicular thyroid neoplasm with papillarylike nuclear features (NIFTPs), and rarely benign nodules. For a definitive diagnosis of PTC, INCIs should always be interpreted in the context of other architectural and cellular features.[1]

Another characteristic morphologic feature of PTC is the longitudinal nuclear groove that is often seen in other entities such as oncocytic neoplasms, NIFTP, and some follicular adenomas. Even though most PTCs show scant colloid, occasional cases can have abundant colloid that can be misinterpreted as a benign thyroid nodule. Once again, careful evaluation of the combination of cellular and nuclear features is essential for making the correct interpretation.

One of the most challenging and common causes of an FP diagnosis of PTC is HTT.[95,96] This rare tumor of follicular cell origin is characterized by trabecular growth, marked stromal hyalinization, and nuclear changes of PTC. Most HTTs are cytologically misinterpreted as PTC or suspicious for malignancy. However, the absence of papillary architecture, and elongated epithelial cells together with acellular stromal hyaline material are subtle microscopic clues of HTT. Ancillary studies that support the diagnosis of HTT include cytoplasmic positivity for MIB-1 and the lack of *BRAF*^{V600E} mutation.

FOLLICULAR VARIANT OF PAPILLARY THYROID CARCINOMA AND NONINVASIVE FOLLICULAR THYROID NEOPLASM WITH PAPILLARYLIKE NUCLEAR FEATURES

The follicular variant of PTC (FVPTC) is completely or almost completely composed of a follicular architecture with atypical nuclear features of PTC.[89–93] FVPTC is the most common variant of PTC, accounting for 15% to 30% of them and including 3 different subtypes: (1) infiltrative FVPTC (I-FVPTC); (2) encapsulated FVPTC (E-FVPTC), and (3) noninvasive encapsulated FVPTC (NI-EFVPTC).[57–65] Although I-FVPTC frequently metastasizes to cervical lymph nodes similar to classic PTC, E-FVPTC behaves in indolent fashion, especially when there is no capsular or vascular invasion (NI-EFVPTC). The Endocrine Pathology Society working group (ESP-WG) reviewed a large series (n = 268) of NI-EFVPTCs and concluded that the absence of invasion was associated with an indolent biological behavior, similar to follicular adenomas, even when patients were treated conservatively with thyroid lobectomy without radioactive iodine therapy.[60] Thus, the ESP-WG introduced the new diagnostic term for NI-FVPTC:NIFTP.[60]

Distinguishing between these 3 follicular-patterned subtypes is not possible by FNA.[57–65] For this reason, a distinction between NIFTP and the other follicular-patterned neoplasms is problematic. Since the introduction of NIFTP, several studies have provided insight to the impact of this new terminology on the interpretation of thyroid lesions.[57–65] If NIFTP was classified as a nonmalignant lesion, the ROM in each diagnostic category of TBSRTC would be reduced, particularly for nodules classified as indeterminate.[57–65] Most NIFTP cases are classified in TBSRTC categories III, IV, and V (**Fig. 6**). Most importantly, to avoid the diagnostic pitfall of interpreting NIFTP as PTC by FNA, cases that are follicular patterned but lack papillary structures should not be diagnosed as malignant.

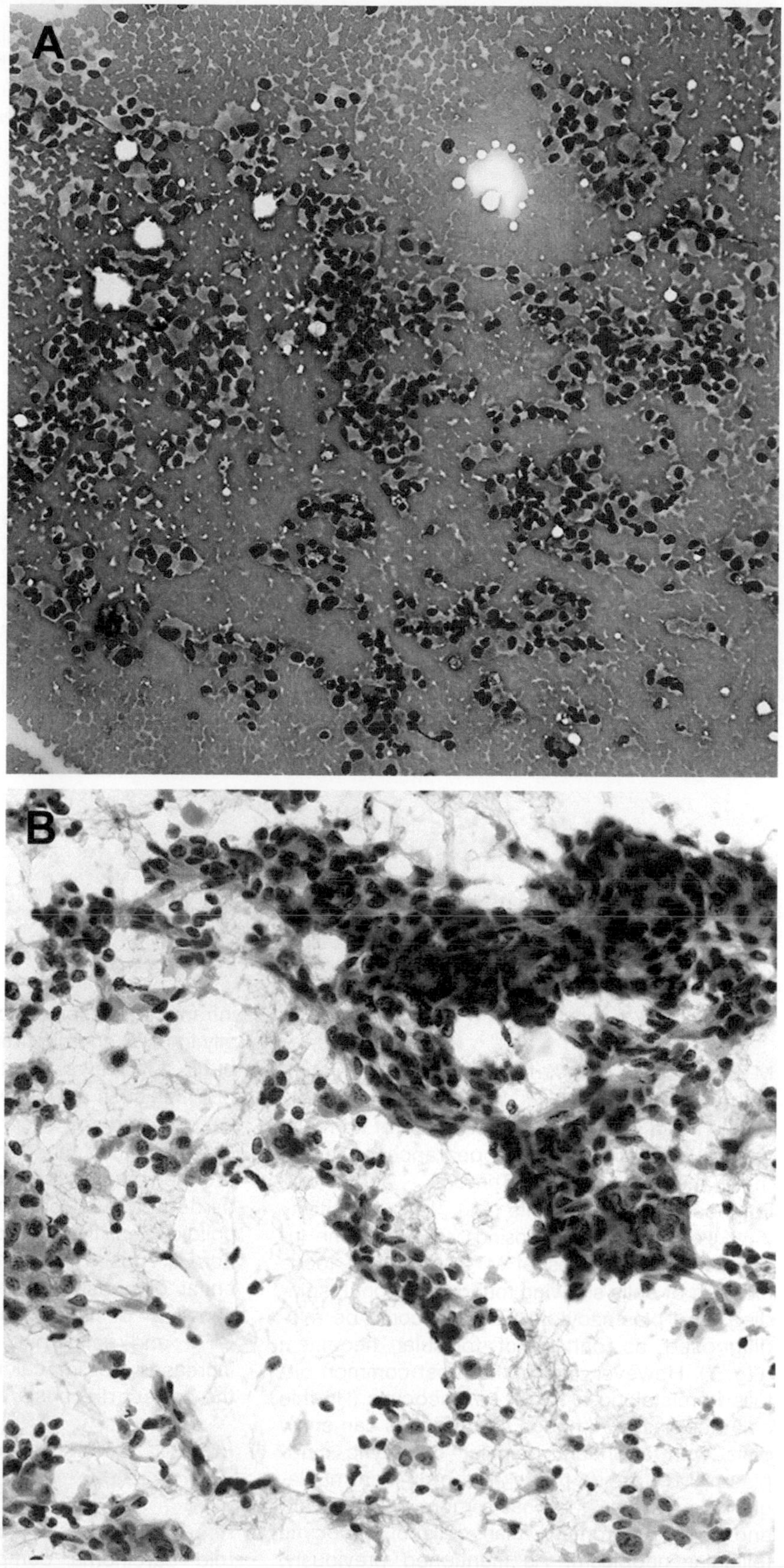

Fig. 7. FNA of MTC. (*A*) Loose clusters and single cells with eccentrically placed nuclei (Diff-Quik stain, original magnification ×200). (*B*) The tumor shows spindling with a pseudopapillary appearance, nuclear elongation, and rare grooves. Single cells are also present in the background (Papanicolaou stain, original magnification ×400).

Fig. 7. (*continued*). (*C*) Tumor cells are immunochemically positive for calcitonin. (Avidin-Biotin complex method, original magnification ×400).

MEDULLARY THYROID CARCINOMA

MTC accounts for 1% to 2% of thyroid cancers in the United States,[97–101] and the FNA diagnosis of MTC can be challenging because of its many different cytomorphologic appearances. A recent meta-analysis from Trimboli and colleagues[1,98,102] highlights the low sensitivity (56%) of FNA for diagnosing MTC. In some instances, the features of MTC, including loose clusters of cells showing round, polygonal, spindled, and plasmacytoid features, could be misdiagnosed as pattern of follicular neoplasm (**Fig. 7**). However, one of the most common pitfalls is mistaking MTC for an oncocytic (Hürthle cell) neoplasm. Although both entities can show cells with abundant granular oncocytic cytoplasm, MTC tends to lack the prominent nucleolus in most cells and has a more delicate salt-and-pepper chromatin than cells of oncocytic follicular neoplasm. As mentioned previously, intranuclear pseudoinclusions occur occasionally in MTC and can raise a differential diagnosis of PTC. However, careful attention to the nuclear qualities such as extensive nuclear grooves, oval shape, and powdery chromatin is needed, because they support a diagnosis of PTC. Another pitfall is that amyloid, identified in one-third of MTCs, can be indistinguishable from colloid, and it is also present in amyloid goiter. For FNA cases in which MTC is part of the differential diagnosis, application of an IHC panel, showing positive staining for synaptophysin, CEA, and calcitonin, or demonstration of an increased serum calcitonin level, can lead to the correct diagnosis.[97–101]

POORLY DIFFERENTIATED THYROID CARCINOMA

Poorly differentiated carcinoma (PDC) is a thyroid carcinoma composed of follicular cells organized in an insular, solid, or trabecular growth pattern.[103–111] Cytologically, PDCs are difficult to recognize prospectively unless the case is associated with apoptosis, mitotic activity, and necrosis. The morphologic features of PDC overlap with those of follicular neoplasms; therefore, most of these cases are classified by FNA as SFN/FN. Nonetheless, insular and/or trabecular clusters of monomorphic atypical follicular cells with increased nuclear/cytoplasm ratio in a necrotic background might suggest a diagnosis of suspicious for malignancy not otherwise specified. Possible pitfalls include MTC, possible metastatic tumors, and lymphoproliferative disorders. The diagnosis of lymphoproliferative disorders is an important pitfall for those cases with predominance of isolated cells.[105–111]

ANAPLASTIC THYROID CARCINOMA AND METASTATIC TUMORS

ATC is an aggressive thyroid carcinoma, easily recognized in cytologic samples as a high-grade malignancy. Tumor cells are pleomorphic and can include both epithelioid and spindle features (**Fig. 8**).[112–118] The cytomorphologic findings combined with characteristic clinical features, including the presence of a rapidly growing mass in a hard nodular thyroid gland, with infiltration into surrounding extrathyroid soft tissue, lead to the correct diagnosis. Given its high-grade undifferentiated appearance, the differential diagnosis includes metastatic malignant tumors, sarcoma, PDC, MTC, and lymphoma. The most common diagnostic pitfall is metastatic tumors, such as melanoma, sarcomatoid renal carcinoma, squamous cell carcinoma, and poorly differentiated adenocarcinoma of the lung.[119–123] IHC studies, including PAX-8 and keratin, are useful when combined with clinical and radiological evidence of a tumor centered in the thyroid gland. Most anaplastic carcinoma are negative for TTF-1 and thyroglobulin, and a subset are negative for keratins. The possibility of a metastatic thyroid tumor should be considered, especially for those patients with a previous history of malignant extrathyroidal neoplasm (**Fig. 9**).

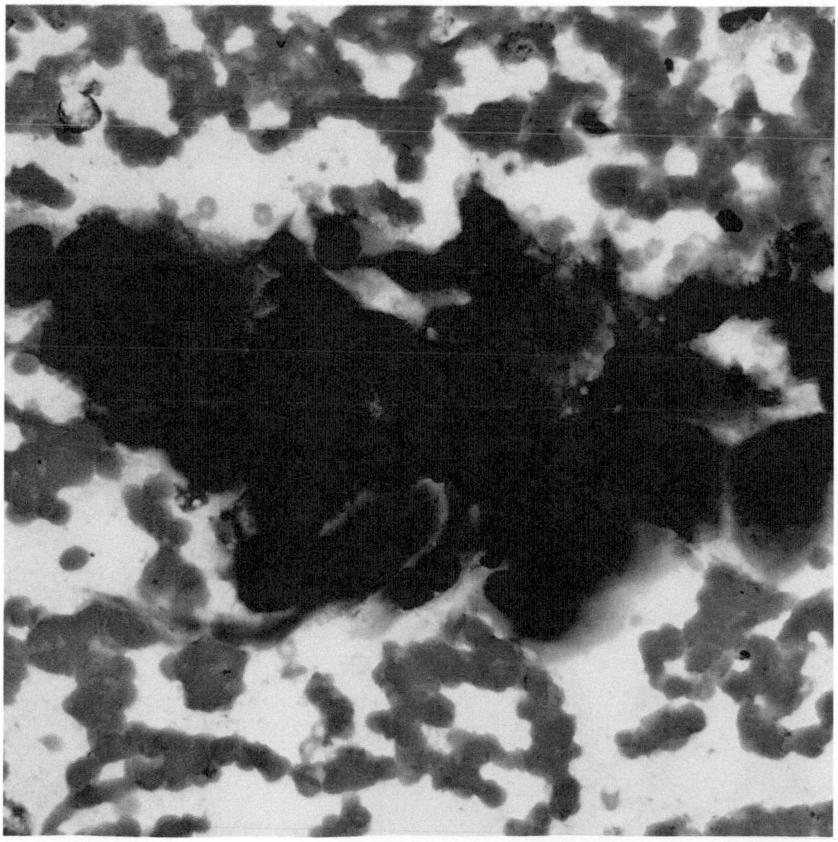

Fig. 8. FNA of ATC showing a dispersed population of markedly atypical cells (Diff-Quik stain, original magnification ×600).

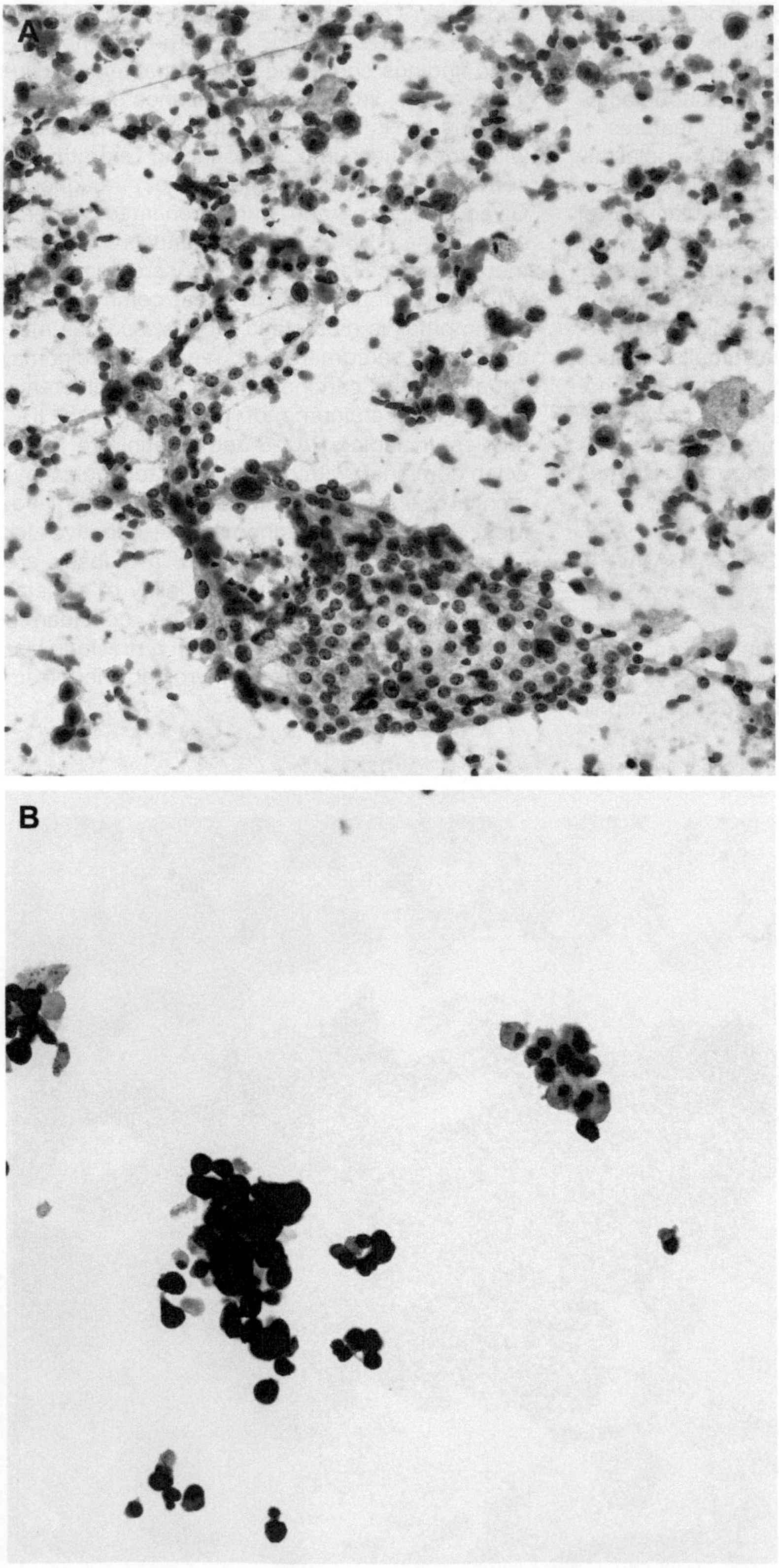

Fig. 9. FNA of metastatic melanoma to the thyroid. (*A*) Infiltrating single cells of melanoma are seen in the background of nonneoplastic follicular cells (Papanicolaou stain, original magnification ×400). (*B*) Melan A immunochemical stain highlighting the tumor cells; the background normal follicular cells are negative. (Original magnification ×400).

SUMMARY

The main goal of thyroid FNA is to triage patients with nodules having a high ROM for surgery while avoiding unnecessary surgical procedures for others. The evaluation of patients with thyroid nodules should be based on a combination of the clinical, radiological, and cytomorphologic findings. Nonetheless, thyroid FNA is challenging and there are many potential diagnostic pitfalls, several of which are discussed in this article. An awareness of these potential diagnostic pitfalls combined with careful attention to cytologic and clinical features, along with judicious use of ancillary studies, can help to reduce errors and lead to more accurate FNA interpretations and improved patient care.

REFERENCES

1. Ali S, Cibas ES. The Bethesda system for reporting thyroid cytopathology. Definitions, criteria and explanatory notes. 2nd edition. Cham (Switzerland): Springer; 2018.
2. Tee YY, Lowe AJ, Brand CA, et al. Fine-needle aspiration may miss a third of all malignancy in palpable thyroid nodules: A comprehensive literature review. Ann Surg 2007;246(5):714–20.
3. Cramer H. Fine-needle aspiration cytology of the thyroid: an appraisal. Cancer 2000;90:325–9.
4. Gharib H, Papini E, Paschke R. Thyroid nodules: a review of current guidelines, practices and prospects. Eur J Endocrinol 2008;159:493–505.
5. Ravetto C, Colombo L, Dottorini ME. Usefulness of fine- needle aspiration in the diagnosis of thyroid carcinomas. A retrospective study in 37,895 patients. Cancer Cytopathol 2000;90: 357–63.
6. Poller DN, Ibrahim AK, Cummings MH, et al. Fine-needle aspiration of the thyroid. Importance of an indeterminate diagnostic category. Cancer Cytopathol 2000;90:239–44.
7. Rossi ED, Morassi F, Santeusanio G, et al. Thyroid fine-needle aspiration cytology processed by Thin Prep: An additional slide decreased the number of inadequate results. Cytopathology 2010;21:97–102.
8. Baloch ZW, LiVolsi VA, Asa SL, et al. Diagnostic terminology and morphologic criteria for cytologic diagnosis of thyroid lesions: a synopsis of the National Cancer Institute Fine-needle aspiration state-of-science Conference. Diagn Cytopathol 2008;36:425–37.
9. Cross P, Chandra A, Giles T, et al. Guidance on the reporting of thyroid cytology specimens. London: The royal college of Pathologists; 2016.
10. Yang J, Schnadig V, Logrono R, et al. Fine needle aspiration of thyroid nodules: A study of 4703 patients with histologic and clinical correlations. Cancer 2007;111:306–15.
11. Alexander EK, Kennedy GC, Baloch ZW, et al. Preoperative diagnosis of benign thyroid nodules with indeterminate cytology. N Engl J Med 2012;367:705–15.
12. Tan YY, Kebebee E, Reiff E, et al. Does routine consultation of thyroid Fine needle aspiration cytology change surgical management? J Am Coll Surg 2007;205(1):8–12.
13. Wong L, Baloch ZW. Analysis of the Bethesda system for reporting thyroid cytopathology and similar precursor thyroid cytopathology reporting schemes. Adv Anat Pathol 2012;19(5):313–9.
14. Lew JI, Snyder RA, Sanchez YM, et al. Fine needle aspiration of the thyroid: correlation with final histopathology in a surgical series of 797 patients. J Am Coll Surg 2011;213:188–94.
15. Cancer Genome Atlas Research Network. Integrated genomic characterization of papillary thyroid carcinoma. Cell 2014;159:676–90.
16. Nikiforova MN, Nikiforov Y. Molecular diagnostics and predictors in thyroid cancer. Thyroid 2009;19: 1351–61.
17. Nikiforov YE, Steward DL, Robinson-Smith TM, et al. Molecular testing for mutations in improving the fine needle aspiration diagnosis of thyroid nodules. J Clin Endocrinol Metab 2009;94:2092–8.
18. Cheung CC, Carydis B, Ezzat S, et al. Analysis of *RET/PTC* gene rearrangements refines the fine needle aspiration diagnosis of thyroid cancer. J Clin Endocrinol Metab 2001;86:2187–90.
19. Moses W, Weng J, Sansano I, et al. Molecular testing for somatic mutations improves the accuracy of thyroid fine needle aspiration biopsy. World J Surg 2010;34:2589–94.
20. Musholt TJ, Fottner C, Weber M, et al. Detection of papillary carcinoma by analysis of *BRAF* and *RET/PTC1* mutations in fine needle aspiration biopsies of thyroid nodules. World J Surg 2010;34: 2595–603.
21. Xing M. *BRAF* mutation in papillary thyroid cancer: pathogenic role, molecular bases, and clinical implications. Endocr Rev 2007;28:742–62.
22. Rorive S, D'Haene N, Fossion C, et al. Ultrasound-guided fine needle aspiration of thyroid nodules: stratification of malignancy risk using follicular proliferation grading , clinical and ultrasonographic features. Eur J Endocrinol 2001;162:1107–15.
23. Bohacek L, Milas M, Mitchell J, et al. Diagnostic accuracy of surgeon-performed ultrasound guided fine needle aspiration of thyroid nodules. Ann Surg Oncol 2012;19:45–51.
24. Piana S, Frasoldati A, Ferrari M, et al. Is a five-category reporting scheme for thyroid fine needle aspiration cytology accurate? Experience of over 18,000 FNAs reported at the same institution during 1998-2007. Cytopathology 2011;22:164–73.

25. Nayar R, Ivanovic M. The indeterminate thyroid fine needle aspiration: experience from an academic center using terminology similar to that proposed in the 2007 National cancer institute thyroid fine needle aspiration state of the science conference. Cancer 2009;117:195–2002.
26. Carr R, Ustun B, Chhieng D, et al. Radiologic and clinical predictors of malignancy in the follicular lesion of undetermined significance of the thyroid. Endocr Pathol 2013;24:62–8.
27. Jaragh M, Carydis VB, MacMillan C, et al. Predictors of malignancy in thyroid fine-needle aspirates "cyst fluid only" cases. Can potential clues of malignancy be identified? Cancer Cytopathol 2009; 120:305–10.
28. Gage H, Hubbard E, Nodit L. Multiple squamous cells in thyroid fine needle aspiration: friends or foes? Diagn Cytopathol 2016;44(8):676–81.
29. Faquin WC, Cibas E, Renshaw AA. Atypical cells in needle aspiration biopsy specimens of benign thyroid cysts. Cancer 2005;105:71–9.
30. Jaffar R, Mohanty SK, Khan A, et al. Hemosiderin laden macrophages and hemosiderin within follicular cells distinguish benign follicular lesions from follicular neoplasms. Cytojournal 2009;6:3.
31. Chen AL, Renshaw AA, Faquin WC, et al. Thyroid FNA biopsies comprised of abundant, mature squamous cells can be reported as benign: A cytologic study of 18 patients with clinical correlation. Cancer Cytopathol 2018;126:336–41.
32. Ryska A, Ludvíková M, Rydlová M, et al. Massive squamous metaplasia of the thyroid gland– report of three cases. Pathol Res Pract 2006;202: 99–106.
33. Richmond BK, Judhan R, Chong B, et al. False-negative results with the Bethesda system of reporting thyroid cytopathology: Predictors of malignancy in thyroid nodules classified as benign by cytopathologic evaluation. Am Surg 2014;80(8): 811–6.
34. Anderson SR, Mandel S, LiVolsi VA, et al. Can cytomorphology differentiate between benign nodules and tumors arising in Graves' disease? Diagn Cytopathol 2004;30(1):64–7.
35. Haugen BR, Alexander E, Bible KC, et al. American Thyroid Association (ATA) Guidelines Taskforce on Thyroid Nodules and Differentiated Thyroid Cancer. 2015 American Thyroid Association management guidelines for adult patients with thyroid nodules and differentiated thyroid cancer. Thyroid 2016; 26:1–133.
36. Belfiore A, Russo D, Vigneri R, et al. Graves' disease, thyroid nodules and carcinoma. Clin Endocrinol 2001;55:711–8.
37. Dobyns BM, Sheline GE, Workman JB, et al. Malignant and benign neoplasm of the thyroid in patients treated for hyperthyroidism: A report of the cooperative thyro-toxicosis therapy follow-up study. J Clin Endocrinol Metab 1974;38:976–98.
38. Anila KR, Nayak Nn, Jayasree K. Cytomorphologic spectrum of lymphocytic thyroiditis and correlation between cytological grading and biochemical parameters. J Cytol 2016;33(3):145–9.
39. Bhatia A, Rajwanshi A, Dash RJ, et al. Lymphocytic thyroiditis-Is cytological grading significant? A correlation of grades with clinical biochemical, ultrasonographic and radionuclide parameters. Cytojournal 2007;4:10.
40. Yi KI, Ahn S, Park DY, et al. False-positive cytopathology results for papillary thyroid carcinoma: a trap for thyroid surgeons. Clin Otolaryngol 2017;42:1153–60.
41. Boi F, Pani F, Mariotti S. Thyroid autoimmunity and thyroid cancer: review focused on cytological studies. Eur Thyroid J 2017;6(4):178–86.
42. Solano JG, Bascunana AG, Perez JS, et al. Fine needle aspiration of subacute granulomatous thyroiditis (De quervain's thyroiditis): a clinic-cytologic review of 36 cases. Diagn Cytopathol 1997;16(3):214–20.
43. Rosa M. Cytologic features of subacute granulomatous thyroiditis can mimic malignancy in liquid-based preparations. Diagn Cytopathol 2016;44(8): 682–4.
44. Anderson CE, Duvall E, Wallace WA. A single ThinPrep slide may not be representative in all head and neck fine needle aspirate specimens. Cytopathology 2009;20:87–90.
45. Vural C, Paksoy N, Gok ND, et al. Subacute granulomatous (De Quervain) thyroiditis: Fine needle aspiration cytology and ultrasonographic characteristics of 21 cases. Cytojournal 2015;12:9.
46. Olah R, Hajos O, Soos Z, et al. De Quervain thyroiditis. Corner point of the diagnosis. Orv Hetil 2014; 155:676–80.
47. Singer PA. Thyroiditis. Acute, subacute and chronic. Med Clin North Am 1991;75:61–77.
48. Baloch ZW, LiVolsi VA. Follicular-patterned afflictions of the thyroid gland: Reappraisal of the most discussed entity in endocrine pathology. Endocr Pathol 2014;25:12–20.
49. Renshaw A, Wang E, Wilbur D, et al. Interobserver agreement on microfollicles in thyroid fine needle aspirates. Arch Path Lab Med 2006;130: 148–52.
50. Broome JT, Solorzano CC. The impact of atypia/follicular lesion of undetermined significance on the rate of malignancy in thyroid fine-needle aspiration: Evaluation of the Bethesda System for Reporting Thyroid Cytopathology. Surgery 2011;150: 1234–9.
51. Shi Y, Ding X, Klein M, et al. Thyroid fine-needle aspiration with atypia of undetermined significance: a necessary or optional category? Cancer 2009;117:298–304.

52. Damiani D, Suciu V, Vielh P. Cytopathology of follicular cell nodules. Endocr Pathol 2015;26:286–91.
53. Nagarkatti SS, Faquin WC, Lubitz CC, et al. Management of thyroid nodules with atypical cytology on fine-needle aspiration biopsy. Ann Surg Oncol 2013;20:60–5.
54. Olson MT, Clark DP, Erozan YS, et al. Spectrum of Risk of Malignancy in Subcategories of 'Atypia of Undetermined Significance'. Acta Cytol 2011;55: 518–25.
55. Horne MJ, Chhieng DC, Theoharis C, et al. Thyroid follicular lesion of undetermined significance: Evaluation of the risk of malignancy using the two-tier sub-classification. Diagn Cytopathol 2012;40: 410–5.
56. Rossi ED, Martini M, Capodimonti S, et al. Morphology combined with ancillary techniques: An algorithm approach for thyroid nodules. Cytopathology 2018;29(5):418–27.
57. Rossi ED, Bizzarro T, Martini M, et al. Cytopathology of Follicular Cell Nodules. Adv Anat Pathol 2017;24(1):45–55.
58. Cibas ES, Ali SZ. The Bethesda System for Reporting Thyroid Cytopathology. Thyroid 2009;9: 1159–65.
59. Baloch Z, LiVolsi VA, Henricks WH, et al. Encapsulated follicular variant of papillary thyroid carcinoma. Am J Clin Pathol 2002;118(4):603–5.
60. Howitt BE, Chang S, Eslinger M, et al. Fine-needle aspiration diagnoses of noninvasive follicular variant of papillary thyroid carcinoma. Am J Clin Pathol 2015;144(6):850–7.
61. Ganly I, Wang L, Tuttle MR, et al. Invasion rather than nuclear features correlates with outcome in encapsulated follicular tumors: further evidence for the reclassification of the encapsulated papillary thyroid carcinoma follicular variant. Hum Pathol 2015;46(5):657–64.
62. Nikiforov YE, Seethala RR, Tallini G, et al. Nomenclature revision for encapsulated follicular variant of papillary thyroid carcinoma: a paradigm shift to reduce overtreatment of indolent tumors. JAMA Oncol 2016;2(8):1023–9.
63. Thompson LD. Ninety-four cases of encapsulated follicular variant of papillary thyroid carcinoma: a name change to noninvasive follicular thyroid neoplasm with papillary like nuclear features would help to prevent overtreatment. Mod Pathol 2016; 29(7):698–707.
64. Bizzarro T, Martini M, Capodimonti S, et al. The morphologic analysis of non-invasive follicular thyroid neoplasm with papillary-like nuclear features (NIFTP) on liquid based cytology: Some insights of their identification in our institutional experience. Cancer Cytopathol 2016;124(10):699–710.
65. Faquin W, Wong L, Afrogheh A, et al. Impact of reclassifying non invasive FVPC on the risk of malignancy in the Bethesda system for reporting thyroid Cytopathology. Cancer Cytopathol 2016; 124(3):181–7.
66. Nikiforov Y, Baloch ZW, Hodak SP, et al. Change in diagnostic criteria for noninvasive follicular thyroid neoplasm with papillary like nuclear features. JAMA Oncol 2018. https://doi.org/10.1001/jamaoncol.2018.1446.
67. Ohori NP, Wolfe J, Carty S, et al. The influence of the noninvasive follicular thyroid neoplasm with papillary-like nuclear features (NIFTP) resection diagnosis on the false-positive thyroid cytology rate relates to quality assurance thresholds and the application of NIFTP criteria. Cancer Cytopathol 2017;125:692–700.
68. Agarwal AM, Bentz JS, Hungerford R, et al. Parathyroid fine needle aspiration cytology in the evaluation of parathyroid adenoma: cytologic findings from 53 patients. Diagn Cytopathol 2009;37: 407–10.
69. Rossi ED, Mulè A, Zannoni GF, et al. Asymptomatic intrathyroidal parathyroid adenoma. Report of a case with a cytologic differential diagnosis including thyroid neoplasms. Acta Cytol 2004; 48(3):437–40.
70. Cho M, Oweity T, Brandler TC, et al. Distinguishing parathyroid and thyroid lesions on ultrasound-guide fine needle aspiration: A correlation of clinical data, ancillary studies and molecular analysis. Cancer Cytopathol 2017;125(9):674–82.
71. Vanderlaan PA, Marqusee E, Krane JF. Usefulness of diagnostic qualifiers for thyroid fine-needle aspirations with atypia of undetermined significance. Am J Clin Pathol 2011;136(4):572–7.
72. Krane JF, Vanderlaan PA, Faquin WC, et al. The atypia of undetermined significance/follicular lesion of undetermined significance: malignant ratio: a proposed performance measure for reporting in The Bethesda System for thyroid cytopathology. Cancer Cytopathol 2012;120(2):111–6.
73. Ohori NP, Nikiforova MN, Schoedel KE, et al. Contribution of molecular testing to thyroid fine needle aspiration cytology of "Follicular lesion of undetermined significance/Atypia of undetermined significance". Cancer Cytopathol 2010;118:17–23.
74. Colanta A, Lin O, Tafe L, et al. BRAF mutation analysis of fine-needle aspiration biopsies of papillary thyroid carcinoma: impact on diagnosis and prognosis. Acta Cytol 2011;55:563–9.
75. Nikiforov YE, Ohori P, Hodack SP, et al. Impact of mutational testing on the diagnosis and management of patients with cytologically indeterminate thyroid nodules: a prospective analysis of 1056 FNA samples. J Clin Endocrinol Metabol 2011;96: 3390–7.
76. Radkay L, Chiosea SI, Seethala RR, et al. Thyroid nodules with KRAS mutations are different from

nodules with NRAS and HRAS mutations with regard to cytopathologic and histopathologic outcome characteristics. Cancer Cytopathol 2014;122:873–82.

77. Rossi ED, Martini M, Capodimonti S, et al. BRAF (V600E) mutation analysis on LBC-processed aspiration biopsies predicts bilaterality and nodal involvement in papillary thyroid microcarcinoma. Cancer Cytopathol 2013;121:291–7.
78. Giorgadze T, Rossi ED, Fadda G, et al. Does the fine-needle aspiration diagnosis of "Hürthle-cell neoplasm/follicular neoplasm with oncocytic features" denote increased risk of malignancy? Diagn Cytopathol 2004;31(5):307–12.
79. Straccia P, Rossi ED, Bizzarro T, et al. A meta-analytic review of the Bethesda System for Reporting Thyroid Cytopathology: Has the rate of malignancy in indeterminate lesions been underestimated? Cancer Cytopathol 2015;123(12):713–22.
80. Rossi ED, Martini M, Straccia P, et al. The cytologic category of oncocytic (Hurthle) cell neoplasm mostly includes low-risk lesions at histology: an institutional experience. Eur J Endocrinol 2013;169(5):649–55.
81. Montone KT, Baloch ZW, LiVolsi VA. The thyroid Hurthle (oncocytic) cell and its associated pathologic conditions: a surgical pathology and cytopathology review. Arch Pathol Lab Med 2008;132:1241–50.
82. Kasper KA, Stewart J, Das K. Fine-needle aspiration cytology of thyroid nodules with hurthle cells: cytomorphologic predictors for neoplasms, improving diagnostic accuracy and overcoming pitfalls. Acta Cytol 2014;58:145–52.
83. Díaz Del Arco C, Fernández Aceñero MJ. Preoperative Diagnosis of Neoplastic or Malignant Hürthle Cell Lesions: A Chimera? Acta Cytol 2018;62(3):193–203.
84. Moreira AL, Waisman J, Cangiarella JF. Aspiration cytology of the oncocytic variant of papillary adenocarcinoma of the thyroid gland. Acta Cytol 2004;48(2):137–41.
85. Maximo V, Rios E, Sobrinho-Simoes M. Oncocytic lesions of the thyroid, kidney, salivary glands, adrenal cortex and parathyroid glands. Int J Surg Pathol 2014;22:33–6.
86. Bai S, Baloch ZW, Samulski TD, et al. Poorly differentiated oncocytic (hürthle cell) follicular carcinoma: an institutional experience. Endocr Pathol 2015;26(2):164–9.
87. Rossi ED, Mule ' A, Miraglia A, et al. Granular cell tumour on conventional cytology and thin-layer smears. Cytopathology 2005;16(5):259–61.
88. Wong YP, Sharifah NA, Tan GC, et al. Intrathyroidal oxyphilic parathyroid carcinoma: A potential diagnostic caveat in cytology? Diagn Cytopathol 2016;44(8):688–92.
89. Khanafshar E, Lloyd RV. The spectrum of papillary thyroid carcinoma variants. Adv Anat Pathol 2011;18:90–7.
90. Albores-Saavedra J, Wu J. The many faces and mimics of papillary thyroid carcinoma. Endocr Pathol 2006;17:1–18.
91. Baloch Z, LiVolsi VA, Tondon R. Aggressive variants of follicular cell derived thyroid carcinoma; the so called "Real Thyroid Carcinomas". J Clin Pathol 2013;66:733–43.
92. Rosai J, Carcangiu ML, DeLellis RA. Tumors of the thyroid gland. Vol 3rd series, fascicle 5. Washington, DC: Armed forces institute of pathology.
93. Llyod RV, Osamura RY, Kloppel G, et al. Tumors of the thyroid gland. In: WHO Classifications of tumors of the endocrine organs. 4th edition; 2017.
94. Hawn WA. The many appearances of papillary carcinoma of the thyroid. Cleve Clin Q 1976;43:207–16.
95. Saglietti C, Piana S, La Rosa S, et al. Hyalinizing trabecular tumor of the thyroid: Fine needle aspiration cytological diagnosis and correlation with histology. J Clin Pathol 2017;70:641–7.
96. Choi WJ, Baek JH, Ha EJ, et al. The ultrasonography features of hyalinizing trabecular tumor of the thyroid gland and the role of fine needle aspiration cytology and core needle biopsy in its diagnosis. Acta Radiol 2015;56(9):1113–8.
97. Wells SA, Asa S, Dralle H, et al. Revised American Thyroid Association Guidelines for the Management of Medullary Thyroid Carcinoma. The American Thyroid Association Guidelines Task Force on Medullary Thyroid Carcinoma. Thyroid 2015;25:567–610.
98. Trimboli P, Treglia G, Guidobaldi L, et al. Detection rate of FNA cytology in medullary thyroid carcinoma: A meta-analysis. Clin Endocrinol 2015;82:280–5.
99. Papaparaskeva K, Nagel H, Droese M. Cytologic diagnosis of medullary carcinoma of the thyroid gland. Diagn Cytopathol 2000;22:351–8.
100. Pusztaszeri M, Bongiovanni M, Faquin WC. Update on the cytological and molecular features of medullary thyroid carcinoma. Adv Anat Pathol 2014;21:26–35.
101. Rossi ED, Raffaelli M, Mulè A, et al. Relevance of immunocytochemistry on thin-layer cytology in thyroid lesions suspicious for medullary carcinoma: a case-control study. Appl Immunohistochem Mol Morphol 2008;16(6):548–53.
102. Baloch ZW, LiVolsi VA. Special types of thyroid carcinoma. Histopathology 2018;72(1):40–52.
103. Carcangiu ML, Zampi G, Rosai J. Poorly differentiated (insular) thryoid carcinoma. A reinterpretation of Langahns " wuchernde struma". Am J Surg Pathol 1984;8:655–68.

104. Volante M, Landolfi S, Chiusa L, et al. Poorly differentiated carcinomas of the thyroid with trabecular, insular, and solid pattern: A clinicopathological study of 183 patients. Cancer 2004;100:950–7.
105. Bongiovanni M, Bloom I, Krane JF, et al. Cytomorphologic features of poorly differentiated thyroid carcinoma: a multi-institutional analysis of 40 cases. Cancer 2009;117:185–94.
106. Kane SV, Sharma TP. Cytologic diagnostic approach to poorly differentiated thyroid carcinoma: A single-institution study. Cancer Cytopathol 2015;123:82–91.
107. Barwad A, Dey P, Nahar Saikia UN, et al. Fine needle aspiration cytology of insular carcinoma of thyroid. Diagn Cytopathol 2012;40:E40–7.
108. Khetrapal S, Rana S, Jetley S, et al. Poorly differentiated carcinoma of thyroid: Case report of an uncommon entity. J Cancer Res Ther 2018;14(5): 1142–4.
109. Purkait S, Agarwal S, Mathur SR, et al. Fine needle aspiration cytology features of poorly differentiated thyroid carcinoma. Cytopathology 2016;27(3): 176–84.
110. Sironi M, Collini P, Cantaboni A. Fine needle aspiration cytology of insular thyroid carcinoma. A report of four cases. Acta Cytol 1992;36(3):435–9.
111. Laforga JB, Cortés VA. Oncocytic poorly differentiated (insular) thyroid carcinoma mimicking metastatic adenocarcinoma. A case report and review of the literature. Diagn Cytopathol 2019. https://doi.org/10.1002/dc.24147.
112. Bauman ME, Tao LC. Cytopathology of papillary carcinoma of the thyroid with anaplastic transformation. A case report. Acta Cytol 1995;39(3): 525–9.
113. Oktay MH, Smolkin MB, Williams M, et al. Metastatic anaplastic carcinoma of the thyroid mimicking squamous cell carcinoma: report of a case of a challenging cytologic diagnosis. Acta Cytol 2006; 50(2):201–4.
114. Maatouk J, Barklow TA, Zakaria W, et al. Anaplastic thyroid carcinoma arising in long-standing multinodular goiter following radioactive iodine therapy: report of a case diagnosed by fine needle aspiration. Acta Cytol 2009;53(5):581–3.
115. Feng G, Laskin WB, Chou PM, et al. Anaplastic thyroid carcinoma with rhabdoid features. Diagn Cytopathol 2015;43(5):416–20.
116. Suh HJ, Moon HJ, Kwak JY, et al. Anaplastic thyroid cancer: ultrasonographic findings and the role of ultrasonography-guided fine needle aspiration biopsy. Yonsei Med J 2013;54(6):1400–6.
117. Guarda LA, Peterson CE, Hall W, et al. Anaplastic thyroid carcinoma: cytomorphology and clinical implications of fine-needle aspiration. Diagn Cytopathol 1991;7(1):63–7.
118. Mehdi G, Ansari HA, Siddiqui SA. Cytology of anaplastic giant cell carcinoma of the thyroid with osteoclast-like giant cells–a case report. Diagn Cytopathol 2007;35(2):111–2.
119. Straccia P, Mosseri C, Brunelli C, et al. Diagnosis and Treatment of Metastases to the Thyroid Gland: a Meta-Analysis. Endocr Pathol 2017;28(2): 112–20.
120. Papi G, Fadda G, Corsello SM, et al. Metastases to the thyroid gland: prevalence, clinicopathological aspects and prognosis: a 10-year experience. Clin Endocrinol (Oxf) 2007;66(4):565–71.
121. Rossi ED, Martini M, Straccia P, et al. Is thyroid gland only a "land" for primary malignancies? role of morphology and immunocytochemistry. Diagn Cytopathol 2015;43(5):374–80.
122. Ciobanu D, Vulpoi C, Găluşcă B, et al. The value of the immunohistochemical exam in the diagnosis of the secondary malignant tumors to the thyroid gland. Rom J Morphol Embryol 2007;48(2):113–9.
123. Shah SS, Faquin WC, Izquierdo R, et al. FNA of misclassified primary malignant neoplasms of the thyroid: Impact on clinical management. Cytojournal 2009;6:1.

Prognostic Parameters in Differentiated Thyroid Carcinomas

Nicole A. Cipriani, MD

KEYWORDS

• Papillary thyroid carcinoma • Follicular thyroid carcinoma • Variants • Extrathyroidal extension • Angioinvasion • Extranodal extension • *BRAF* V600E • *TERT* promoter

Key points

- The AJCC staging system and the ATA risk prediction system are the best predictors of mortality and recurrence, respectively, in differentiated thyroid carcinoma.
- Pathologic reporting should include: aggressive variants of PTC; extrathyroidal extension; angioinvasion; number, location, and size of lymph node metastases; extranodal extension; genetics (if known).
- Reporting of these key features may prompt more aggressive treatment in some cases and provide more accurate risk expectations for patients.

ABSTRACT

Differentiated thyroid carcinomas make up most thyroid malignancies. The AJCC staging system and the ATA risk prediction system are the best predictors of mortality and recurrence, respectively. Key factors to be identified and reported by pathologists are reviewed in this article and include: (1) aggressive histologic variants of papillary thyroid carcinoma (including tall cell, columnar cell, and hobnail variants); (2) presence of gross extrathyroidal extension (into skeletal muscle or adjacent organs); (3) angioinvasion (including number of foci); (4) number, anatomic level, and size of lymph node metastases; (4) extranodal extension; (5) genetics (especially *BRAF* V600E or *TERT* promoter mutation).

OVERVIEW

Thyroid carcinoma represents 3% of new cancer diagnoses in the United States, with an estimated 54,000 new cases and 2000 cancer-related deaths in 2018.[1] Women are affected 3 times more frequently than men. The median age at diagnosis is 51 years, and the median age at death is 73 years. Although incidence in thyroid carcinoma has more than tripled since the 1970s, mortality rates have remained relatively unchanged. Overall 5-year survival of thyroid carcinoma is greater than 90%.[1] Most differentiated thyroid carcinomas (DTCs) arising from follicular cells are histologically well-differentiated papillary thyroid carcinomas (PTCs) (>80% of all thyroid cancers) followed by follicular thyroid carcinomas (FTCs) and Hürthle cell carcinomas (HCCs) (up to 5%–10% combined).[2,3] The best predictors of mortality have been shown to be the American Joint Committee on Cancer (AJCC) TNM staging system and the Mayo Clinic MACIS (metastasis, age, completeness of resection, invasion, and size) system.[4,5] Predicting disease recurrence has proven challenging; however, the American Thyroid Association (ATA) has developed an Initial Risk Stratification System (on a spectrum from low to intermediate to high) using several clinical, pathologic, and genetic factors to aid in prediction of

Disclosure: The author has nothing to disclose.

Department of Pathology, The University of Chicago, 5841 South Maryland Avenue, MC 6101, Chicago, IL 60637, USA
E-mail address: nicole.cipriani@uchospitals.edu
twitter: @NICOLECIPRIANI (N.A.C.)

Surgical Pathology 12 (2019) 883–900
https://doi.org/10.1016/j.path.2019.07.001
1875-9181/19/

recurrence and to guide postoperative treatment.[4] Identification and reporting of these key factors by pathologists is necessary for active risk stratification of patients as well as ongoing studies to refine predictive and prognostic criteria.[6]

MORTALITY IN DIFFERENTIATED THYROID CARCINOMA

Various systems were developed to predict risk of mortality in DTC. The first, published in 1979, was developed by the European Organization for Research on Treatment of Cancer and included 5 variables: age, sex, extrathyroidal extension (ETE), distant metastasis, and cell type (specifically differentiating between follicular-derived, medullary, and anaplastic).[7] The scoring system assigned patients to 1 of 5 risk groups, with 5-year survivals ranging from 95% in group 1, to 51% in group 3, to 5% in group 5. Throughout the 1980s and 1990s, other systems were developed to address additional risk factors (tumor size, multifocality, histologic "grade," lymph node involvement, and margin status): the 1987 AGES (age, grade, extent, and size) system,[8] the 1988 AMES (age, metastases, extent, and size) system,[9] the 1993 MACIS system,[10] the 1994 OSU (Ohio State University) system,[11] the 1995 MSKCC (Memorial Sloan-Kettering Cancer Center) system,[12] and the 1998 NTCTCS (National Thyroid Cancer Treatment Cooperative Study) system.[13] The MACIS system developed at the Mayo Clinic is considered to be one of the better predictors, with 20-year survivals ranging from 99% in low-risk groups to 24% in high-risk groups.[10] It takes into account metastasis, age, completeness of resection, invasion, and size (**Table 1**).

Since then, the AJCC TNM staging system has almost superseded previous systems and is considered to be one of the best predictors of mortality in DTC[4,5] (**Table 2**). In comparing the AMES, MACIS, and TNM systems, Voutilainen and colleagues[14] found TNM to be the best differentiator of mortality rates in high-risk versus low-risk patients, and it had a high proportion of explained variance (in other words, statistically, TNM was relatively good at predicting mortality when applied to a broad range of patient cohorts with intrinsic variability). Important changes from the 7th to 8th editions include the downstaging of patients with low-risk disease to more accurately estimate their high rates of survival.[15] First, the 8th edition necessitates the distinction of gross from microscopic ETE, which is thought to impact recurrence but not mortality in DTC. Only gross (not microscopic) ETE is staged as T3. ETE is discussed in detail subsequently. Second, level VII (superior mediastinal) lymph node involvement, previously N1b disease, is now staged along with central neck lymph nodes (N1a disease), also downstaging many patients. Involvement of lateral cervical lymph nodes (levels I through V) is thought to portend worse prognosis compared with involvement of only central neck or superior mediastinal nodes (levels VI and VII). However, it is unclear whether other features such as size of nodal deposits, number of positive nodes, or presence of extranodal extension (ENE) are potentially confounding. Finally, age at diagnosis is an important prognostic factor in the stage groups. In previous editions, diagnosis at age 45 years or above was considered a negative prognostic indicator. However, on retrospective review, patients between the ages of 45 and

Table 1
MACIS system

Parameter	Numeric Value	Final MACIS Score	15–20-y Disease-Specific Survival (%)
Metastasis	+1 if metastatic	<6	99
Age	If ≤39: 3.1 × age in years If ≥40: 0.8 × age in years	≥6 and <7 ≥7 and <8	84–89 56–74
Completeness of resection	+1 if incompletely resected	≥8	24–51
Invasion	+1 if locally invasive (extrathyroidal invasion)		
Size	0.3 × size in cm		

Data from Hay ID, Bergstralh EJ, Goellner JR, Ebersold JR, Grant CS. Predicting outcome in papillary thyroid carcinoma: Development of a reliable prognostic scoring system in a cohort of 1779 patients surgically treated at one institution during 1940 through 1989. *Surgery.* 1993;114(6):1050-1058; and Voutilainen PE, Siironen P, Franssila KO, Sivula A, Haapiainen RK, Haglund CH. AMES, MACIS and TNM prognostic classifications in papillary thyroid carcinoma. *Anticancer Research.* 2003;23(5b):4283-4288.

Table 2
American Joint Committee on Cancer TNM staging system

T stage	Size	T1a ($\leq$1 cm) T1b (>1 to $\leq$2 cm) T2 (>2 to $\leq$4 cm) T3a (>4 cm)
	Gross extrathyroidal invasion	T3b (strap muscles) T4a (subcutis, larynx, trachea, esophagus, recurrent laryngeal nerve) T4b (prevertebral fascia, encasing carotid/ mediastinal vessels)
N stage	Lymph nodes negative	N0a (cytologically/ histologically confirmed negative) N0b (radiographically/ clinically negative)
	Lymph nodes positive, location	N1a (levels VI–VII) N1b (levels I–V or retropharyngeal)
M stage	Distant metastasis present	M1

Data from Amin MB, Edge S, Greene F, et al., eds. *AJCC Cancer Staging Manual.* 8 ed. Springer International Publishing; 2017.

55 years were frequently upstaged without significant differences in mortality compared with younger patients.[15] Therefore, the current 8th edition incorporates the modified TNM system and an age cutoff of 55 years to stratify patients into groups with differing survivals (**Table 3**). This age change alone is estimated to downstage approximately 12% of patients.[16] Taking into account all changes including age, lymph node levels, ETE, and modifications of stage groupings, estimated 10-year disease-specific survival decreases significantly in stages III and IV, because patients with low-risk disease are more appropriately included in lower-stage groups with good relative prognoses.[17]

RECURRENCE IN DIFFERENTIATED THYROID CARCINOMA

Estimated rates of recurrence in DTC vary, with most studies estimating approximately 20% recurrence overall, ranging from less than 1% in very low-risk patients to greater than 50% in high-risk patients.[4,18] The 2009 Risk Stratification System conceived by the ATA took into account various clinical and pathologic features thought to predict cancer recurrence, and grouped patients into low, intermediate, and high risk. Using these groups, recurrence rates in the patient cohort who underwent total thyroidectomy with radioactive iodine (RAI) ablation were 9% to 22%, 37% to 48%, and 69% to 86%, respectively.[4] Of those who did not undergo RAI ablation, recurrence rates were 1% to 2% and up to 8% in the low-risk and intermediate-risk

Table 3
American Joint Committee on Cancer prognostic stage groups

Group	I	II		III	IVA	IVB
<55 y	T any N any M0	T any N any *M1*		n/a	n/a	n/a
$\geq$55 y	T1/T2 N0/NX M0	T1/T2 *N1* M0	*T3a/T3b* N any M0	*T4a* N any M0	*T4b* N any M0	T any N any *M1*
Expected 10-y DSS (8th edition)	98%–100%	85%–95%		60%–70%	<50%	
Previous 10-y DSS (7th edition)	97%–100%	95%–99%		88%–95%	50%–75%	

Abbreviation: DSS, disease-specific survival.
Data from Amin MB, Edge S, Greene F, et al., eds. *AJCC Cancer Staging Manual.* 8 ed. Springer International Publishing; 2017; and Tuttle RM, Haugen B, Perrier ND. Updated American Joint Committee on Cancer/Tumor-Node-Metastasis Staging System for Differentiated and Anaplastic Thyroid Cancer (Eighth Edition): What Changed and Why? *Thyroid.* 2017;27(6):751-756. https://doi.org/10.1089/thy.2017.0102.

Table 4
American Thyroid Association initial risk stratification for differentiated thyroid carcinomas

	Low Risk[a]	Intermediate Risk	High Risk
Clinical features	• Complete macroscopic resection	• RAI-avid metastatic foci in the neck (if I-131 is given)	• Incomplete macroscopic resection • Distant metastases • Postoperative serum thyroglobulin suggestive of distant metastases
Nodal features	• cN0 • pN1 (≤5 LNs, tumor foci <0.2 cm) • pN1 (≤3 LNs, without ENE)	• cN1 • pN1 (>5 LNs, tumor foci <3 cm)	• pN1 (≥3 cm) • pN1 (>3 LNs, with ENE)
Pathologic features	• Intrathyroidal low-risk tumors: ○ Encapsulated PTC-FV ○ FTC with capsular invasion and <4 foci angioinvasion ○ PTC <4 cm ○ PTMC (any no. of foci)	• Aggressive variants of PTC (tall cell, hobnail, columnar cell) • PTC with angioinvasion • Microscopic extrathyroidal invasion in: ○ PTC ○ FTC ○ PTMC	• Macroscopic extrathyroidal invasion • FTC with >4 foci of angioinvasion
Treatment	• RAI not recommended	• RAI considered	• RAI recommended

Abbreviations: ENE, extranodal extension; FTC, follicular thyroid carcinoma; FV, follicular variant; LN, lymph node; PTC, papillary thyroid carcinoma; PTMC, papillary thyroid microcarcinoma; RAI, radioactive iodine.

[a] Features that must be absent in low-risk PTC: local or distant metastases; loco-regional invasion; aggressive histologic variant; RAI-avid metastatic foci outside the thyroid bed (if I-131 is given); angioinvasion.

Data from Haugen BR, Alexander EK, Bible KC, et al. 2015 American Thyroid Association Management Guidelines for Adult Patients with Thyroid Nodules and Differentiated Thyroid Cancer: The American Thyroid Association Guidelines Task Force on Thyroid Nodules and Differentiated Thyroid Cancer. *Thyroid*. 2016;26(1):1-133. https://doi.org/10.1089/thy.2015.0020.

groups. The 2015 modification of the system introduced additional risk factors and recommended considering risk as a spectrum rather than 3 discrete groups.[4] The implication is that RAI is not recommended for patients on the low end, it should be considered for those in the intermediate range, and RAI is recommended for patients on the high end (**Table 4**). In addition, the National Comprehensive Cancer Network (NCCN) clinical practice guidelines provide algorithms for treatment of DTC based on a variety of clinical and pathologic features.[19] Salient features that should be reported by pathologists are discussed individually, and include: aggressive histologic variants of PTC, ETE, angioinvasion, lymph node metastasis, ENE, and genetic profile, if known.

PAPILLARY THYROID CARCINOMA VARIANTS

Recurrence in the smallest variant, papillary thyroid microcarcinoma (PTMC), is low, ranging from 1% to 2% in unifocal intrathyroidal PTMC to 4% to 6% in multifocal PTMC with ETE and *BRAF* V600E mutation.[4] Some studies have found multifocality, ETE or peripheral tumor location, fibrosis, and/or *BRAF* V600E mutation to predict recurrence in PTMC.[20,21] Therefore, any of these high-risk features in PTMC should be reported just as in larger PTCs. In carcinomas of larger size, 2 and 4 cm are considered to represent clinically significant size cutoffs. Postoperative RAI ablation is considered in carcinomas between 2 and 4 cm and is routinely recommended by the NCCN in carcinomas greater than 4 cm, because increasing size is thought to linearly correlate with recurrence and mortality.[11,19] In PTCs greater than 1 cm in size, several histologic variants are thought to portend worse prognosis, and RAI should be considered in otherwise low-risk patients who manifest these variants. Tall cell, columnar cell, and hobnail variants (HNVs) are highlighted by the ATA and/or NCCN.

> **Key Points**
> **AGGRESSIVE HISTOLOGIC VARIANTS OF PAPILLARY THYROID CARCINOMA**
>
> - Tall cell variant: at least 30% of cells 2 to 3 times taller than wide; eosinophilic cytoplasm; "tram-track" follicles; exaggerated nuclear features of PTC (can report as "tall cell features" if minimal criteria not met)
> - Columnar cell variant: architectural heterogeneity; pseudostratified columnar cells with sub- or supranuclear vacuoles; elongated nuclei with coarse chromatin (should report as circumscribed vs invasive)
> - Hobnail variant: at least 30% of cells with apically located nuclei bulging into the lumen; eosinophilic cytoplasm; papillary or micropapillary architecture (can report as "hobnail features" if minimal criteria not met)

TALL CELL VARIANT

The tall cell variant (TCV) is the most common histologic variant of PTC (after excluding classic type, microcarcinomas, and follicular variants).[3] It is defined by the World Health Organization (WHO) as tumors of which at least 30% of cells are 2 to 3 times taller than they are wide and have abundant eosinophilic cytoplasm.[2] However, in practice, diagnosis of TCV is highly variable, with some pathologists considering a height:width ratio of 3:1 (others 2:1) with tall cells occupying at least 30% (but up to 50%) of the tumor volume.[22] Additional features used to identify TCV include elongated "tram-track" follicles and exaggerated nuclear features of PTC[22] (**Fig. 1**A, B). Given the inconsistency in identification and reporting of TCV (incidence ranging from 4% to 17% of PTCs),[23] the clinical and prognostic significance may come into question. Nevertheless, many studies have shown that carcinomas meeting the various definitions of TCV (including as low as 10% tall cells) have increased size, increased rates of multifocality, higher TNM stage, increased frequency of ETE, increased angioinvasion, increased lymph node and distant metastasis, higher recurrence and mortality rates, higher frequency of transformation to poorly differentiated or anaplastic carcinoma, increased rates of *BRAF* V600E mutation, and potentially decreased RAI avidity.[24–28] On the other hand, some studies have shown that TCV is not an independent risk factor for recurrence and mortality, and when using controls matched for age, sex, tumor size, lymph node metastasis, and ETE, differences in disease-free survival disappear.[29–32] In a Surveillance, Epidemiology, and End Results data analysis of TCV, disease-related mortality was 6.3% in TCV compared with 2.6% in classic PTC, but the ICD coding did not distinguish between TCV and columnar cell variant (CCV) (discussed below).[33] Although the data are conflicting and long-term controlled studies are warranted, tall cell features (possibly including the percent of tumor volume occupied by tall cells) should be included in pathology reports to allow surgeons, endocrinologists, and patients to individualize therapy.

COLUMNAR CELL VARIANT

The CCV is described by WHO as containing papillae or follicles lined by pseudostratified columnar cells without overt conventional nuclear features of PTC.[2] Various architectural patterns may be present, including trabeculae, cribriform spaces, solid areas, or complex branching glands.[34] CCV often resembles endometrial or intestinal carcinoma and may have subnuclear or supranuclear vacuoles. Nuclear features of PTC may be minimal, but nuclei often show enlargement, elongation, and coarse dark chromatin[35] (**Fig. 1**C, D). Immunopositivity for CDX2 has been reported, but is of no known prognostic significance.[36,37] CCV is rare, representing less than 1% of PTCs. When circumscribed, it tends to behave in an indolent fashion.[34] However, when diffusely infiltrative, CCV may show increased ETE, nodal metastasis, and disease recurrence and mortality.[32,35,38] In a study comparing classic PTC and CCV (matching for age, sex, tumor size, lymph node metastasis, and ETE), CCV had up to 50% recurrence compared with 22% for classic PTC.[32] Identification of CCV, as well as reporting circumscription versus invasion, is important for risk stratification and possible therapeutic modification.

HOBNAIL VARIANT

The HNV of PTC is described by WHO as having at least 30% of tumor volume composed of papillae and micropapillae lined by somewhat dyscohesive cells with eosinophilic cytoplasm and apically located nuclei with prominent nucleoli that create an apical bulge into the lumen[2,35] (**Fig. 1**E, F). Early reports of this very rare variant (up to 1% of PTCs) documented high rates of angioinvasion, lymph node metastasis (76%), local recurrence, distant metastasis (63%), and death (50%), especially in

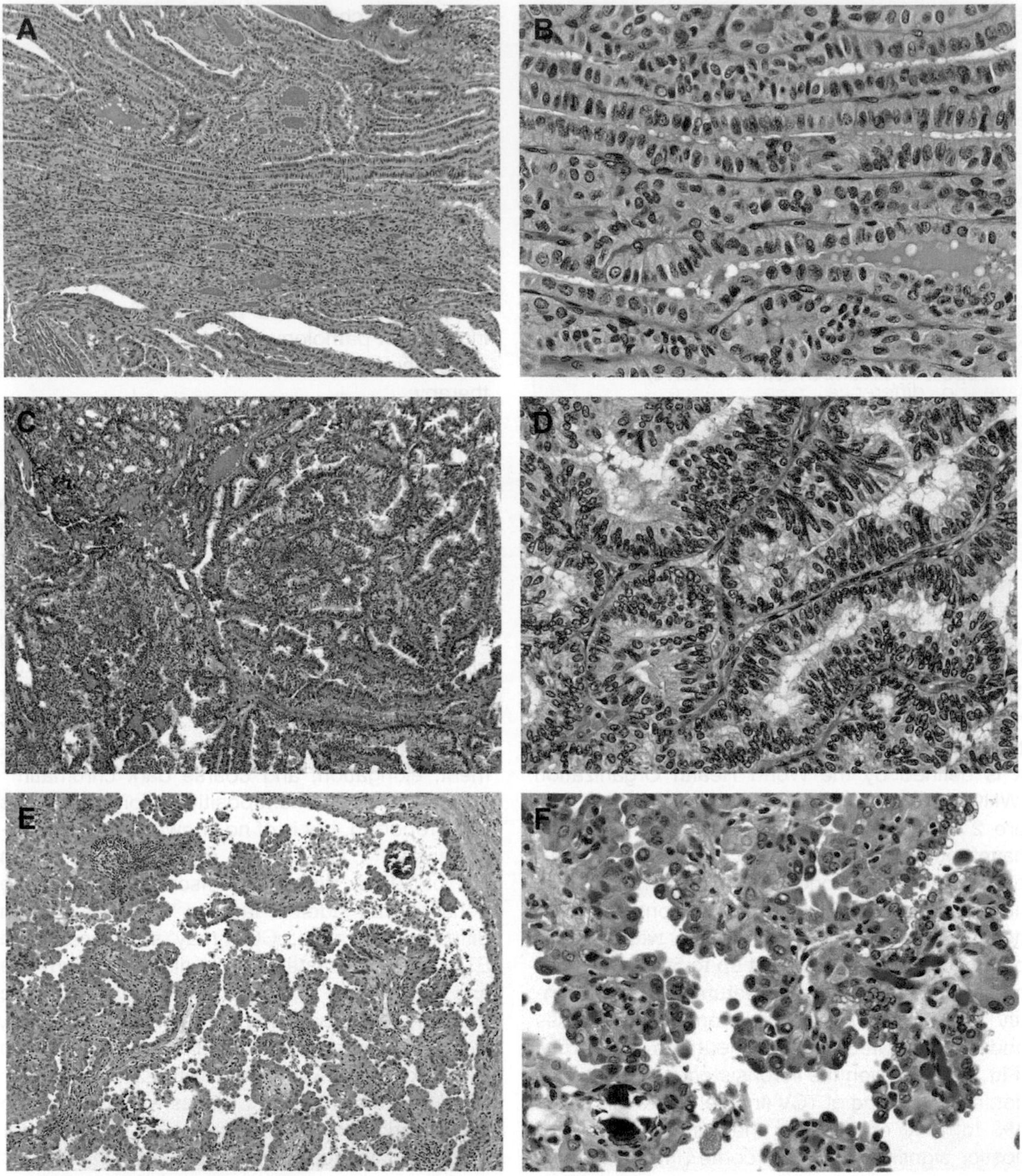

Fig. 1. Aggressive histologic variants of PTC. Tall cell variant of PTC often contains long "tram-track" follicles and appears eosinophilic on low power (*A*). The height of the cells is 2 to 3 times the width, the cytoplasm is densely eosinophilic, and nuclear features of PTC are prominent, including elongation, grooves, and pseudoinclusions (*B*). Columnar cell variant of PTC contains various architectural patterns, including branching glands, and appears basophilic on low power (*C*). The cells are usually tall with elongated nuclei, dark chromatin (unusual for PTC), pale cytoplasm, and may contain subnuclear or supranuclear vacuoles (*D*). Hobnail variant of PTC contains branching papillae and micropapillae, and also appears eosinophilic (*E*). The nuclei are oriented toward the apices of the cells causing the luminal border to undulate, and they have classic nuclear features of PTC including pseudoinclusions (*F*).

those with greater than 30% hobnail features.[39,40] Subsequent studies showed higher rates of HNV associated with poorly differentiated (22%) and anaplastic thyroid carcinoma (4%) compared with classic PTC (1%).[41] In a recent review of the nearly 100 reported HNV cases, mortality rates were 20%, possibly related to decreased responsiveness to radioiodine.[42] Whereas these data seem to suggest increased aggressiveness in HNV, controlled studies or multivariate analyses of HNV compared with classic PTC have not been performed. Nevertheless, the presence and percentage of a tumor occupied by hobnail features should be reported to potentially change patient management and guide future understanding of this disease.

EXTRATHYROIDAL EXTENSION

In the 8th edition of AJCC, T stage takes into account not only tumor size but also gross ETE. Patients with microscopic ETE alone are thought to have no difference in recurrence or survival compared with those without ETE, perhaps related to high interobserver variation in histologic identification of ETE.[15,43] Indicators of microscopic ETE may include skeletal muscle involvement (especially in the lateral lobes rather than isthmus), perithyroidal perineural invasion, and proximity to thick-walled vessels.[43] However, only gross ETE into strap muscles qualifies for an increase in T stage to pT3 (**Fig. 2**). Furthermore, extensive extrathyroidal invasion of adjacent structures beyond the strap muscles (subcutis, larynx, trachea, esophagus, or recurrent laryngeal nerve) results in a designation of pT4 (see **Table 2**). The specific extent of ETE thought to impact recurrence is somewhat controversial. Gross ETE is defined as clinical/surgical evidence of extrathyroidal invasion. Many studies report that patients with gross ETE identified intraoperatively (without distinction between muscle, cartilage, and so forth) had higher recurrence rates (29%–52%) than patients with microscopic ETE only identified histologically (also without distinction between fat, muscle, and so forth) and patients with no ETE (10%–21%).[44–48] Similarly, patients with clinical intrathyroidal (cT1/T2) tumors with and without microscopic ETE had similar recurrence and survival rates.[49] However, a recent study by Amit and colleagues[50] suggests that even gross ETE into strap muscle alone is insufficient to predict worse disease-free or overall survival compared with patients with ETE into fibroadipose tissue or microscopic ETE into skeletal muscle. Patients with ETE into skeletal muscle alone (without distinction between gross versus microscopic identification) may have similar recurrence rates as those with ETE into perithyroidal adipose tissue and those without ETE (<5%–10%).[51,52] Those with ETE into subcutis, larynx, trachea, esophagus, or recurrent laryngeal nerve had significantly increased recurrence (up to 30%) and decreased survival (85%).[51,52] Therefore, it is unclear whether gross ETE into skeletal muscle alone is predictive of increased recurrence: studies that group gross skeletal muscle invasion (T3) with gross cartilage/subcutaneous invasion (T4) show increased recurrence compared with patients without gross ETE, but studies that separate skeletal muscle from cartilage/subcutaneous invasion show no differences in recurrence between gross skeletal muscle invasion and absence of gross invasion (regardless of microscopic invasion). Nevertheless, for staging purposes, gross ETE does qualify for increase in T stage. During gross examination of thyroidectomies, prosectors should report the presence or absence of gross tumor invasion outside the thyroid (because it is likely an indication of clinically relevant gross ETE), including involvement of skeletal (strap) muscle, or other anatomic structures such as skin, trachea, esophagus, or recurrent laryngeal nerve. In addition, the operative report should be reviewed for surgical perception of ETE and taken into account for staging.

Key Points
EXTRATHYROIDAL EXTENSION

- If only microscopic extrathyroidal invasion is present (usually into fibroadipose tissue alone), stage is based on size
- If gross extrathyroidal invasion is present into strap muscles based on intraoperative evaluation and/or pathologic examination, stage is pT3b
- Extensive gross extrathyroidal invasion is pT4: into subcutis, larynx, trachea, esophagus, or recurrent laryngeal nerve (pT4a); prevertebral fascia or carotid/mediastinal vessels (pT4b)

ANGIOINVASION

Invasion of blood vessels (usually venous vascular invasion, ie, angioinvasion) is distinguished from lymphatic invasion in thyroid carcinomas, because it is thought to predict increased recurrence in PTC[53–55] and FTC.[56] Whereas lymphatic invasion is very common in PTC, angioinvasion is less frequent (5%–30% of PTC).[55] Conversely, lymphatic invasion is not common in FTC, but angioinvasion has been reported to occur in 30% to 80% of cases.[57] The definition of angioinvasion has changed over time, such that proposed histologic criteria have become increasingly strict. Previous definitions

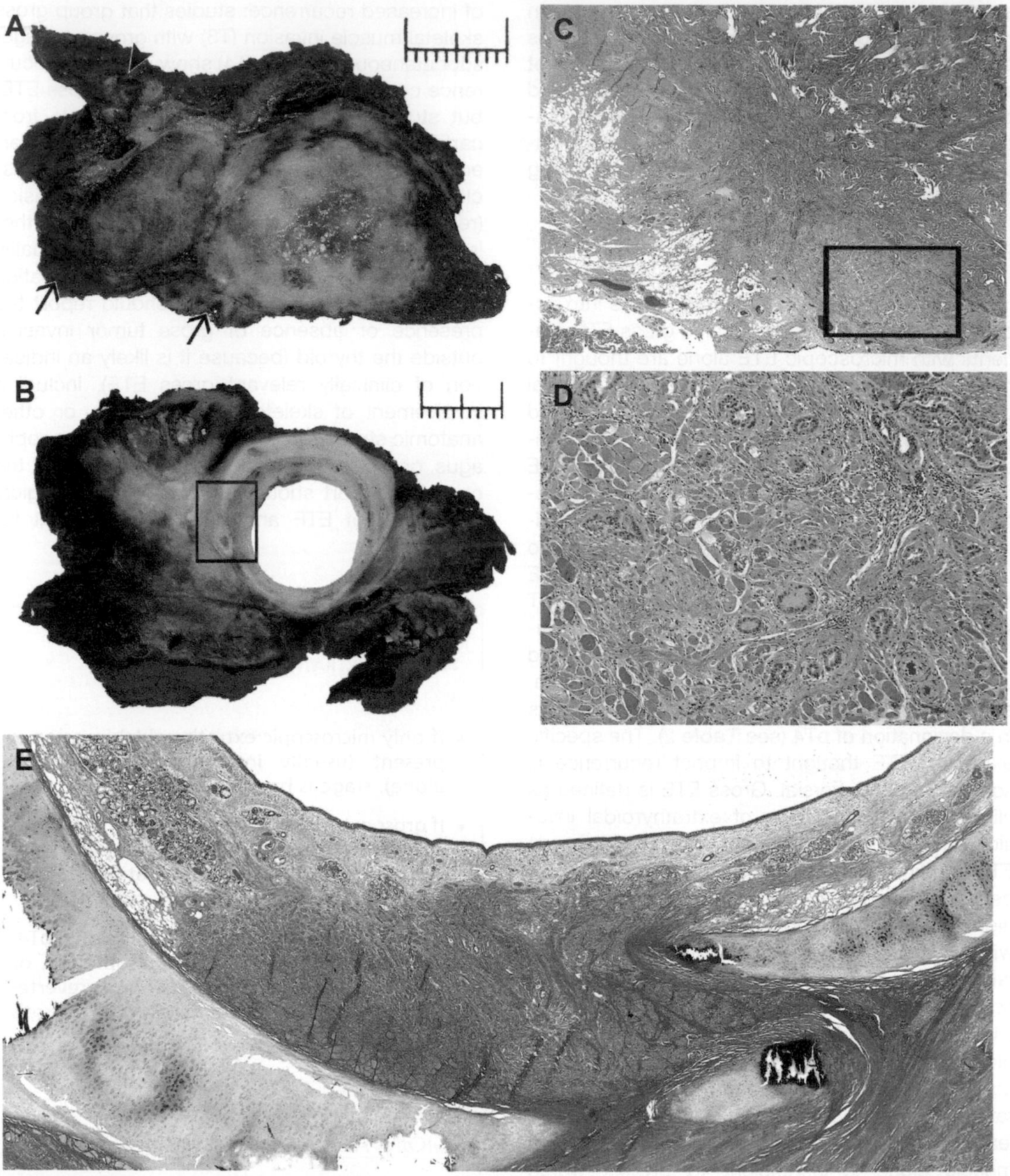

Fig. 2. Extrathyroidal extension in papillary thyroid carcinoma. Gross examination of thyroidectomies should include examination of the extrathyroidal tissues to assess for invasion into skeletal (strap) muscle. Presence of large vessels (*arrowhead*) and skeletal muscle (*arrows*) indicates a wider surgical resection field, suggesting that extrathyroidal extension may have been clinically or radiographically present (*A*). In the same case, extrathyroidal invasion into adipose tissue and skeletal muscle is evident on low power (*C*). The box highlighted in (*C*) is magnified in (*D*), confirming neoplastic glands within skeletal muscle (*D*). The stage is pT3b, and the clinical impression of skeletal muscle invasion should be confirmed by reading the operative report or discussion with the surgeon. In rare cases, laryngectomies for tracheal or laryngeal invasion by thyroid carcinoma are performed (*B*). Sectioning the specimen transversely allows for good visualization of the extent of invasion. The box highlighted in (*B*) is seen histologically in (*E*), confirming invasion through the intercartilaginous soft tissue plane into the respiratory mucosa of the trachea and cricoid (*E*). The pathologic stage here is pT4a.

of angioinvasion have included direct extension of tumor cells into the vascular lumen or tumor nests covered by endothelium, with or without attached thrombi, all restricted to various-sized vessels within or just outside the tumor capsule.[58] Vessels within the tumor mass have been uniformly excluded from analysis, as have dislodged clusters of nonendothelialized tumor cells not associated with fibrin and not attached to the vessel wall. Some studies using less stringent criteria demonstrated no difference in outcome related to extent of angioinvasion in either PTC or FTC.[57–59] However, others reported increasingly poor prognosis in FTCs with angioinvasion (80% 10-year survival) compared with those with capsular invasion alone (98% 10-year survival) and those with diffuse intrathyroidal and extrathyroidal invasion (38% 10-year survival).[56] In addition, the number of angioinvasive foci in FTC as well as HCC have been suggested to be prognostically important: involvement of 4 or more vessels has been suggested by some authors to predict increased recurrence.[60–63] Any number of angioinvasive foci in PTC may also be associated with increased distant recurrence, specifically when excluding lymphatic invasion and matching for age, gender, histologic variants, TNM stage, and follow-up time.[53]

When using increasingly strict morphologic criteria for diagnosis of angioinvasion, the quantity of foci may less be prognostically important than their presence in any number.[64] Interestingly, manual manipulation of postmortem benign thyroid glands resulted in small groups of follicular cells in vascular spaces as well as subendothelial bulging by tumor cells with an intact overlying endothelium, without fibrin thrombi. In ex vivo thyroid glands removed surgically, additional artifactual or "pseudo-invasive" features included reactive endothelial proliferation at sites of previous biopsy as well as prominent subendothelial bulging. When cut transversely, subendothelial bulging may occasionally manifest as a nodule of tumor within a vessel covered by intact endothelium without associated fibrin thrombi[64] (**Fig. 3**A, B). These features did not correlate to development of distant metastases. However, clinically significant angioinvasion was represented by tumor cells directly invading through a vessel wall into the intraluminal space as well as intravascular tumor nests with associated adherent thrombus (**Fig. 3**C, D). Using these criteria, one-third of angioinvasive DTCs developed distant metastasis.[64]

The 2016, 2017, and 2019 College of American Pathologists (CAP) *Protocol for the Examination of Specimens From Patients With Carcinomas of the Thyroid Gland* acknowledged these conflicting data and outlined proposed diagnostic criteria for angioinvasion in DTC: (1) vessels should be located within the capsule, outside the capsule, or outside the tumor; (2) vessels should be vascular rather than lymphatic (CD31 and D2-40 immunostains could be used if desired); and (3) tumor should be present within the vascular lumen and be accompanied by fibrin thrombus.[65–67] Conversely, pseudo-vascular invasion is represented by: (1) irregular intraluminal floating tumor fragments; (2) subendothelial tumor bulging indenting the vessel wall; and (3) intraluminal endothelialized tumor nodule not adherent to the wall, all without thrombosis (see **Fig. 3**). Any of these atypical findings may prompt examination of at least 3 deeper histologic sections to exclude definitive angioinvasion. Finally, intraluminal endothelialized tumor nodule adjacent/adherent to the wall without thrombosis is contentious.[65,66] However, the AFIP Atlas of Tumor Pathology supports diagnosis of vascular invasion in the setting of endothelialized tumor nests protruding in the vascular lumen, hypothesizing that this phenomenon is analogous to thrombus organization and recanalization.[68] Whereas separate reporting of angioinvasion and lymphatic invasion are recommended by CAP, the presence of lymphatic invasion (most frequently in PTC) has no known prognostic significance or treatment implication. Therefore, identification and reporting of vascular (angio-) invasion into blood vessels at the periphery of the tumor is most crucial. Currently, CAP recommends reporting focal (<4 foci) versus extensive ($\geq$4 foci) angioinvasion. The ATA remains conservative, also using a 4-vessel cutoff to isolate low-risk from high-risk FTCs, and any angioinvasion to identify intermediate risk PTCs.[4] On the other hand, WHO regards as "encapsulated angioinvasive" an FTC with any number of foci of angioinvasion, compared with "minimally invasive" (an FTC with capsular invasion alone) and "widely invasive" (an FTC with diffuse intrathyroidal and extrathyroidal invasion).[2] As CAP, AJCC, and WHO regard the number of angioinvasive foci differently, pathologists should consider reporting the number of foci of angioinvasion. Endocrinologists may also consider angioinvasion on a spectrum with other negative prognostic indicators, rather than simply a binary factor. Because there still exits variability in diagnosis by pathologists and incomplete understanding of the significance of angioinvasion, treatment decisions may be individualized based on a variety of risk factors.

> **Key Points**
> **ANGIOINVASION**
>
> - Must be present in intracapsular, pericapsular, or peritumoral vessels rather than intratumoral vessels
> - Vessels should be blood vessels rather than lymphatic vessels
> - Tumor should be associated with fibrin thrombus or endothelialized and adherent to the vessel wall
> - Number of foci should be reported (4 may be an important clinical cutoff)

LYMPH NODE INVOLVEMENT AND EXTRANODAL EXTENSION

The AJCC TNM staging of thyroid cancers with positive lymph nodes seems relatively simple: patients with clinically, radiographically, or pathologically negative nodes are N0; those with positive lymph nodes are N1, separated into N1a and N1b by location.[15] It has been suggested that this staging system may overestimate the risk of recurrence in N1 patients with clinically inapparent microscopic lymph node metastases, while not taking into account possibly high-risk nodal features such as size, number, or ENE.[69] Tasked by the *ATA Surgical Affairs Committee's Taskforce on Thyroid Cancer Nodal Surgery*, Randolph and colleagues[69] performed an extensive evaluation of published data on the clinical significance of lymph node metastasis in DTC. They found low rates of

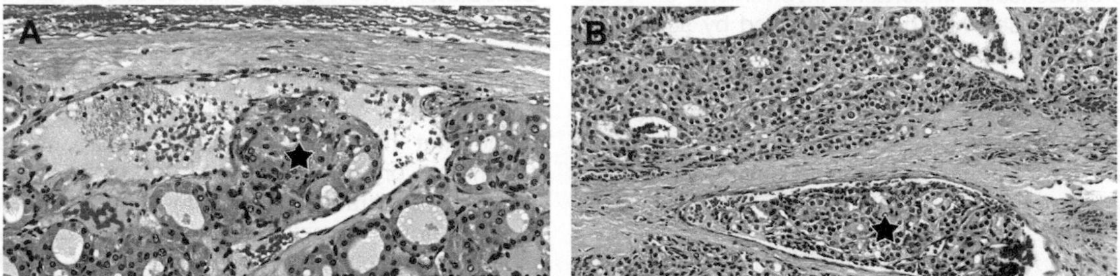

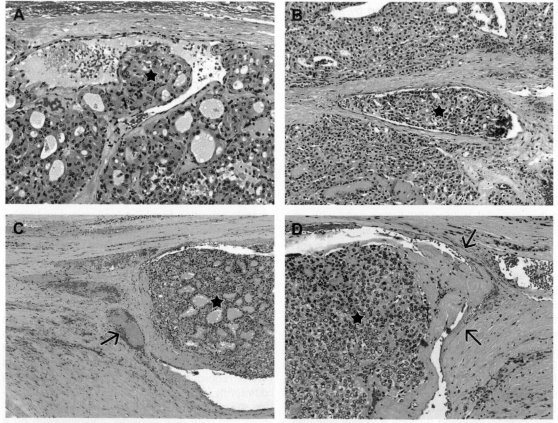

Fig. 3. Angioinvasion. The histologic definition of angioinvasion has become increasingly strict, as some authors (including the College of American Pathologists) advocate that subendothelial tumor bulging without thrombosis (*A*) and intraluminal endothelialized tumor nodules without mural adherence or thrombosis (*B*) should not be considered as angioinvasion. The tumor follicles (*A, star*) bulge into the vascular lumen but the base of the tumor is contained within stroma and there is no intraluminal thrombosis. If this type of focus were cut transversely, it may appear as an intraluminal endothelialized nodule (*B, star*), also without mural adherence or thrombosis. Although these strict definitions are controversial, most agree that an intraluminal tumor nodule (*C, D, star*) with thrombosis (C, *arrow*) and/or fibrous attachment to the vascular wall (*D, arrows*) are diagnostic of angioinvasion.

recurrence (<5%) in pN1 disease if the lymph nodes were clinically undetectable (cN0), if the sizes of the metastatic foci were small (especially <0.2 cm), and if the number of involved nodes was ≤5. Conversely, higher rates of recurrence (>20%) occurred in pN1 disease if the lymph nodes were clinically detectable (cN1), if the sizes of the metastatic foci were large (especially >3 cm), and if the number of involved nodes was greater than 5.[69] Extranodal extension can occur in lymph nodes of all sizes; however, the size of the metastatic focus is thought to be directly proportional to the likelihood of ENE[70] (**Fig. 4**). Recurrence rates in the presence of ENE are estimated to

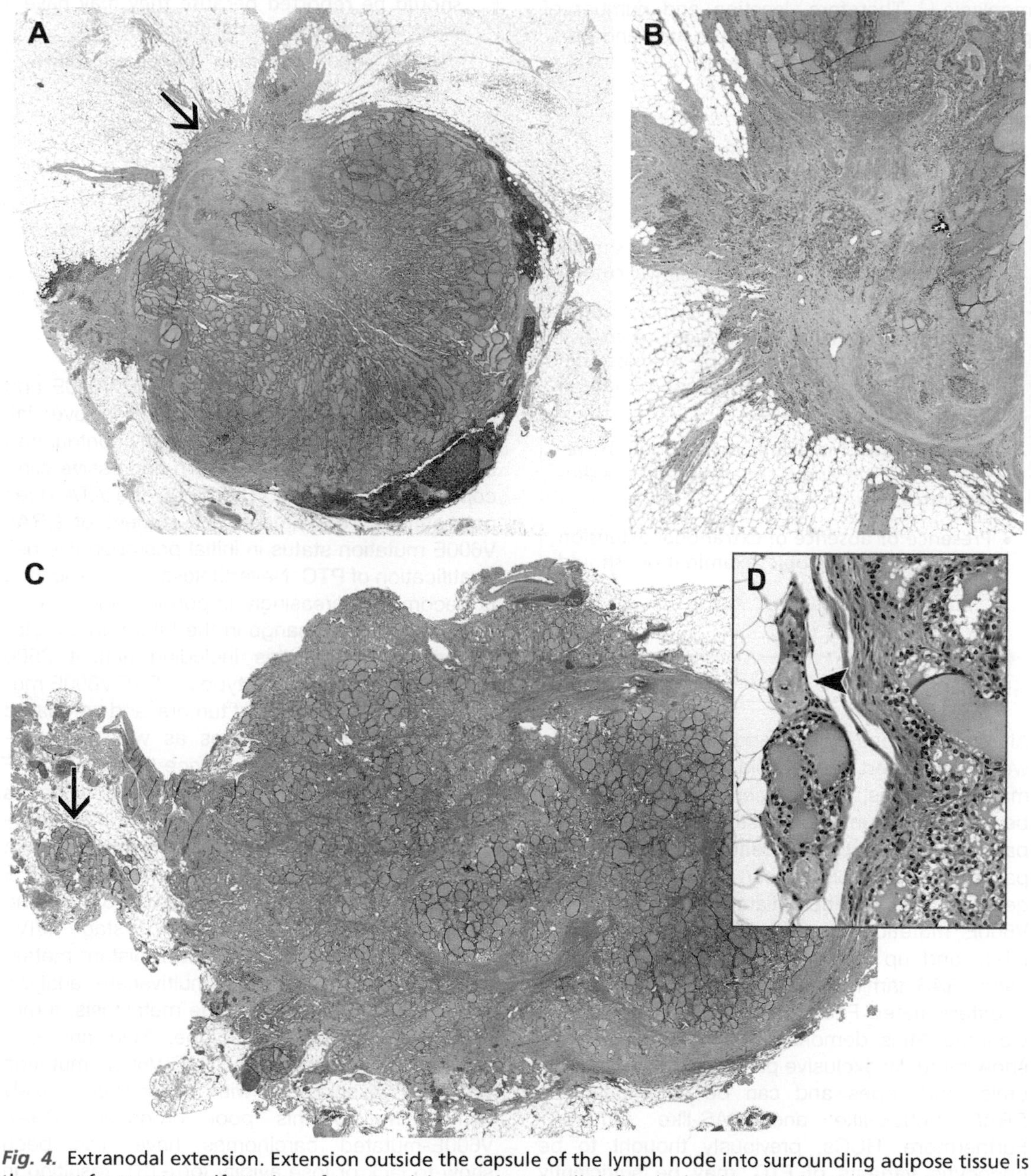

Fig. 4. Extranodal extension. Extension outside the capsule of the lymph node into surrounding adipose tissue is the most frequent manifestation of extranodal extension. An ill-defined edge (*A, arrow*) is visible on low power. On higher power, nests of tumor with associated fibrous stromal reaction outside the border of the lymph node are identified (*B*). This lymph node is completely effaced by metastatic carcinoma (*C*). Whereas the right border of the node is circumscribed, the left border shows tongue-like invasion into adipose tissue, including a satellite nodule in fat (*C, arrow*). Occasionally, perinodal lymphovascular invasion (*D, arrowhead*) could be overinterpreted as extranodal extension.

be higher than without, although data are somewhat limited and perhaps confounded by high interobserver variation in histologic identification of ENE.[69,71] Involvement of perinodal adipose tissue is considered, by most pathologists, to be the best indicator of ENE; however, additional features might include perinodal perineural invasion, skeletal muscle involvement, or extranodal desmoplasia.[71] Therefore, location and number of positive nodes, size of metastatic foci, and presence of ENE should be reported.

Key Points
LYMPH NODE METASTASES

- Total number of positive lymph nodes should be reported (5 is an important clinical cutoff)
- Anatomic level of positive lymph nodes should be reported: involvement of central neck (level VI) and superior mediastinum (level VII) is pN1a; involvement of lateral neck (levels I–V) is pN1b
- Size of largest metastatic focus should be reported (0.2 cm and 3 cm are important clinical cutoffs)
- Presence or absence of extranodal extension based on microscopic examination should be reported

GENETICS

Although various clinical and histologic features were evaluated in thyroid carcinomas over many decades, only recently have genetics become sufficiently understood as to become part of the workup and treatment algorithms of patients with thyroid cancer. The most common genetic driver in differentiated PTC is the *BRAF* V600E mutation, present in up to 65% of all PTCs and up to 95% of TCVs. On the other hand, *RAS* family mutations are most common in differentiated FTCs (up to 50%).[3] The Cancer Genome Atlas demonstrated that most tumors show mutually exclusive pan-genomic and proteomic landscapes and can be separated into *BRAF* V600E-like and *RAS*-like tumors.[72] Furthermore, HCCs, previously thought to be oncocytic variants of FTC, may be sufficiently genetically distinct as to be considered a separate category of thyroid tumors. Specifically, they show relatively decreased rates of *RAS* mutation, increased *TP53* and *PTEN* mutations, and mitochondrial DNA mutation.[3]

Key Points
GENETICS

- Genetic testing is not routinely recommended for initial postoperative risk stratification
- However, if known, the following mutations should be reported because they may have prognostic or treatment implications
  - *BRAF* V600E mutation (by immunohistochemistry or sequencing)
  - *TERT* promoter mutation
  - Combined *BRAF* V600E and *TERT* promoter mutation
  - Combined *RAS* and *TERT* promoter mutation

BRAF V600E

The prognostic significance of *BRAF* V600E and other genetic driver mutations is controversial, not entirely understood, and possibly confounded by the presence of other known aggressive clinicopathologic features. Therefore, the ATA does not routinely recommend assessment of *BRAF* V600E mutation status in initial postoperative risk stratification of PTC. Nevertheless, its significance is becoming increasingly important, and recommendations may change in the future. In a meta-analysis of 14 studies including almost 2500 PTCs of all histologic subtypes, *BRAF* V600E mutation was found in 45% of tumors, and correlated to various high-risk features as well as recurrence.[73] Specifically, recurrence rates in *BRAF* V600E-mutated patients (24.9%) was twice as high as in *BRAF* wild-type patients (12.6%). However, *BRAF*-mutated patients were also at increased risk of lymph node metastasis (54.1% versus 36.8%), ETE (46.2% versus 23.6%), and higher stage (35.4% versus 19.6% stage III/IV). There was no difference in risk of distant metastasis (8% overall).[73] In a multivariate analysis adjusting for ETE, lymph node metastasis, tumor stage, and histologic subtype, Xing and colleagues[74] found that the *BRAF* V600E mutation was still associated with recurrence. Likely contributing to this poor prognosis, *BRAF* V600E-mutated carcinomas have also been show to lack or lose avidity for I-131, resulting in relative RAI resistance.[74]

Only few studies have examined the influence of *BRAF* V600E in isolation. Huang and colleagues[75] evaluated recurrence rates in solitary, intrathyroidal, nonmetastatic PTCs, greater than 1 and

≤4 cm, with and without the *BRAF* V600E mutation, and demonstrated increased recurrence in the *BRAF* V600E-mutated group (9.5% versus 3.4%). The risk discrepancy was most pronounced in tumors greater than 3 and ≤4 cm (30% *BRAF* V600E-mutated versus 1.9% *BRAF* wild type). In addition, recurrence rates approached those in solitary PTCs with lymph node metastasis or extrathyroidal invasion, even after controlling for RAI treatment.[75] In a similar study, Elisei and colleagues[76] demonstrated recurrence rates of 16% in *BRAF* V600E-mutated intrathyroidal, nonmetastatic PTCs ≤4 cm (compared with 3.3% in BRAF wild-type patients). In this regard, *BRAF* V600E mutation could be an additional negative prognostic indicator in patients with low-risk tumors who may not otherwise be considered for RAI remnant ablation. In these studies, the prevalence of *BRAF* V600E mutation in the intrathyroidal PTCs was 33% to 34%.[75,76] If used in practice, mutational testing could identify a significant number of patients who may benefit from additional treatment. Although sequencing of all low-risk PTCs could be prohibitively expensive and potentially not reimbursed, immunostain detecting the *BRAF* V600E mutant protein product is relatively inexpensive and highly accurate (**Fig. 5**). In a recent meta-analysis of studies comparing *BRAF* V600E immunostain to mutational analysis, concordance rates of immunopositive and immunonegative cases were 92.1% and 89.4%, respectively.[77] Pooled sensitivity and specificity were relatively high at 97% and 78%.[77] Cases with negative immunostaining are highly likely to be *BRAF* wild type, and those with moderate to strong staining are likely to be mutated. It has been suggested that equivocal cases (those with a low proportion and intensity of positive cells) may benefit from confirmatory molecular testing.[78] There are currently no recommendations for global *BRAF* V600E testing in thyroid cancer; therefore, practices can be customized toward institutional preferences.

TERT PROMOTER

Other genes are emerging as possible sentinels of aggressive behavior in DTC. Specifically, mutations

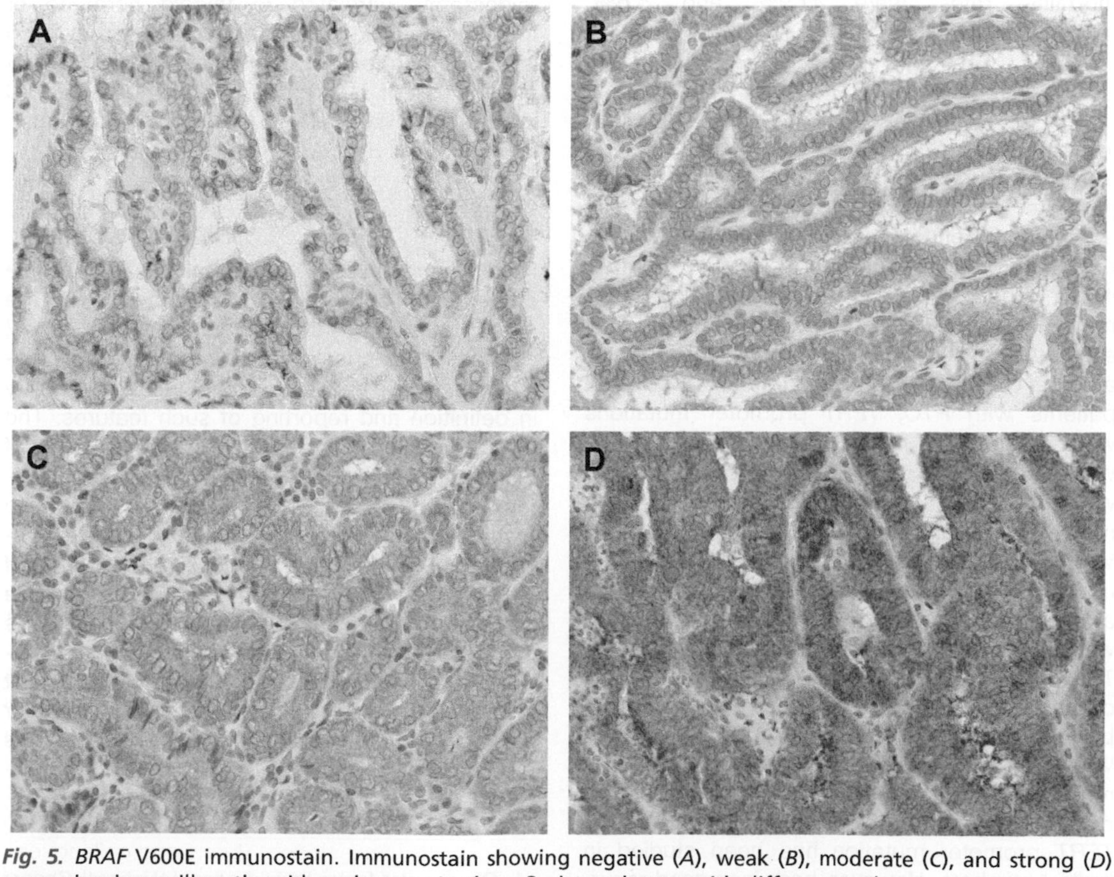

Fig. 5. *BRAF* V600E immunostain. Immunostain showing negative (*A*), weak (*B*), moderate (*C*), and strong (*D*) expression in papillary thyroid carcinomas. In these 3 pictured cases with diffuse cytoplasmic expression, *BRAF* V600E mutation was present using next-generation sequencing.

in the promoter region of the *TERT* gene are implicated in prognosis of PTC and FTC.[79,80] Mutations in either of the hotspots (C228T or C250T) increase the expression of telomerase reverse transcriptase, leading to lengthening of telomeres and promoting cellular longevity.[3,81] *TERT* is not thought to be expressed in significant amounts in nonneoplastic or benign thyroid, and *TERT* promoter mutations are so infrequently found in benign-behaving thyroid lesions that they are thought to be considered a marker of malignancy.[82] In recent meta-analyses, the prevalence of *TERT* promoter mutation is estimated to be 10% to 12% in PTC, 17% in FTC, and 14% in HCC.[24,82,83] The prevalence in poorly differentiated and anaplastic thyroid carcinomas is higher, at approximately 40%.[81] In addition to associating with male sex, older age, increased tumor size, extrathyroidal invasion, vascular invasion, lymph node metastasis (albeit weakly), and higher stage, *TERT* promoter mutation was significantly associated with distant metastasis, persistent or recurrent disease, and mortality.[82,83] Namely, rates of distant metastasis in mutated versus wild-type DTCs were 33.2% and 10.5%, respectively; recurrence rates were 52.1% and 18.7%, respectively; mortality rates were 41.9% and 5.6%, respectively.[81]

SYNERGISM

Whereas isolated *TERT* promoter mutation may be a useful prognostic tool in DTC, combined *TERT* promoter and *BRAF* V600E mutations may have a synergistic effect, representing an even more powerful predictor of cancer-specific mortality.[84,85] The prevalence of coexistent *TERT* promoter and *BRAF* V600E mutations in PTC is estimated to be 5% to 8%.[86,87] In a meta-analysis of 13 studies including greater than 4000 patients with PTC, *TERT* promoter mutations were present in a higher percentage of patients with *BRAF* V600E mutation (11.4%) versus those without (6.3%).[87] Compared with *BRAF* V600E mutation alone, combined *TERT* and *BRAF* V600E was associated with older age, male sex, higher TNM stage, ETE, lymph node metastasis, and distant metastasis. Interestingly, compared with *TERT* promoter mutation alone, combined *TERT* and *BRAF* V600E was associated with all of the above factors except distant metastasis.[87] Lastly, patients with combined *TERT* and *BRAF* V600E mutations had the highest risk of recurrence and cancer-specific mortality.[86,87] The possible synergistic effect of combined *RAS* and *TERT* promoter mutation has been studied in limited numbers. However, both increased recurrence and disease-specific mortality have been demonstrated for coexistent *RAS* and *TERT* promoter mutations.[88,89] Additional studies are warranted.

PATIENT PERSPECTIVE

As most thyroid cancers are indolent, their potential psychosocial impact on patients with cancer may be underestimated by treating physicians. The North American Thyroid Cancer Survivorship Study reported that patients with thyroid cancer of all stages have lower self-reported quality of life scores compared with patients with other cancers, including colorectal, breast, and glial.[90,91] The investigators hypothesized that patients may feel that their concerns are being minimized by physicians and family members who perceive thyroid cancer as a relatively "good" cancer.[90] Quality of life is negatively impacted by fear of cancer recurrence, fear of metastasis, and fear of development of a second cancer.[91] A survey of Swedish patients with thyroid cancer found that 75% of patients had fear of cancer recurrence at diagnosis, and that these patients had worse quality of life scores at 1 year after thyroidectomy, unrelated to thyroid hormone or thyroid-stimulating hormone suppression levels.[92] Therefore, systems that more accurately predict risk of recurrence and mortality in DTC may help alleviate patient fear and increase quality of life.

SUMMARY

Predicting recurrence and mortality in DTC can be challenging, especially given changes in the nomenclature of thyroid tumors over time, changes in diagnostic criteria for various pathologic features, and high interobserver variability in definition and reporting of such features. The AJCC system is considered the best predictor of mortality, whereas the ATA risk stratification system is the best predictor of recurrence. Pathologic features taken into account in either of these systems include aggressive histologic variants of PTC, gross ETE, angioinvasion, lymph node metastasis, ENE, and genetics. As most DTC is indolent, identification and reporting of key features may facilitate more aggressive treatment for patients at high risk, spare patients at lower risk, and provide more accurate risk expectations for patients.

REFERENCES

1. Cancer stat facts: thyroid cancer. National Cancer Institute Surveillance, Epidemiology, and End

Results Program. Available at: https://seer.cancer.gov/statfacts/html/thyro.html. Accessed February 17, 2019.
2. Lloyd RV, Osamura RY, Klöppel G, et al, editors. WHO classification of tumours of endocrine organs, vol. 10, 4th edition. Lyon: IARC Press; 2017.
3. Giordano TJ. Genomic hallmarks of thyroid neoplasia. Annu Rev Pathol 2018;13:141–62.
4. Haugen BR, Alexander EK, Bible KC, et al. 2015 American Thyroid Association Management guidelines for adult patients with thyroid nodules and differentiated thyroid cancer: the American Thyroid Association guidelines task force on thyroid nodules and differentiated thyroid cancer. Thyroid 2016; 26(1):1–133.
5. Hahn LD, Kunder CA, Chen MM, et al. Indolent thyroid cancer: knowns and unknowns. Cancers Head Neck 2017;2(1):1.
6. Janovitz T, Barletta JA. Clinically relevant prognostic parameters in differentiated thyroid carcinoma. Endocr Pathol 2018;29(4):357–64.
7. Byar DP, Green SB, Dor P, et al. A prognostic index for thyroid carcinoma. A study of the E.O.R.T.C. Thyroid Cancer Cooperative Group. Eur J Cancer 1979; 15(8):1033–41.
8. Hay ID, Grant CS, Taylor WF, et al. Ipsilateral lobectomy versus bilateral lobar resection in papillary thyroid carcinoma: a retrospective analysis of surgical outcome using a novel prognostic scoring system. Surgery 1987;102(6):1088–95.
9. Cady B, Rossi R. An expanded view of risk-group definition in differentiated thyroid carcinoma. Surgery 1988;104(6):947–53.
10. Hay ID, Bergstralh EJ, Goellner JR, et al. Predicting outcome in papillary thyroid carcinoma: development of a reliable prognostic scoring system in a cohort of 1779 patients surgically treated at one institution during 1940 through 1989. Surgery 1993;114(6):1050–8.
11. Mazzaferri EL, Jhiang SM. Long-term impact of initial surgical and medical therapy on papillary and follicular thyroid cancer. Am J Med 1994; 97(5):418–28.
12. Shaha AR, Loree TR, Shah JP. Prognostic factors and risk group analysis in follicular carcinoma of the thyroid. Surgery 1995;118(6):1131–6, [discussion:1136–8].
13. Sherman SI, Brierley JD, Sperling M, et al. Prospective multicenter study of thyroid carcinoma treatment. Cancer 1998;83(5):1012–21.
14. Voutilainen PE, Siironen P, Franssila KO, et al. AMES, MACIS and TNM prognostic classifications in papillary thyroid carcinoma. Anticancer Res 2003;23(5b): 4283–8.
15. Amin MB, Edge S, Greene F, et al, editors. AJCC cancer staging manual. 8th edition. Switzerland: Springer International Publishing; 2017.
16. Nixon IJ, Wang LY, Migliacci JC, et al. An international multi-institutional validation of age 55 years as a cutoff for risk stratification in the AJCC/UICC staging system for well-differentiated thyroid cancer. Thyroid 2016;26(3):373–80.
17. Tuttle RM, Haugen B, Perrier ND. Updated American Joint Committee on cancer/tumor-node-metastasis staging system for differentiated and anaplastic thyroid cancer (eighth edition): what changed and why? Thyroid 2017;27(6):751–6.
18. Zhao Y, Zhang Y, Liu X. Prognostic factors for differentiated thyroid carcinoma and review of the literature. Tumori 2018;98(2):233–7.
19. NCCN clinical practice guidelines in oncology (NCCN guidelines). Available at: https://www.nccn.org/professionals/physician_gls/pdf/thyroid.pdf. Accessed February 17, 2019.
20. Niemeier LA, Kuffner Akatsu H, Song C, et al. A combined molecular-pathologic score improves risk stratification of thyroid papillary microcarcinoma. Cancer 2012;118(8):2069–77.
21. Siddiqui S, White MG, Antic T, et al. Clinical and pathologic predictors of lymph node metastasis and recurrence in papillary thyroid microcarcinoma. Thyroid 2016;26(6):807–15.
22. Hernandez-Prera JC, Machado RA, Asa SL, et al. Pathologic reporting of tall-cell variant of papillary thyroid cancer: have we reached a consensus? Thyroid 2017;27(12):1498–504.
23. Ghossein R, LiVolsi VA. Papillary thyroid carcinoma tall cell variant. Thyroid 2008;18(11):1179–81.
24. Liu Z, Zeng W, Chen T, et al. A comparison of the clinicopathological features and prognoses of the classical and the tall cell variant of papillary thyroid cancer: a meta-analysis. Oncotarget 2017;8(4): 6222–32.
25. Shi X, Liu R, Basolo F, et al. Differential clinicopathological risk and prognosis of major papillary thyroid cancer variants. J Clin Endocrinol Metab 2016; 101(1):264–74.
26. Ganly I, Ibrahimpasic T, Rivera M, et al. Prognostic implications of papillary thyroid carcinoma with tall-cell features. Thyroid 2014;24(4):662–70.
27. Dettmer MS, Schmitt A, Steinert H, et al. Tall cell papillary thyroid carcinoma: new diagnostic criteria and mutations in BRAF and TERT. Endocr Relat Cancer 2015;22(3):419–29.
28. Ghossein RA, Leboeuf R, Patel KN, et al. Tall cell variant of papillary thyroid carcinoma without extrathyroid extension: biologic behavior and clinical implications. Thyroid 2007;17(7):655–61.
29. Michels JJ, Jacques M, Henry-Amar M, et al. Prevalence and prognostic significance of tall cell variant of papillary thyroid carcinoma. Hum Pathol 2007; 38(2):212–9.
30. Prendiville S, Burman KD, Ringel MD, et al. Tall cell variant: an aggressive form of papillary thyroid

carcinoma. Otolaryngol Head Neck Surg 2000; 122(3):352–7.
31. Russo M, Malandrino P, Moleti M, et al. Tall cell and diffuse sclerosing variants of papillary thyroid cancer: outcome and predicting value of risk stratification methods. J Endocrinol Invest 2017;40(11): 1235–41.
32. Song E, Jeon MJ, Oh H-S, et al. Do aggressive variants of papillary thyroid carcinoma have worse clinical outcome than classic papillary thyroid carcinoma? Eur J Endocrinol 2018;179(3): 135–42.
33. Kazaure HS, Roman SA, Sosa JA. Aggressive variants of papillary thyroid cancer: incidence, characteristics and predictors of survival among 43,738 patients. Ann Surg Oncol 2012;19(6):1874–80.
34. Chen J-H, Faquin WC, Lloyd RV, et al. Clinicopathological and molecular characterization of nine cases of columnar cell variant of papillary thyroid carcinoma. Mod Pathol 2011;24(5):739–49.
35. Nath MC, Erickson LA. Aggressive variants of papillary thyroid carcinoma: hobnail, tall cell, columnar, and solid. Adv Anat Pathol 2018;25(3):172–9.
36. Enriquez ML, Baloch ZW, Montone KT, et al. CDX2 expression in columnar cell variant of papillary thyroid carcinoma. Am J Clin Pathol 2012;137(5): 722–6.
37. Sujoy V, Pinto A, Nosé V. Columnar cell variant of papillary thyroid carcinoma: a study of 10 cases with emphasis on CDX2 expression. Thyroid 2013; 23(6):714–9.
38. Jiang C, Cheng T, Zheng X, et al. Clinical behaviors of rare variants of papillary thyroid carcinoma are associated with survival: a population-level analysis. Cancer Manag Res 2018;10:465–72.
39. Asioli S, Erickson LA, Sebo TJ, et al. Papillary thyroid carcinoma with prominent hobnail features: a new aggressive variant of moderately differentiated papillary carcinoma. A clinicopathologic, immunohistochemical, and molecular study of eight cases. Am J Surg Pathol 2010;34(1):44–52.
40. Asioli S, Erickson LA, Righi A, et al. Papillary thyroid carcinoma with hobnail features: histopathologic criteria to predict aggressive behavior. Hum Pathol 2013;44(3):320–8.
41. Amacher AM, Goyal B, Lewis JS, et al. Prevalence of a hobnail pattern in papillary, poorly differentiated, and anaplastic thyroid carcinoma: a possible manifestation of high-grade transformation. Am J Surg Pathol 2015;39(2):260–5.
42. Ambrosi F, Righi A, Ricci C, et al. Hobnail variant of papillary thyroid carcinoma: a literature review. Endocr Pathol 2017;28(4):293–301.
43. Su HK, Wenig BM, Haser GC, et al. Inter-observer variation in the pathologic identification of minimal extrathyroidal extension in papillary thyroid carcinoma. Thyroid 2016;26(4):512–7.
44. Arora N, Turbendian HK, Scognamiglio T, et al. Extrathyroidal extension is not all equal: implications of macroscopic versus microscopic extent in papillary thyroid carcinoma. Surgery 2008;144(6):942–7, [discussion: 947–8].
45. Hay ID, Johnson TR, Thompson GB, et al. Minimal extrathyroid extension in papillary thyroid carcinoma does not result in increased rates of either cause-specific mortality or postoperative tumor recurrence. Surgery 2016;159(1):11–9.
46. Park SY, Kim HI, Kim JH, et al. Prognostic significance of gross extrathyroidal extension invading only strap muscles in differentiated thyroid carcinoma. Br J Surg 2018;105(9):1155–62.
47. Radowsky JS, Howard RS, Burch HB, et al. Impact of degree of extrathyroidal extension of disease on papillary thyroid cancer outcome. Thyroid 2014; 24(2):241–4.
48. Rivera M, Ricarte-Filho J, Tuttle RM, et al. Molecular, morphologic, and outcome analysis of thyroid carcinomas according to degree of extrathyroid extension. Thyroid 2010;20(10):1085–93.
49. Nixon IJ, Ganly I, Patel S, et al. The impact of microscopic extrathyroid extension on outcome in patients with clinical T1 and T2 well-differentiated thyroid cancer. Surgery 2011; 150(6):1242–9.
50. Amit M, Boonsripitayanon M, Goepfert RP, et al. Extrathyroidal extension: does strap muscle invasion alone influence recurrence and survival in patients with differentiated thyroid cancer? Ann Surg Oncol 2018;25(11):3380–8.
51. Jin BJ, Kim MK, Ji YB, et al. Characteristics and significance of minimal and maximal extrathyroidal extension in papillary thyroid carcinoma. Oral Oncol 2015;51(8):759–63.
52. Ito Y, Tomoda C, Uruno T, et al. Prognostic significance of extrathyroid extension of papillary thyroid carcinoma: massive but not minimal extension affects the relapse-free survival. World J Surg 2006; 30(5):780–6.
53. Cao J, Hu J-L, Chen C, et al. Vascular invasion is an independent prognostic factor for distant recurrence-free survival in papillary thyroid carcinoma: a matched-case comparative study. J Clin Pathol 2016;69(10):872–7.
54. Falvo L, Catania A, D'Andrea V, et al. Prognostic importance of histologic vascular invasion in papillary thyroid carcinoma. Ann Surg 2005;241(4): 640–6.
55. Wreesmann VB, Nixon IJ, Rivera M, et al. Prognostic value of vascular invasion in well-differentiated papillary thyroid carcinoma. Thyroid 2015;25(5): 503–8.
56. D'Avanzo A, Treseler P, Ituarte PHG, et al. Follicular thyroid carcinoma: histology and prognosis. Cancer 2004;100(6):1123–9.

57. Furlan JC, Bedard YC, Rosen IB. Clinicopathologic significance of histologic vascular invasion in papillary and follicular thyroid carcinomas. J Am Coll Surg 2004;198(3):341–8.
58. Thompson LD, Wieneke JA, Paal E, et al. A clinicopathologic study of minimally invasive follicular carcinoma of the thyroid gland with a review of the English literature. Cancer 2001;91(3): 505–24.
59. Goldstein NS, Czako P, Neill JS. Metastatic minimally invasive (encapsulated) follicular and Hurthle cell thyroid carcinoma: a study of 34 patients. Mod Pathol 2000;13(2):123–30.
60. Lang W, Choritz H, Hundeshagen H. Risk factors in follicular thyroid carcinomas. A retrospective follow-up study covering a 14-year period with emphasis on morphological findings. Am J Surg Pathol 1986; 10(4):246–55.
61. Collini P, Sampietro G, Pilotti S. Extensive vascular invasion is a marker of risk of relapse in encapsulated non-Hürthle cell follicular carcinoma of the thyroid gland: a clinicopathological study of 18 consecutive cases from a single institution with a 11-year median follow up. Histopathology 2004; 44(1):35–9.
62. Ghossein RA, Hiltzik DH, Carlson DL, et al. Prognostic factors of recurrence in encapsulated Hurthle cell carcinoma of the thyroid gland: a clinicopathologic study of 50 cases. Cancer 2006;106(8): 1669–76.
63. Xu B, Wang L, Tuttle RM, et al. Prognostic impact of extent of vascular invasion in low-grade encapsulated follicular cell-derived thyroid carcinomas: a clinicopathologic study of 276 cases. Hum Pathol 2015;46(12):1789–98.
64. Mete O, Asa SL. Pathological definition and clinical significance of vascular invasion in thyroid carcinomas of follicular epithelial derivation. Mod Pathol 2011;24(12):1545–52.
65. Seethala RR, Asa SL, Carty SE, et al. College of American Pathologists protocol for the examination of specimens from patients with carcinomas of the thyroid gland. 2016. Available at: https://www.cap.org/protocols-and-guidelines/cancer-reporting-tools. Accessed February 18, 2019.
66. Seethala RR, Asa SL, Bullock MJ, et al. College of American Pathologists protocol for the examination of specimens from patients with carcinomas of the thyroid gland. 2017. Available at: https://www.cap.org/protocols-and-guidelines/cancer-reporting-tools. Accessed February 18, 2019.
67. Mete O, Seethala RR, Asa SL, et al. College of American Pathologists protocol for the examination of specimens from patients with carcinomas of the thyroid gland 2019. Available at: https://www.cap.org/protocols-and-guidelines/cancer-reporting-tools. Accessed August 16, 2019.
68. Rosai J, Delellis RA, Carcangiu ML, et al. In: Silverberg SG, Delellis RA, Sobin LH, editors. AFIP Atlas of Tumor Pathology. Fourth Series. Fascicle 21. Tumors of the Thyroid and Parathyroid Glands. Silver Spring, MD: ARP Press; 2014.
69. Randolph GW, Duh Q-Y, Heller KS, et al. The prognostic significance of nodal metastases from papillary thyroid carcinoma can be stratified based on the size and number of metastatic lymph nodes, as well as the presence of extranodal extension. Thyroid 2012;22(11):1144–52.
70. Rowe ME, Ozbek U, Machado RA, et al. The prevalence of extranodal extension in papillary thyroid cancer based on the size of the metastatic node: adverse histologic features are not limited to larger lymph nodes. Endocr Pathol 2018;29(1):80–5.
71. Du E, Wenig BM, Su HK, et al. Inter-observer variation in the pathologic identification of extranodal extension in nodal metastasis from papillary thyroid carcinoma. Thyroid 2016;26(6):816–9.
72. Cancer Genome Atlas Research Network. Integrated genomic characterization of papillary thyroid carcinoma. Cell 2014;159(3):676–90.
73. Tufano RP, Teixeira GV, Bishop J, et al. BRAF mutation in papillary thyroid cancer and its value in tailoring initial treatment: a systematic review and meta-analysis. Medicine (Baltimore) 2012;91(5):274–86.
74. Xing M, Westra WH, Tufano RP, et al. BRAF mutation predicts a poorer clinical prognosis for papillary thyroid cancer. J Clin Endocrinol Metab 2005;90(12): 6373–9.
75. Huang Y, Qu S, Zhu G, et al. BRAF V600E mutation-assisted risk stratification of solitary intrathyroidal papillary thyroid cancer for precision treatment. J Natl Cancer Inst 2018;110(4):362–70.
76. Elisei R, Viola D, Torregrossa L, et al. The BRAF(V600E) mutation is an independent, poor prognostic factor for the outcome of patients with low-risk intrathyroid papillary thyroid carcinoma: single-institution results from a large cohort study. J Clin Endocrinol Metab 2012;97(12):4390–8.
77. Pyo J-S, Sohn JH, Kang G. BRAF immunohistochemistry using clone VE1 is strongly concordant with BRAF V600E mutation test in papillary thyroid carcinoma. Endocr Pathol 2015;26(3):211–7.
78. Kim YH, Choi S-E, Yoon SO, et al. A testing algorithm for detection of the B-type Raf kinase V600E mutation in papillary thyroid carcinoma. Hum Pathol 2014;45(7):1483–8.
79. Melo M, da Rocha AG, Vinagre J, et al. TERT promoter mutations are a major indicator of poor outcome in differentiated thyroid carcinomas. J Clin Endocrinol Metab 2014;99(5):E754–65.
80. Bournaud C, Descotes F, Decaussin-Petrucci M, et al. TERT promoter mutations identify a high-risk group in metastasis-free advanced thyroid carcinoma. Eur J Cancer 2019;108:41–9.

81. Liu R, Xing M. TERT promoter mutations in thyroid cancer. Endocr Relat Cancer 2016;23(3):R143–55.
82. Alzahrani AS, Alsaadi R, Murugan AK, et al. TERT promoter mutations in thyroid cancer. Horm Cancer 2016;7(3):165–77.
83. Yin D-T, Yu K, Lu R-Q, et al. Clinicopathological significance of TERT promoter mutation in papillary thyroid carcinomas: a systematic review and meta-analysis. Clin Endocrinol (Oxf) 2016;85(2):299–305.
84. Liu R, Bishop J, Zhu G, et al. Mortality risk stratification by combining BRAF V600E and TERT promoter mutations in papillary thyroid cancer: genetic duet of BRAF and TERT promoter mutations in thyroid cancer mortality. JAMA Oncol 2017;3(2):202–8.
85. Xing M, Liu R, Liu X, et al. BRAF V600E and TERT promoter mutations cooperatively identify the most aggressive papillary thyroid cancer with highest recurrence. J Clin Oncol 2014;32(25):2718–26.
86. Vuong HG, Duong UNP, Altibi AMA, et al. A meta-analysis of prognostic roles of molecular markers in papillary thyroid carcinoma. Endocr Connect 2017;6(3):R8–17.
87. Moon S, Song YS, Kim YA, et al. Effects of coexistent BRAFV600E and TERT promoter mutations on poor clinical outcomes in papillary thyroid cancer: a meta-analysis. Thyroid 2017;27(5):651–60.
88. Song YS, Lim JA, Choi H, et al. Prognostic effects of TERT promoter mutations are enhanced by coexistence with BRAF or RAS mutations and strengthen the risk prediction by the ATA or TNM staging system in differentiated thyroid cancer patients. Cancer 2016;122(9):1370–9.
89. Shen X, Liu R, Xing M. A six-genotype genetic prognostic model for papillary thyroid cancer. Endocr Relat Cancer 2017;24(1):41–52.
90. Aschebrook-Kilfoy B, James B, Nagar S, et al. Risk factors for decreased quality of life in thyroid cancer survivors: initial findings from the North American Thyroid Cancer Survivorship Study. Thyroid 2015; 25(12):1313–21.
91. Applewhite MK, James BC, Kaplan SP, et al. Quality of life in thyroid cancer is similar to that of other cancers with worse survival. World J Surg 2016;40(3):551–61.
92. Hedman C, Djärv T, Strang P, et al. Fear of recurrence and view of life affect health-related quality of life in patients with differentiated thyroid carcinoma: a prospective Swedish population-based study. Thyroid 2018. https://doi.org/10.1089/thy.2018.0388.

Thyroid Tumors You Don't Want to Miss

Kristine S. Wong, MD, Justine A. Barletta, MD*

KEYWORDS

- Anaplastic thyroid carcinoma • Poorly differentiated thyroid carcinoma
- Rare papillary thyroid carcinoma subtypes • Medullary thyroid carcinoma • NIFTP
- Cowden syndrome

Key points

- A diagnosis of anaplastic thyroid carcinoma (ATC) can be challenging when the anaplastic component comprises a small percentage of the tumor.
- A diagnosis of poorly differentiated thyroid carcinoma (PDTC) can be missed if mitotic activity and necrosis are overlooked. All follicular thyroid carcinomas and Hürthle cell carcinomas with solid/trabecular/insular growth should be evaluated for increased mitotic activity and necrosis.
- Rare papillary thyroid carcinoma (PTC) subtypes are aggressive. In addition to familiarity with specific morphologic features, evaluating for increased mitotic activity and tumor necrosis can help identify these aggressive PTC.
- Most non-invasive follicular thyroid neoplasm with papillary-like nuclear features (NIFTP) are easily diagnosed; however, it is important to be aware of NIFTP mimics, including follicular-predominant classic PTC and subtle infiltrative follicular variant of PTC 2.
- Thyroidectomy findings may be the first indication of a hereditary tumor syndrome.

ABSTRACT

This article examines more uncommon thyroid entities, including anaplastic thyroid carcinoma, poorly differentiated thyroid carcinoma, rare papillary thyroid carcinoma variants, medullary thyroid carcinoma, non-invasive follicular thyroid neoplasm with papillary-like nuclear features (NIFTP), and multiple adenomatous nodules in the setting of Cowden syndrome. These entities were chosen based on their clinical significance and because they can be diagnostically challenging due to their morphologic diversity and overlap with other thyroid tumors. This article addresses the diagnostic features of each entity, focusing on how to avoid potential pitfalls and mimics while also highlighting the clinical implications of each diagnosis.

OVERVIEW

The most common finding in thyroidectomy specimens is nodular hyperplasia, followed by malignant neoplasms, benign neoplasms, and other benign findings, such as thyroiditis.[1] Of malignancies, the most common type is papillary thyroid carcinoma (PTC), which comprises approximately 85% of all thyroid cancers when including microcarcinomas.[2] The most common types of PTC are classic type and follicular variant, whereas tall cell variant (TCV) comprises approximately 6% to 8% of PTC, and other less common variants encompass the small subset of remaining cases.[2–4] Anaplastic thyroid carcinoma (ATC), poorly differentiated thyroid carcinoma (PDTC), and medullary thyroid carcinoma (MTC) comprise approximately 10% of thyroid

Disclosure Statement: No disclosures.
Department of Pathology, Brigham and Women's Hospital, Harvard Medical School, 75 Francis Street, Boston, MA 02115, USA
* Corresponding author.
E-mail address: jbarletta@bwh.harvard.edu

Surgical Pathology 12 (2019) 901–919
https://doi.org/10.1016/j.path.2019.08.008

carcinomas combined.[2] Although most thyroid malignancies are diagnostically straight forward, these uncommon tumors may be more difficult to recognize given their rarity and morphologic diversity. In addition, the spectrum of benign and malignant neoplasia has become increasingly complex due to changing criteria and the introduction of new nomenclature, such as non-invasive follicular thyroid neoplasm with papillary-like nuclear features (NIFTP). Moreover, the recognition of tumor-predisposition syndromes has also contributed to the complexity of thyroid pathology. Tumors examined in this review include ATC, PDTC, rare PTC variants, MTC, NIFTP, and multiple adenomatous nodules in the setting of Cowden syndrome (CS). These entities are all important for pathologists to recognize because of the clinical implications of the diagnoses.

UNDIFFERENTIATED (ANAPLASTIC) THYROID CARCINOMA

ATC accounts for approximately 2% of all thyroid carcinomas in the United States.[5] There is a female predominance (2:1 female-to-male ratio), and the mean age at diagnosis is 60 to 70 years.[6,7] Most patients present with regional or distant metastases and die within a year.[7] There is considerable variation in the microscopic appearance of ATC, although there are 3 main patterns: spindle cell, pleomorphic giant cell, and epithelioid/squamoid.[8] Characteristic features of ATC include marked pleomorphism, a high proliferative rate, and invasive/infiltrative growth, with most tumors demonstrating extensive vascular invasion and significant extrathyroidal extension.[8] Compared with PDTC, ATC shows increased pleomorphism and proliferative activity. Between 25% and 75% of ATC are found in association with a differentiated thyroid carcinoma.[9–13] Based on studies demonstrating that tumors with a minor/focal anaplastic component have an improved survival compared with patients with tumors with a major anaplastic component,[6,14–18] the College of American Pathologists indicates that ATC should be characterized as comprising a major component of the tumor or a minor component without extrathyroidal extension (although the maximum percentage of tumor that is allowable for the term *focal* to be applied is unclear at this point).[19] In addition, T staging for ATC has changed in the eighth edition of the American Joint Committee on Cancer staging manual, with the T stage now based on the same criteria as those for differentiated thyroid carcinomas.[20] This change was made to reflect the observation that patients with less invasive ATC may have improved survival compared with patients with tumors with gross extrathyroidal extension.[7] However, all ATC are still categorized as stage group IV (IVA: intrathyroidal, IVB: gross extrathyroidal extension or lymph node metastasis, or IVC: distant metastasis).[20]

Although the diagnosis of ATC is often apparent, ATC may be overlooked when (1) the primary tumor is large and the anaplastic component comprises only a small percentage of the tumor, or (2) when the anaplastic component is present in lymph nodes only (either at the time of the initial thyroidectomy or as recurrent disease). In these cases, the prior fine needle aspiration (FNA) often does not sample the dedifferentiated component (ie, the preceding FNA diagnosis may be PTC) and the aggressive nature of the tumor may not be clinically apparent. Patients with tumors with a minor/focal component of ATC have a variable clinical course. Some patients die of disease rapidly, whereas others have a more protracted clinical course but eventually die of disease, and a small subset are long-term survivors.[6]

Focal dedifferentiation may be subtle when the anaplastic component has a spindle cell or spindle cell squamous morphology (**Figs. 1** and **2**), the latter of which has been well described in association with TCV of PTC and can be mistaken for a laryngeal squamous cell carcinoma.[21] All aggressive differentiated tumors should be carefully evaluated for areas of increased cytologic atypia and mitotic activity to exclude ATC. Special attention should be paid to the periphery of the tumor (where the focal component of ATC often arises) to ensure that apparent "fibrosis" does not actually represent spindle cell ATC. It is important to be aware of the fact that, although most ATC with a spindle cell pattern demonstrate marked pleomorphism, some may appear relatively bland (though readily identifiable mitoses can serve as a clue to the diagnosis). In such cases, immunohistochemistry (IHC) should be considered to evaluate for a potential anaplastic component (discussed below). Squamous metaplasia (a finding that can be seen in association with PTC) also should be examined to ensure the absence of marked cytologic atypia or mitotic activity, that is, findings that would instead suggest ATC. Finally, pure ATC can be difficult to differentiate from other aggressive malignancies, including head and neck squamous cell carcinoma (SCC), undifferentiated carcinoma of other primary sites, and sarcoma.

In challenging cases, IHC may be used to support an ATC diagnosis. Approximately 80% of ATC are PAX8 positive.[22] PAX8 staining may be especially helpful when the differential is a squamoid ATC

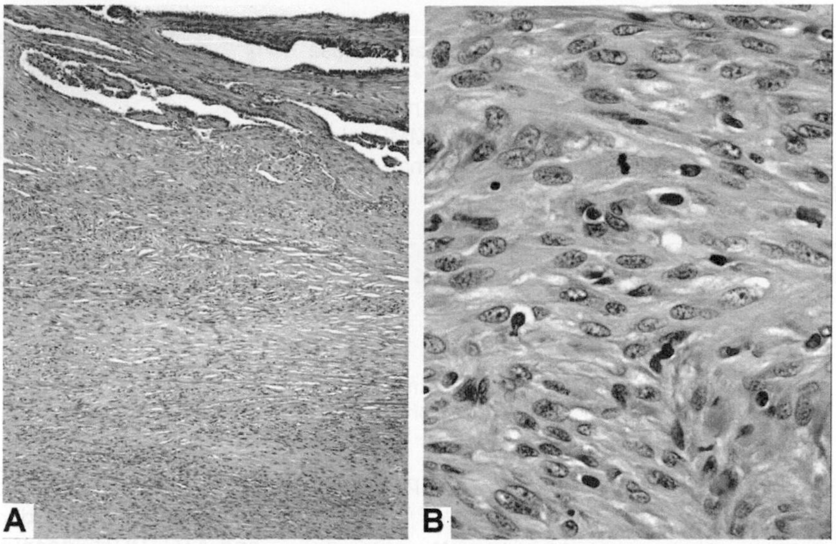

Fig. 1. Low-power photomicrograph of ATC with a spindle cell morphology (*A*). The anaplastic component is a minor component of the tumor and could be mistaken for fibrosis adjacent to a large PTC. On high power, the anaplastic component lacks marked pleomorphism, but mitoses are evident (*B*).

versus a head and neck SCC because PAX8 expression is seen in the vast majority of squamoid ATC (more than 80%) and is essentially absent in head and neck SCC.[22] Cytokeratin staining may be variable but is at least focally positive in most ATC cases,[23] a finding that can support the diagnosis of spindle cell pattern of ATC. p63/p40 can be used to highlight squamous differentiation in squamoid ATC, although it will also be positive in squamous metaplasia and in head and neck SCC. Thyroglobulin is negative in ATC, and TTF-1 is usually negative, with focal weak TTF-1 expression reported in approximately 15% of tumors.[23–25] Loss of thyroglobulin and TTF-1 expression can be used to support histologic evidence of dedifferentiation. One of the most helpful stains is Ki67, because the proliferative index is essentially always markedly elevated (>30%) in ATC.[26] Similarly, because approximately 60% of ATC harbor a *TP53* mutation (in contrast to most other thyroid tumors),[26–28] overexpression of p53 also can be used to support an ATC diagnosis. Finally, because a subset (roughly one-third) of ATC have a *BRAF* V600E mutation, BRAF V600E positivity may be used to support a diagnosis of ATC over other undifferentiated malignancies in the appropriate clinical setting, such as in a patient with a rapidly growing neck mass. BRAF V600E IHC status also may be used to guide therapy because *BRAF* V600E-mutant ATC may be treated with selective BRAF inhibitors alone or in

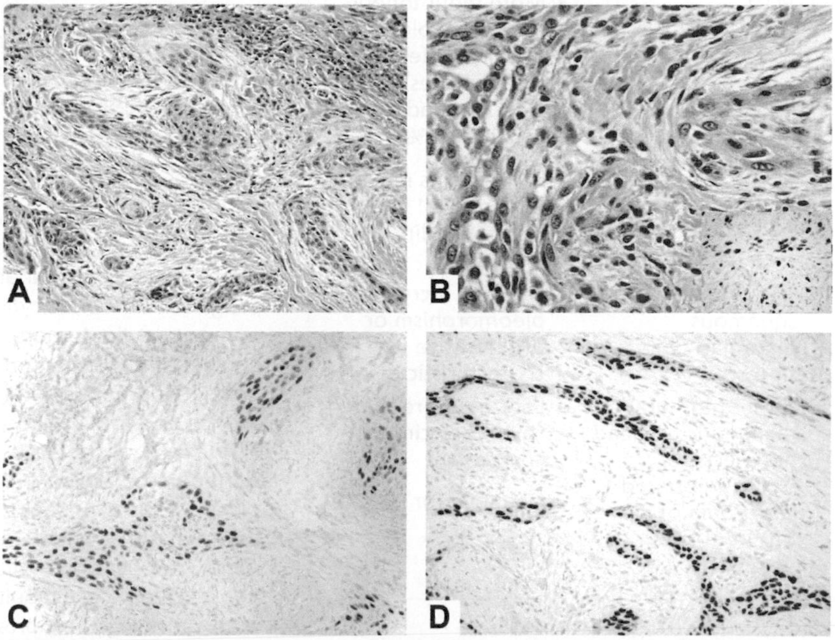

Fig. 2. Low-power photomicrograph of ATC with a spindle cell squamous morphology that was present as a minor component of a TCV of PTC (*A*). The anaplastic component has cells with vesicular chromatin, variably prominent nucleoli, and increased mitotic activity (inset: MIB1 confirms the increased proliferative index of the anaplastic component) (*B*). A p63 stain highlights the anaplastic component (*C*). PAX8 is also strongly positive (*D*).

combination with a MEK inhibitor.[29–31] Mismatch repair (MMR) IHC also could be considered because 10% to 15% of ATC are MMR-deficient,[27,28,32] with some evidence that these tumors may have improved survival compared with MMR-intact ATC.[32] In addition, MMR status may guide therapy.[32]

Pathologic Key Features

1. Variable morphology, including spindle cell, pleomorphic giant cell, and epithelioid/squamoid
2. Typically demonstrate marked pleomorphism and invasive growth
3. May arise in association with differentiated thyroid carcinoma
4. Most cases positive for PAX8
5. Negative for thyroglobulin and usually negative for TTF-1
6. Demonstrate a high Ki67 proliferative index (>30%)

Differential Diagnosis

Entity	Distinguishing Features
1. PDTC	• More monotonous cytomorphology and lower proliferative rate (mitoses less frequent and Ki67 usually <30%) • PDTC shows maintained TTF-1 and thyroglobulin expression
2. PTC with associated squamous metaplasia or fibrosis	• Lack the increased pleomorphism or proliferative rate characteristic of ATC
3. Other high-grade malignancies: head and neck SCC, undifferentiated carcinoma of different sites, sarcoma	• Lack a differentiated thyroid carcinoma component • Negative for PAX8

Pitfall

! ATC can be overlooked when it is a minor component of the tumor or is present in lymph node metastases only. It is important to closely evaluate aggressive PTC for progression to ATC.

POORLY DIFFERENTIATED THYROID CARCINOMA

The histologic features and clinical outcome of PDTC are intermediate between those of differentiated follicular-cell–derived thyroid carcinomas and ATC. PDTC accounts for approximately 2% of thyroid malignancies in the United States.[33] The average patient age is 55 to 63 years, and there is a slight female predominance.[33–35] Distant metastases are common, and the 5-year and 10-year survivals are approximately 70% and 50%, respectively. The 2017 Endocrine World Health Organization (WHO) defines PDTC using the criteria initially established in the Turin proposal,[36] that is, PDTC is defined as a tumor with conventional characteristics of malignancy (capsular or vascular invasion) that shows a solid, insular, or trabecular growth pattern, an absence of nuclear features of PTC, and at least 1 of the following: convoluted nuclei, a mitotic count of $\geq$3 per 10 high-power fields (HPFs), or tumor necrosis (**Fig. 3**).[26] Although convoluted nuclei are included in the definition of PDTC (and many PDTC demonstrate convoluted nuclei), studies published after the Turin proposal have found that convoluted nuclei fail to provide prognostic value,[33,34] and many endocrine pathologists (including the authors of this review) reserve a diagnosis of PDTC for tumors showing increased mitotic activity and/or necrosis. The criteria for PDTC also can be applied to oncocytic tumors.[33] There have been variable results regarding the prognosis of oncocytic PDTC compared with non-oncocytic tumors. Asioli and colleagues[33] showed that both tumors have a similar prognosis, whereas Dettmer and colleagues[37] and Wong and colleagues[38] found that oncocytic PDTC are associated with a worse outcome. Although the clinical behavior of tumors with focal progression to PDTC has not been established, there is some evidence that tumors with even a minor poorly differentiated component can be aggressive.[39] As a result, the 2017 WHO indicates that pathology reports should document any

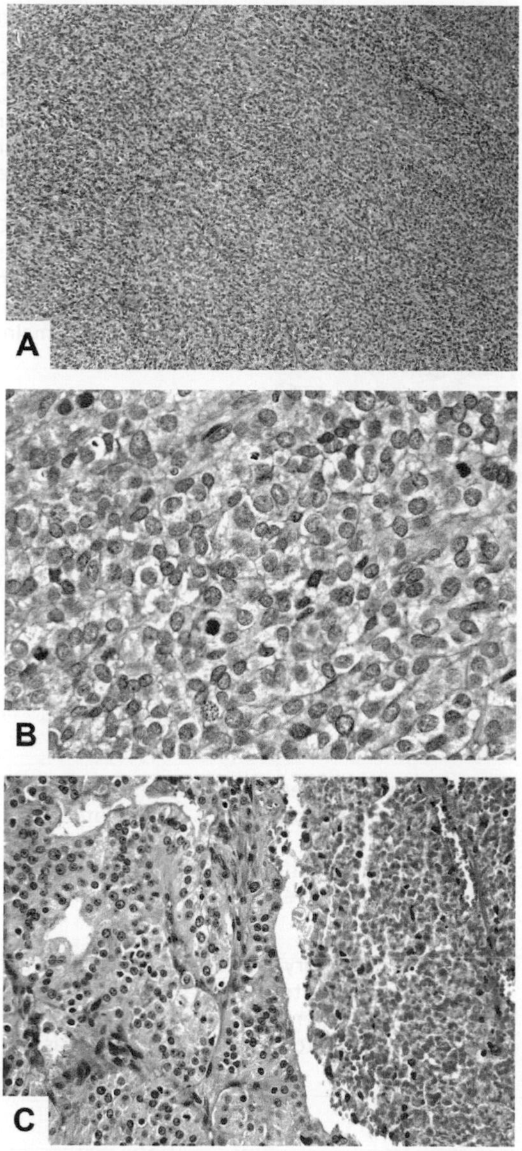

Fig. 3. Low-power photomicrograph of a PDTC with a solid architecture (*A*). On high power, the tumor is composed of fairly uniform cells with small dark nuclei (no nuclear features of PTC) and increased mitotic activity (*B*). An oncocytic PDTC with necrosis (*C*). Mitoses numbered 28 per 10 HPFs in this tumor.

poorly differentiated component (with the percentage of tumor demonstrating a poorly differentiated morphology recorded).[8] Our group has recently reported that the extent of invasion is prognostic in PDTC. Based on these findings, we suggest that the extent of invasion for PDTC should be documented as follows: encapsulated with capsular penetration only, encapsulated with focal vascular invasion (fewer than 4 foci), encapsulated with extensive vascular invasion (4 or more foci), or widely invasive.[38]

The diagnosis of PDTC can be challenging.[40] The aggressive nature of the tumor may be missed if the increased mitotic activity of the tumor is not appreciated. All follicular thyroid carcinomas and Hürthle cell carcinomas that demonstrate solid, trabecular, or insular growth should be carefully evaluated for increased mitotic activity and necrosis. It is important to recognize that proliferative activity may not be uniform throughout the tumor, so all slides should be evaluated for increased mitotic activity. Although necrosis is seen in approximately half of PDTC,[33,38] necrosis is not always indicative of PDTC. Necrosis can occur secondary to FNA, especially in Hürthle cell tumors. Thus, a Hürthle cell tumor with necrosis (and capsular and/or vascular invasion) may represent a Hürthle cell carcinoma with necrosis secondary to FNA or an oncocytic PDTC. Hürthle cell tumors with necrosis secondary to FNA should not show increased proliferative activity (although Ki67 may be elevated in macrophages adjacent to the area of FNA-induced necrosis). One of the main entities in the differential diagnosis for PDTC is solid variant of PTC (**Fig. 4**). In contrast to PDTC, solid variant of PTC has more cytoplasm and maintained nuclear features of PTC. The distinction between solid variant of PTC and PDTC is significant because, although solid variant of PTC has been reported to have a slightly higher frequency of distant metastases than classic PTC, the prognosis is significantly better than that of PDTC.[41] Finally, because PDTC tend to be monomorphic and often lack associated colloid, MTC may be considered in the differential diagnosis. MTC usually can be morphologically distinguished from PDTC based on the spindled or plasmacytoid cytomorphology, stippled chromatin, and associated amyloid.

The diagnosis of PDTC is primarily based on morphologic features; however, IHC can be used to support the diagnosis. PDTC are positive for PAX8, TTF-1, and thyroglobulin, although the

Pathologic Key Features

1. Conventional criteria of malignancy (capsular or vascular invasion)
2. Solid, insular, or trabecular growth
3. Absence of nuclear features of PTC
4. At least 1 of the following: convoluted nuclei, mitotic count $\geq$3 per 10 HPFs, coagulative tumor necrosis

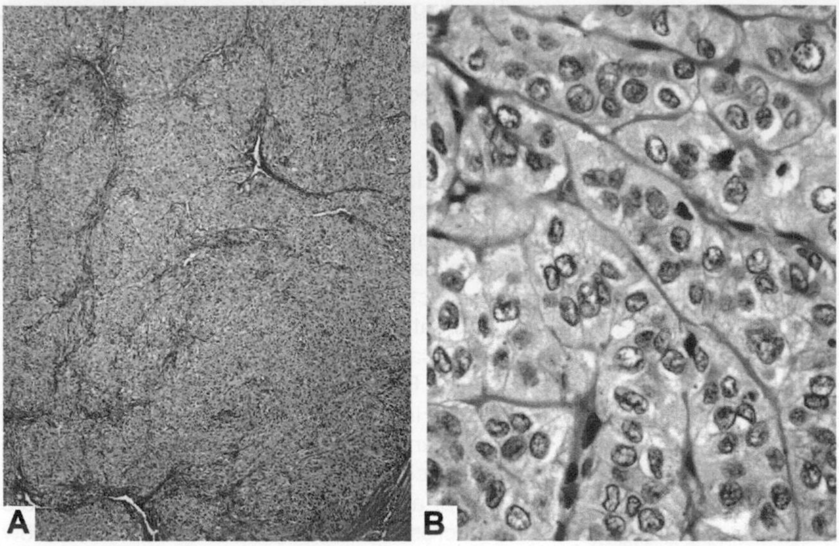

Fig. 4. One of the main tumors in the differential diagnosis for PDTC is solid variant of PTC, seen here at low power (*A*). Although the tumor has solid growth, the cells have more cytoplasm than most PDTC so the tumor appears less blue. In addition, on high power, nuclear features of PTC are maintained (*B*).

expressions of TTF-1 and thyroglobulin are generally weaker than seen with differentiated follicular-cell–derived thyroid tumors. In addition, thyroglobulin staining often has a dot-like paranuclear pattern. The Ki67 proliferative index is usually elevated (>5%) but less than that of ATC (ie, <30%).[8]

ΔΔ Differential Diagnosis

Entity	Distinguishing Features
1. Follicular carcinoma/ Hürthle cell carcinoma	• Absence of necrosis or increased mitotic rate
2. Solid variant of PTC	• More cytoplasm, nuclear features of PTC are maintained
3. MTC	• Associated amyloid deposition, spindled or plasmacytoid cytomorphology, stippled ("salt and pepper") chromatin • Mitotic rate is usually low • Positive for calcitonin, chromogranin, synaptophysin

Pitfalls

! PDTC may be missed if increased mitotic activity or focal necrosis is not appreciated. All follicular thyroid carcinomas and Hürthle cell carcinomas with solid growth should be examined for increased proliferative activity or necrosis.

! Necrosis secondary to FNA in oncocytic tumors can be misinterpreted as tumor necrosis. Evaluate whether the tumor has increased mitotic activity to support the diagnosis of PDTC.

UNCOMMON VARIANTS OF PAPILLARY THYROID CARCINOMA

The most common types of PTC are classic type and follicular variant, whereas TCV comprises approximately 6% to 8% of PTCs.[2–4] This section of the review focuses on rare PTC variants that have profound clinical implications but can be challenging to recognize because of lack of familiarity with histologic features of these rare tumors and overlapping morphology with more common thyroid tumors.

HOBNAIL VARIANT

Hobnail variant of PTC is a recently described rare PTC subtype associated with an aggressive clinical course. These tumors are associated with a high rate of distant metastases, are difficult to treat because of lack of radioactive iodine uptake, and result in death in a significant proportion of patients (with many patients dying within the first 5 years of diagnosis).[42,43] They are usually large, invasive tumors with complex papillary or micropapillary architecture (seen in approximately half of cases) (**Fig. 5**), with areas of follicular architecture also described in a small subset of cases.[43] They are characterized by nuclear pseudostratification, cellular discohesion, and loss of cell polarity with enlarged nuclei protruding from the apical surface. The nuclei are often more atypical than those of classic PTC; however, nuclear features of PTC are maintained. Mitotic rate is elevated, with a mean mitotic rate approaching 5 per 10 HPFs.[43] The 2017 Endocrine WHO indicates that a diagnosis of hobnail variant should be rendered when the hobnail component accounts for more than 30% of the tumor,[8] as it has been shown that tumors with greater than 30% hobnail morphology pursue an aggressive clinical course.[42] However, tumors with as little as 10% hobnail morphology also can act aggressively.[42] Thus, the presence of any hobnail component should be indicated in the pathology report.[8] Because hobnail variant has a high rate of dedifferentiation,[44] these tumors should be sampled generously for histologic evaluation and examined carefully for focal progression to PDTC or ATC.

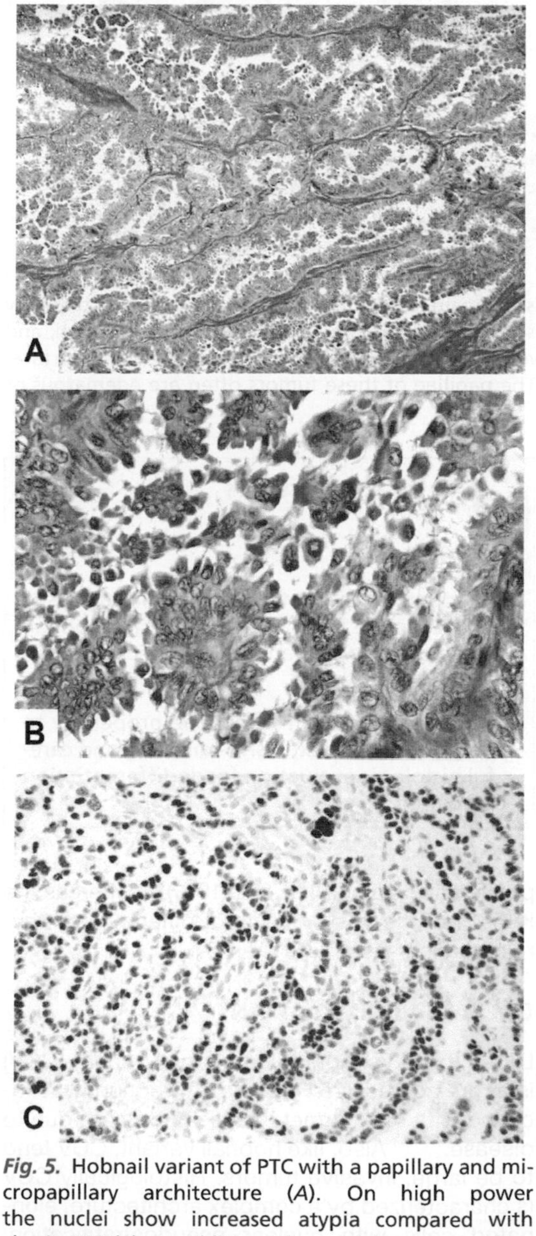

Fig. 5. Hobnail variant of PTC with a papillary and micropapillary architecture (*A*). On high power the nuclei show increased atypia compared with classic PTC (*B*). In addition, the nuclei are protruding out from the apical surface and there is cellular discohesion. A subset of hobnail variant harbor *TP53* mutations and show strong diffuse p53 expression (*C*).

The main entity in the differential diagnosis for hobnail variant is classic/conventional PTC. Differentiating these tumors is essential because PTC overall is associated with disease-specific survival rates of 98% and 93% at 5 and 10 years, respectively,[45] whereas most patients with hobnail variant die of their disease.[42,43] Because hobnail variant (like classic PTC) has a papillary architecture and nuclear features of PTC, it can be mistaken for classic PTC (especially because classic PTC is much more common than hobnail variant). Conversely, a subset of classic PTC has a hobnail-like cytomorphology secondary to degenerative/ischemic change that may mimic hobnail variant (**Fig. 6**). However, whereas hobnail variant is a large, invasive tumor with increased mitotic activity, classic PTC with hobnailing secondary to degenerative/ischemic change are smaller cystic tumors that lack increased proliferative activity. IHC is helpful to support a diagnosis of hobnail variant. Hobnail variant is positive for PAX8, TTF-1, and thyroglobulin (although thyroglobulin may show variable staining or may be lost in metastatic disease).[46] Between 20% and 50% of hobnail variants harbor *TP53* mutations (whereas classic PTC lack *TP53* mutations),[47–49] thus overexpression of p53 (strong, diffuse positivity) would support the diagnosis of hobnail variant. Finally, Ki67 is especially helpful in supporting a diagnosis of hobnail variant, because most have a Ki67 proliferative index (PI) greater than 5% (mean reported Ki67

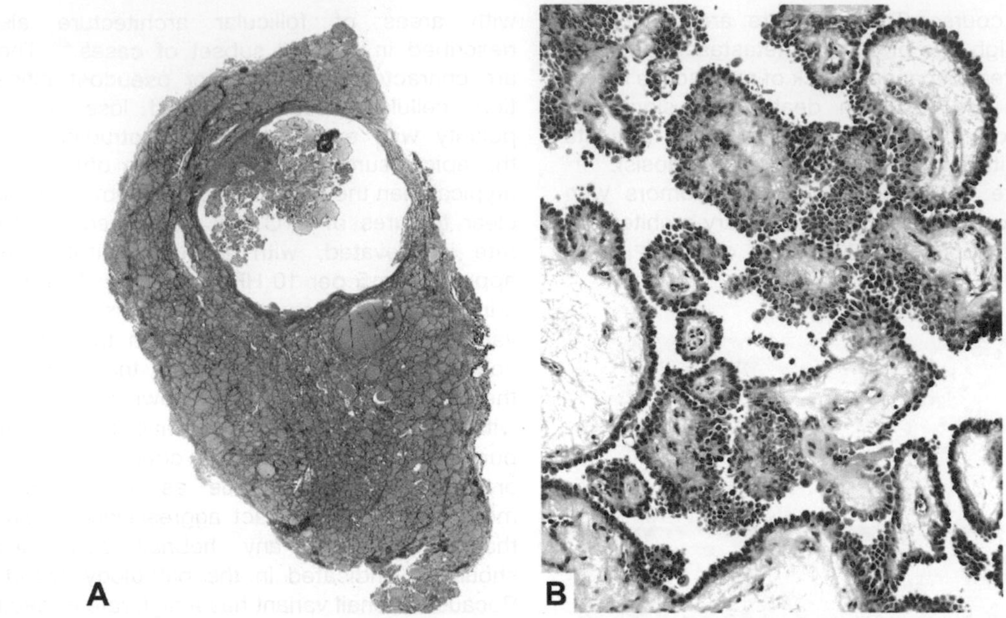

Fig. 6. Classic PTC that has a hobnail-like cytomorphology is the main differential for hobnail variant of papillary thyroid carcinoma. In contrast to true hobnail variant, these tumors are smaller, show less invasive growth, and tend to be cystic, as seen in this example (*A*). On high power, the nuclei are jutting out from the apical surface, but this is reflective of degenerative/ischemic change (*B*). The papillae of these tumors often are edematous or hyalinized.

Pathologic Key Features

1. Complex papillary and/or micropapillary architecture
2. Nuclear pseudostratification, loss of cell polarity, cellular discohesion
3. Enlarged nuclei that protrude from apical surface
4. Elevated Ki67 proliferative index

Pitfalls

! Histopathologic features are similar to classic PTC. Examine large, invasive PTC for hobnail cytomorphology and increased mitotic activity.

! Hobnail variant of PTC has the propensity to dedifferentiate. Extensive sampling and careful histologic evaluation for dedifferentiation is advised.

Differential Diagnosis

Entity	Distinguishing Features
1. Classic PTC	• Usually smaller, less invasive tumors without the increased cytologic atypia or elevated proliferative rate • Ki67 <5%, p53 wild-type staining

proliferative index (PI) is 8%–10%),[43] whereas the Ki67 PI of the vast majority of differentiated thyroid carcinomas is less than 5%.[50]

COLUMNAR CELL VARIANT

Like hobnail variant, columnar cell variant (CCV) is a rare aggressive PTC variant frequently associated with distant metastases and death due to disease.[51–53] Also, like hobnail variant, CCV tend to be large, invasive tumors. Histologically CCV is characterized by a complex architecture, elongated cells with nuclear pseudostratification, and subnuclear and supranuclear vacuoles (**Fig. 7**).[51–53] Nuclear features of PTC may be subtle. On low power these tumors appear bluer

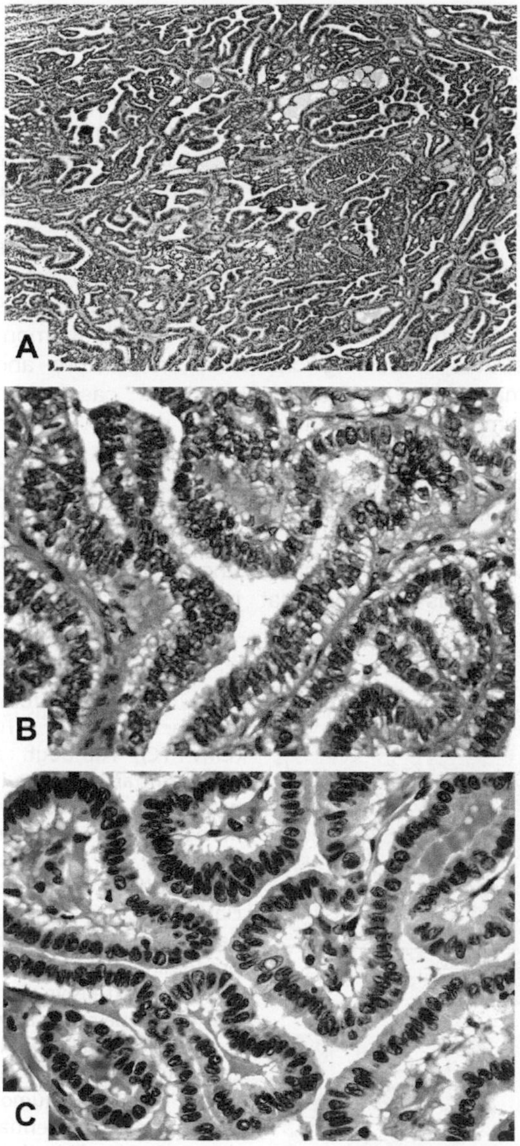

Fig. 7. CCV PTC often has a complex architecture (*A*). On low power these tumors appear bluer than classic PTC due to their high nuclear to cytoplasmic ratio and clear (as opposed to eosinophilic) cytoplasm. At high power, the elongated cytomorphology is evident, as is the nuclear pseudostratification and subnuclear vacuoles (*B*). One of the main tumors in the differential diagnosis for CCV is TCV of PTC (*C*). In contrast to CCV, TCV has cells with brightly eosinophilic cytoplasm and pronounced nuclear features of PTC, often including readily identifiable pseudoinclusions.

than classic PTC because of their high nuclear to cytoplasmic ratio and their blue (vs eosinophilic) cytoplasm. In fact, as a result of their unusual morphology, CCV may not be recognized as a thyroid primary. Consistent with the aggressive nature of this variant, mitoses are elevated, often numbering ≥5 per 10 HPFs, and tumor necrosis may be present. A clinically indolent subset of CCV has been described; however, unlike aggressive CCV, these tumors are histologically encapsulated or well-circumscribed and would not be expected to show increased mitotic activity or necrosis.[53,54]

The main entities in the differential diagnosis for CCV are TCV and metastases. Although TCV can also be large and invasive tumors with elongated tumor cells, TCV are composed of cells with brightly eosinophilic cytoplasm and pronounced nuclear features of PTC (often with numerous pseudoinclusions). In addition, although the mitotic count is elevated in a subset of TCV, the mitotic rate is generally not as high as that of CCV. Although both TCV and CCV are considered aggressive subtypes of PTC (along with hobnail variant) according to the American Thyroid Association guidelines,[55] differentiating CCV and TCV has important clinical implications: the cause-specific death rate is roughly 8% for TCV,[4] whereas most patients with CCV die of disease in less than 5 years.[51,52] Metastatic colorectal adenocarcinoma or endometrial adenocarcinoma may be considered in the differential with CCV based on the architecture of CCV (which may be reminiscent of the rambling glands of endometrial adenocarcinoma) and the elongated cells and nuclei. As a result, it is important to recognize that CCV, although positive for TTF-1 and thyroglobulin, may be positive for CDX2.[56–58]

ΔΔ Differential Diagnosis

Entity	Distinguishing Features
1. TCV	• Eosinophilic cytoplasm, more pronounced nuclear features of PTC (often including frequent pseudoinclusions) • Lacks nuclear pseudostratification
2. Metastatic colorectal adenocarcinoma	• "Dirty necrosis" often seen in association with colorectal adenocarcinoma • Negative for PAX8, TTF-1, and thyroglobulin
3. Metastatic endometrial adenocarcinoma	• Negative for thyroglobulin and usually negative for TTF-1[a]

[a] Approximately 20% of endometrial adenocarcinomas are TTF-1 positive.[59]

Pitfall

! CCV has the propensity to dedifferentiate. Extensive sampling and careful histologic evaluation for dedifferentiation is advised.

CRIBRIFORM MORULAR VARIANT OF PAPILLARY THYROID CARCINOMA

Cribriform morular variant of PTC (CMv-PTC) accounts for less than 1% of thyroid tumors[60] but is important to recognize due to its association with familial adenomatous polyposis (FAP) in approximately 40% of cases.[61–65] It is important for the pathologist to alert the surgeon or endocrinologist of this association, because it may be the first manifestation of FAP (and has been reported to be the first manifestation of FAP in 40% of patients).[61–65] FAP-associated CMv-PTC occurs almost exclusively in women, is often multifocal, and has a favorable clinical course.[60,62–64,66] In contrast, sporadic CMv-PTC can occur in men and is usually unifocal.[60,62–64,66] Rare cases of CMv-PTC pursue an aggressive clinical course.[62,67]

The morphology of CMv-PTC is variable (**Fig. 8**).[60,62–64] In most instances, the tumor is encapsulated or well-circumscribed. As the name implies, CMv-PTC usually demonstrates a striking cribriform architecture and may have morules (in some cases the tumor may be nearly entirely morular, and in other cases morules are absent). A very helpful clue to the diagnosis is a lack of colloid in the cribriform areas. Cells can range from cuboidal to columnar. Nuclear features are also variable. In some cases, the nuclei show conspicuous clearing that is more exaggerated

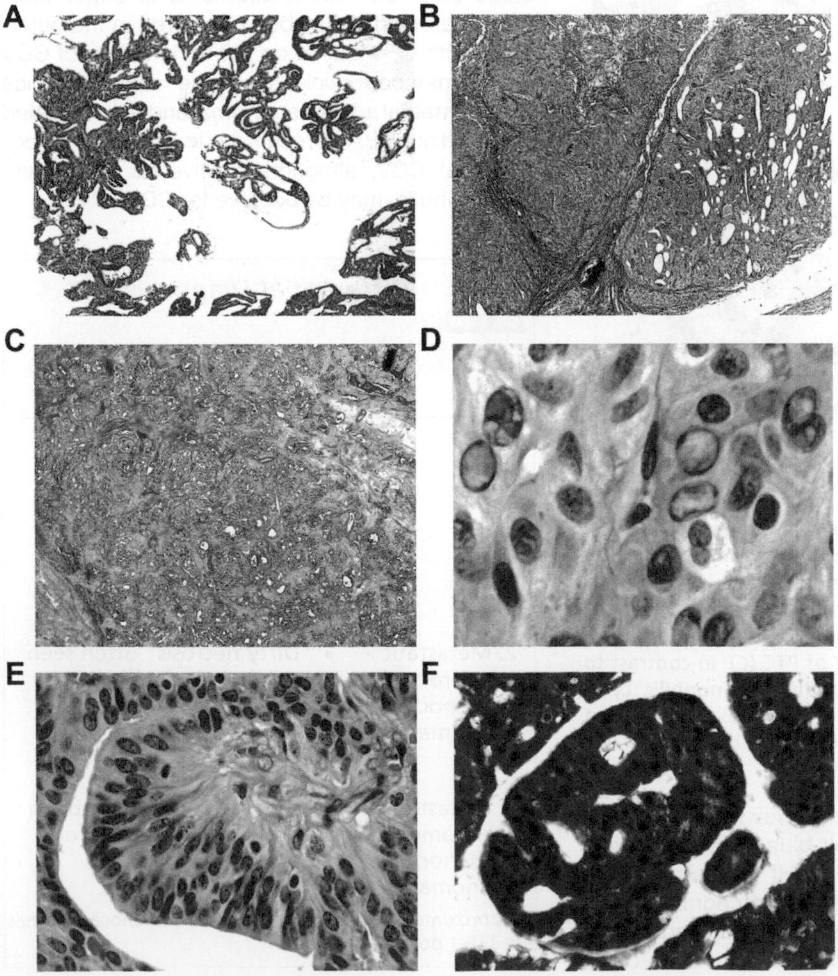

Fig. 8. Cribriform morular variant of PTC (CMv-PTC). Although a cribriform architecture is present (at least focally) in nearly all cases, the cribriform architecture may be difficult to appreciate in cases in which a papillary architecture predominates (*A*) and in cases with extensive morules (*B*). Some cases show extensive stromal hyalinization (*C*), bringing hyalinizing trabecular tumor into the differential diagnosis. Nuclear features of CMv-PTC are variable. Some cases have nuclear features of PTC and have conspicuous nuclear clearing that is, more exaggerated than classic PTC (*D*). Other cases entirely lack nuclear features of PTC (*E*). Nuclear and cytoplasmic (as opposed to membranous) beta-catenin staining confirms a diagnosis of CMv-PTC (*F*).

Pathologic Key Features

1. Usually multifocal/bilateral in FAP (unifocal in sporadic cases)
2. Tumor foci are often well-circumscribed or encapsulated
3. Mixed cribriform, papillary, and solid architecture
4. Morules are variably present
5. Colloid is scarce to absent
6. Stroma may be hyalinized
7. Nuclear features of PTC may be pronounced, subtle, or absent

ΔΔ Differential Diagnosis

Entity	Distinguishing Features
1. Classic PTC	• Absence of cribriform architecture and morules • Membranous beta-catenin
2. CCV of PTC	• Usually large, invasive tumors • Frequently demonstrate increased mitotic activity and tumor necrosis • Membranous beta-catenin, elevated Ki67
3. Hyalinizing trabecular tumor	• Composed of trabeculae or nests of polygonal to elongated cells with abundant eosinophilic to clear cytoplasm (sometimes with faint yellow granules, termed yellow bodies) and with nuclei with clearing, contour irregularities, grooves, and pseudoinclusions • Cells are usually oriented perpendicular to the axis of the trabecula • Membranous beta-catenin, membranous MIB1

than classic PTC,[63] whereas in other cases, the tumor essentially lacks nuclear features of PTC. CMv-PTC can be challenging to recognize when morules are absent, the cribriform architecture is focal or subtle, or when a papillary architecture predominates. In such cases, the main pitfall is rendering a diagnosis of classic PTC. Other tumors in the differential include CCV (if the cells are elongated) and hyalinizing trabecular tumor (when extensive stromal hyalinization is present). If a diagnosis of CMv-PTC is being considered, beta-catenin IHC should be performed. CMv-PTC is associated with alterations in the Wnt signaling pathway.[66] FAP-associated CMv-PTC has an underlying germline *APC* mutation, whereas sporadic CMv-PTC may have a somatic *APC* mutation or a mutation in other genes in the Wnt signaling pathway, including *CTNNB1* (the gene that encodes beta-catenin).[61,66,68,69] As a result of these mutations, there is nuclear and cytoplasmic (as opposed to membranous) localization of beta-catenin in CMv-PTC. Cytoplasmic and nuclear beta-catenin staining has been shown to be both sensitive and specific for CMv-PTC.[70]

Pitfall

! CMv-PTC can have overlapping features with other thyroid tumors; therefore, a low threshold for considering CMv-PTC as a potential diagnosis (and performing beta-catenin IHC) is advised.

MEDULLARY THYROID CARCINOMA

MTC is usually a well-circumscribed tumor with a solid or nested architecture with round, polygonal, plasmacytoid, or spindled cells in a background of hyalinized stroma or amyloid. However, MTC can exhibit a broad range of histologic appearances, such as papillary (**Fig. 9**), oncocytic, clear cell, giant cell, angiosarcoma-like, tubular/follicular, and paraganglioma-like, among others. MTC also can entrap non-neoplastic thyroid follicles, which may make the diagnosis more challenging because it appears the tumor is associated with colloid. In comparison with follicular cells, however, the nuclei of MTC should have coarse "salt and pepper" chromatin and often demonstrate binucleation and greater pleomorphism, occasionally with bizarre

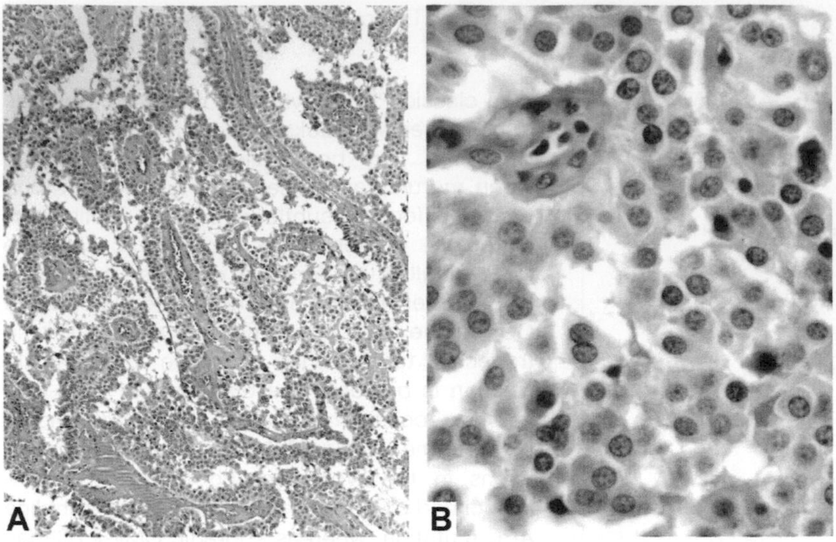

Fig. 9. MTC with a predominantly papillary architecture (*A*). At high power the "salt and pepper" chromatin characteristic of MTC (and neuroendocrine tumors in general) is apparent (*B*).

cells. MTC also can be diagnostically challenging in lymph node metastases, especially in small biopsies in which the tumor is crushed. If only TTF-1 IHC is performed, the tumor can potentially be misdiagnosed as metastatic lung adenocarcinoma. In a patient without clinical or radiographic evidence of a lung primary, calcitonin IHC should be considered. The clinical ramifications of incorrectly diagnosing a metastasis of MTC as lung adenocarcinoma are significant, as treatments differ greatly. MTC is treated surgically when possible, after which targeted treatments based on the presence of an underlying *RET* mutation would be considered.[71] In addition, given the association of MTC with germline *RET* mutations (ie, in multiple endocrine neoplasia type 2), patients with MTC should be referred to genetic counseling.[71]

Pathologic Key Features

1. Variable architectural patterns including solid, trabecular, papillary, and follicular
2. Hyalinized stroma with amyloid deposition
3. Cells with plasmacytoid, spindled, or polygonal morphology
4. Stippled "salt and pepper" chromatin
5. Positive for TTF-1 and calcitonin; PAX8 is also positive in most cases (~75%)[24]

Differential Diagnosis

Entity	Distinguishing Features
1. PTC/follicular thyroid carcinoma/ Hürthle cell carcinoma	• PTC will demonstrate chromatin clearing, nuclear pseudoinclusions, and nuclear membrane irregularities • PTC, follicular thyroid carcinoma, and Hürthle cell carcinoma are positive for thyroglobulin, and negative for calcitonin, synaptophysin, and chromogranin
2. PDTC	• Morphologic evidence of follicular differentiation, positive for thyroglobulin, negative for calcitonin • Increased mitotic activity
3. Paraganglioma	• Zellballen architecture with S100-positive sustentacular cells • Negative for calcitonin and cytokeratins

4. Metastatic lung adenocarcinoma (generally a differential only in lymph node biopsies)	• Clinical or radiologic evidence of a lung tumor • Negative for PAX8, calcitonin, synaptophysin, and chromogranin
5. Metastatic lung carcinoid	• Clinical or radiologic evidence of a lung tumor • Negative for PAX8 and usually negative for calcitonin (a small subset can show some degree of calcitonin expression)[72,73]

Pitfalls

! Unusual morphology or entrapped follicles may lead to an incorrect diagnosis of a follicular-cell derived tumor

! May be misinterpreted as lung adenocarcinoma or a lung carcinoid in small/crushed TTF-1 positive lymph node metastases.

NON-INVASIVE FOLLICULAR THYROID NEOPLASM WITH PAPILLARY-LIKE NUCLEAR FEATURES (NIFTP)

NIFTP was recently introduced to recognize the indolent behavior of thyroid neoplasms previously classified as non-invasive encapsulated follicular variant of PTC (FVPTC).[74] Because NIFTP has very low metastatic potential and recurrence risk, lobectomy instead of total thyroidectomy has been advocated.[74] Resection is still recommended for NIFTP, as it may be a precursor to a more aggressive tumor. Histologic evaluation is also required to assess for infiltrative or invasive growth, which would exclude a diagnosis of NIFTP (ie, a NIFTP diagnosis cannot be rendered on FNA).[75]

The differential diagnosis for NIFTP includes follicular adenoma, adenomatous/hyperplastic nodule, infiltrative or invasive FVPTC, and follicular-predominant classic PTC. NIFTP are encapsulated or well-circumscribed tumors, with an entirely follicular architecture, nuclear features of PTC (including nuclear enlargement, clearing, grooves, and contour irregularities; pseudoinclusions are absent to rare), less than 30% solid growth, and a lack of high-grade features (ie, mitoses number <3 per 10 HPFs and there is no tumor necrosis) (**Fig. 10**). Although there is no upper limit in terms of nuclear atypia of NIFTP, most NIFTP show mild to moderate atypia that is variably present through the tumor. As a result, a diagnosis of follicular adenoma or adenomatous/hyperplastic nodule is often considered when histologically evaluating an NIFTP. Because the clinical implications and treatment (ie, lobectomy only) are similar for NIFTP and follicular adenoma and adenomatous/hyperplastic nodule, the authors of this review would not consider differences in interpretation between these entities a major diagnostic discrepancy. However, because a NIFTP diagnosis implies an exceptionally indolent course, differentiating NIFTP from PTC is more important. Tumors with nuclear features of PTC and any papillary architecture should be considered classic PTC. Although the original NIFTP criteria had a cutoff of 1% for papillae, there has been evolution in the NIFTP diagnosis, moving toward a requirement for the complete absence of papillae.[76] Although NIFTP are variably encapsulated, all have a sharp interface between the tumor and benign parenchyma. If neoplastic cells are seen trickling between benign follicles, a diagnosis of infiltrative FVPTC is appropriate. Finally, it is essential that the periphery of a potential NIFTP is entirely submitted for histologic evaluation. If capsular and/or vascular invasion is identified, a diagnosis of encapsulated FVPTC with invasion should be rendered. In cases with areas suspicious for invasion, level sections should be examined. If, after levels are performed, the question of potential invasion still exists, the 2017 Endocrine WHO indicates that pathologists can use the terminology of well-differentiated tumor of uncertain malignant potential (although this diagnosis should be reserved for rare cases).[8] Although differentiating NIFTP from the previously described NIFTP mimics relies nearly entirely on histologic evaluation, IHC may occasionally be helpful. Because NIFTP lack the *BRAF* V600E mutation, in contrast to infiltrative follicular variant and follicular-predominant classic PTC, which can harbor the *BRAF* V600E mutation, interrogation for the *BRAF* V600E mutation (by molecular testing or IHC) can aid in the evaluation of these tumors.[77,78] Although a negative BRAF V600E stain is not specific for NIFTP, positive BRAF V600E staining suggests that the tumor is likely not a NIFTP.

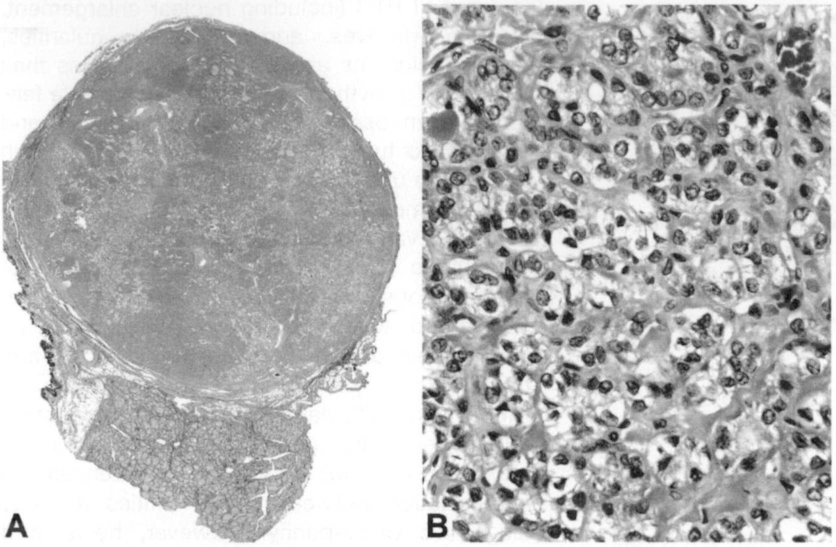

Fig. 10. All non-invasive follicular thyroid neoplasm with papillary-like nuclear features (NIFTP) are encapsulated or well circumscribed (*A*). NIFTP have an entirely follicular architecture and enlarged nuclei with variable contour irregularities, grooves, and clearing (*B*).

Pathologic Key Features

1. Entirely follicular architecture (no papillae)
2. Nuclear features of PTC
3. Encapsulated or partially encapsulated/well-circumscribed
4. Absence of *BRAF* V600E (although molecular testing is not required for the diagnosis)

Pitfalls

! Infiltration into adjacent thyroid parenchyma may be subtle. The periphery of the tumor should be closely evaluated.

! The periphery of the tumor should be entirely submitted to evaluate for capsular/vascular invasion that is focal.

Differential Diagnosis

Entity	Distinguishing Features
1. Infiltrative FVPTC	Infiltration into surrounding thyroid parenchyma
2. Encapsulated FVPTC with invasion	Capsular or vascular invasion
3. Follicular-predominant classic PTC	Has areas of papillary architecture
4. Follicular adenoma or adenomatous/hyperplastic nodule	Absence of nuclear features of PTC

MULTIPLE ADENOMATOUS NODULES IN THE SETTING OF COWDEN SYNDROME

CS is an autosomal dominant disorder caused by a germline mutation in the phosphatase and tensin homolog (*PTEN*) tumor suppressor gene.[79] CS is a multisystem disease characterized by the development of multiple hamartomas (commonly involving the skin, mucosa, and gastrointestinal tract), as well as increased risk for carcinomas of the thyroid, breast, and uterus.[79] The most common malignancy in CS is breast cancer, with a lifetime risk of approximately 25% to 50% in women.[79–81] Early recognition of CS can ensure that patients are appropriately triaged for genetic counseling and cancer screening.

Multiple adenomatous nodules/follicular adenomas with or without nodular hyperplasia, follicular thyroid carcinoma, C cell hyperplasia, and lymphocytic thyroiditis should raise suspicion for CS (**Fig. 11**).[82,83] The lifetime risk of developing thyroid cancer among those with *PTEN* germline

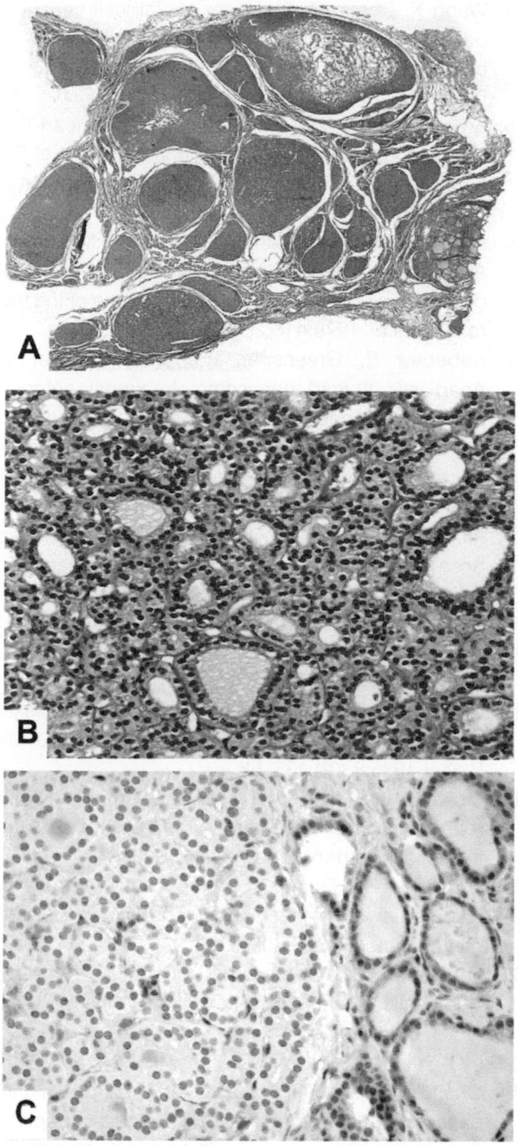

Fig. 11. Multiple adenomatous nodules associated with CS (*A*). Higher power of one of the adenomatous nodules shows a lack of nuclear atypia (*B*). Loss of PTEN staining in the CS-associated adenomatous nodules (with intact nuclear and cytoplasmic staining seen in the adjacent thyroid tissue and in endothelial cells within the adenomatous nodules) (*C*).

Pathologic Key Features

1. Multiple adenomatous nodules or follicular adenomas
2. Additional findings: follicular carcinoma, nodular hyperplasia, lymphocytic thyroiditis, C cell hyperplasia, PTC

mutations has been estimated at approximately 3% to 10%.[84] Both follicular thyroid carcinoma and PTC may develop in patients with CS, although follicular thyroid carcinoma more specifically appears to be overrepresented in CS.[85] Although the presence of these histologic findings suggests CS, they are not specific. Multiple adenomatous nodules and follicular adenomas can be seen in the setting of prior irradiation. However, in contrast to thyroidectomy specimens from patients with CS, which tend to be larger/heavier than normal,[86] thyroidectomy specimens with changes linked to prior radiation tend to be atrophic and weigh less than a normal thyroid gland. In addition, the parenchyma is often more fibrotic than in CS, and there may be radiation-induced nuclear atypia. Some cases of nodular hyperplasia also can show extensive adenomatous change. Although the thyroid manifestations of CS may be subtle in some cases, most cases (or at least most that we recognize) have numerous adenomatous nodules, including numerous small adenomatous nodules that are generally not seen in nodular hyperplasia. If prior clinical or genetic workup is limited or unavailable in cases of suspected CS, PTEN IHC can be informative in

ΔΔ *Differential Diagnosis*

Entity	Distinguishing Features
1. Radiation-induced changes	• Thyroid is small/atrophic, thyroid parenchyma is fibrotic, may show pronounced nuclear atypia
2. Nodular hyperplasia with adenomatous change	• Lack the numerous small adenomatous nodules often seen with CS
3. Other familial tumor syndromes	• Lack a germline *PTEN* mutation • Other currently unidentified germline mutations may be associated with thyroid histology identical to CS (these patients may benefit from referral to a genetic counselor for germline testing)

Pitfalls

! Histologic findings associated with CS are nonspecific and may be seen in patients without CS.
! PTEN IHC may show heterogeneous loss of expression in CS.

thyroidectomy specimens.[86] Loss of PTEN expression by IHC in adenomatous nodules (in contrast to the nuclear and cytoplasmic staining seen in background thyroid parenchyma and in adenomatous nodules from patients without CS) has been found to be both sensitive and specific for CS. Approximately one-third of CS cases show heterogeneous loss of expression in the adenomatous nodules, with some nodules showing complete loss but others with intact expression.[86] In these cases, performing PTEN IHC on multiple blocks may be helpful. Ultimately, genetic testing and clinical assessment are needed to confirm the diagnosis of CS.

SUMMARY

The diagnoses in this review highlight the impact pathologists have when reviewing thyroidectomy specimens. Recognizing the aggressive nature of a rare PTC variant or finding an area of tumor dedifferentiation ensures that the patient receives the appropriate aggressive treatment. Rendering a NIFTP diagnosis (instead of cancer) avoids overtreatment and spares patients the anxiety of a cancer diagnosis. Finally, as a result of identifying thyroidectomy findings associated with hereditary syndromes, patients (and their families) can undergo appropriate genetic counseling and screening.

REFERENCES

1. Sun GH, DeMonner S, Davis MM. Epidemiological and economic trends in inpatient and outpatient thyroidectomy in the United States, 1996–2006. Thyroid 2012;23:727–33.
2. Fagin JA, Wells SA. Biologic and clinical perspectives on thyroid cancer. N Engl J Med 2016; 375(11):1054–67.
3. Jung CK, Little MP, Lubin JH, et al. The increase in thyroid cancer incidence during the last four decades is accompanied by a high frequency of BRAF mutations and a sharp increase in RAS mutations. J Clin Endocrinol Metab 2014;99(2):E276–85.
4. Wang X, Cheng W, Liu C, et al. Tall cell variant of papillary thyroid carcinoma: current evidence on clinicopathologic features and molecular biology. Oncotarget 2016;7(26):40792–9.
5. Smallridge RC, Ain KB, Asa SL, et al. American Thyroid Association Guidelines for Management of Patients with Anaplastic Thyroid Cancer. Thyroid 2012;22:1104–39.
6. Aldinger KA, Samaan NA, Ibanez M, et al. Anaplastic carcinoma of the thyroid. A review of 84 cases of spindle and giant cell carcinoma of the thyroid. Cancer 1978;41:2267–75.
7. Kebebew E, Greenspan FS, Clark OH, et al. Anaplastic thyroid carcinoma: treatment outcome and prognostic factors. Cancer 2005;103:1330–5.
8. Lloyd RV, Osamura RY, Kloppel G, et al. WHO classification of tumours of endocrine organs. 4th edition. Lyon (France): IARC Publications; 2017.
9. Albores-Saavedra J, Hernandez M, Sanchez-Sosa S, et al. Histologic variants of papillary and follicular carcinomas associated with anaplastic spindle and giant cell carcinomas of the thyroid: an analysis of rhabdoid and thyroglobulin inclusions. Am J Surg Pathol 2007;31(5):729–36.
10. Carcangiu ML, Steeper T, Zampi G, et al. Anaplastic thyroid carcinoma. A study of 70 cases. Am J Clin Pathol 1985;83(2):135–58.
11. McIver B, Hay ID, Giuffrida DF, et al. Anaplastic thyroid carcinoma: a 50-year experience at a single institution. Surgery 2001;130(6):1028–34.
12. Nishiyama RH, Dunn EL, Thompson NW. Anaplastic spindle-cell and giant-cell tumors of the thyroid gland. Cancer 1972;30(1):113–27.
13. Venkatesh YS, Ordonez NG, Schultz PN, et al. Anaplastic carcinoma of the thyroid. A clinicopathologic study of 121 cases. Cancer 1990;66(2): 321–30.
14. Choi JY, Hwang BH, Jung KC, et al. Clinical significance of microscopic anaplastic focus in papillary thyroid carcinoma. Surgery 2013;154(1):106–10.
15. Han JM, Bae Kim W, Kim TY, et al. Time trend in tumour size and characteristics of anaplastic thyroid carcinoma. Clin Endocrinol 2012;77(3):459–64.
16. Lee DY, Won JK, Choi HS, et al. Recurrence and survival after gross total removal of resectable undifferentiated or poorly differentiated thyroid carcinoma. Thyroid 2016;26(9):1259–68.
17. Spires JR, Schwartz MR, Miller RH. Anaplastic thyroid carcinoma. Association with differentiated thyroid cancer. Arch Otolaryngol Head Neck Surg 1988;114(1):40–4.
18. Sugitani I, Kasai N, Fujimoto Y, et al. Prognostic factors and therapeutic strategy for anaplastic carcinoma of the thyroid. World J Surg 2001;25(5): 617–22.
19. Mete O, Seethala R, Asa SL, et al. College of American Pathologists Protocol for the examination of

specimens from patients with carcinomas of the thyroid gland 2017.
20. Amin MB. AJCC cancer staging manual. 8th edition. New York: springer international publishing; 2017.
21. Gopal PP, Montone KT, Baloch Z, et al. The variable presentations of anaplastic spindle cell squamous carcinoma associated with tall cell variant of papillary thyroid carcinoma. Thyroid 2011;21(5):493–9.
22. Bishop JA, Sharma R, Westra WH. PAX8 immunostaining of anaplastic thyroid carcinoma: a reliable means of discerning thyroid origin for undifferentiated tumors of the head and neck. Hum Pathol 2011;42:1873–7.
23. Miettinen M, Franssila KO. Variable expression of keratins and nearly uniform lack of thyroid transcription factor 1 in thyroid anaplastic carcinoma. Hum Pathol 2000;31:1139–45.
24. Nonaka D, Tang Y, Chiriboga L, et al. Diagnostic utility of thyroid transcription factors Pax8 and TTF-2 (FoxE1) in thyroid epithelial neoplasms. Mod Pathol 2008;21:192–200.
25. Weissferdt A, Moran CA. Anaplastic thymic carcinoma: a clinicopathologic and immunohistochemical study of 6 cases. Hum Pathol 2012;43(6):874–7.
26. Khan SA, Ci B, Xie Y, et al. Unique mutation patterns in anaplastic thyroid cancer identified by comprehensive genomic profiling. Head Neck 2019;41(6): 1928–34.
27. Kunstman JW, Juhlin CC, Goh G, et al. Characterization of the mutational landscape of anaplastic thyroid cancer via whole-exome sequencing. Hum Mol Genet 2015;24(8):2318–29.
28. Landa I, Ibrahimpasic T, Boucai L, et al. Genomic and transcriptomic hallmarks of poorly differentiated and anaplastic thyroid cancers. J Clin Invest 2016; 126(3):1052–66.
29. Prager GW, Koperek O, Mayerhoefer ME, et al. Sustained response to vemurafenib in a BRAF(V600E)-mutated anaplastic thyroid carcinoma patient. Thyroid 2016;26(10):1515–6.
30. Rosove MH, Peddi PF, Glaspy JA. BRAF V600E inhibition in anaplastic thyroid cancer. N Engl J Med 2013;368(7):684–5.
31. Subbiah V, Kreitman RJ, Wainberg ZA, et al. Dabrafenib and trametinib treatment in patients with locally advanced or metastatic BRAF V600-mutant anaplastic thyroid cancer. J Clin Oncol 2018;36(1):7–13.
32. Wong KS, Lorch JH, Alexander EK, et al. Clinicopathologic features of mismatch repair-deficient anaplastic thyroid carcinomas. Thyroid 2019;29(5): 666–73.
33. Asioli S, Erickson LA, Righi A, et al. Poorly differentiated carcinoma of the thyroid: validation of the Turin proposal and analysis of IMP3 expression. Mod Pathol 2010;23(9):1269–78.
34. Gnemmi V, Renaud F, Do Cao C, et al. Poorly differentiated thyroid carcinomas: application of the Turin proposal provides prognostic results similar to those from the assessment of high-grade features. Histopathology 2014;64:263–73.
35. Volante M, Collini P, Nikiforov YE, et al. Poorly differentiated thyroid carcinoma: the Turin proposal for the use of uniform diagnostic criteria and an algorithmic diagnostic approach. Am J Surg Pathol 2007;31(8):1256–64.
36. Volante M, Collini P, Nikiforov YE, et al. Poorly differentiated thyroid carcinoma: the Turin proposal for the use of uniform diagnostic criteria and an algorithmic diagnostic approach. Am J Surg Pathol 2007;31:1256–64.
37. Dettmer M, Schmitt A, Steinert H, et al. Poorly differentiated oncocytic thyroid carcinoma–diagnostic implications and outcome. Histopathology 2012;60(7): 1045–51.
38. Wong KS, Lorch J, Alexander EK, et al. Prognostic significance of extent of invasion in poorly differentiated thyroid carcinoma. Thyroid 2019, [Epub ahead of print].
39. Dettmer M, Schmitt A, Steinert H, et al. Poorly differentiated thyroid carcinomas: how much poorly differentiated is needed? Am J Surg Pathol 2011;35(12): 1866–72.
40. Dettmer MS, Schmitt A, Komminoth P, et al. Poorly differentiated thyroid carcinoma: an underdiagnosed entity. Pathologe 2019, [Epub ahead of print].
41. Nikiforov YE, Erickson LA, Nikiforova MN, et al. Solid variant of papillary thyroid carcinoma: incidence, clinical-pathologic characteristics, molecular analysis, and biologic behavior. Am J Surg Pathol 2001;25(12):1478–84.
42. Asioli S, Erickson LA, Righi A, et al. Papillary thyroid carcinoma with hobnail features: histopathologic criteria to predict aggressive behavior. Hum Pathol 2013;44(3):320–8.
43. Asioli S, Erickson LA, Sebo TJ, et al. Papillary thyroid carcinoma with prominent hobnail features: a new aggressive variant of moderately differentiated papillary carcinoma. A clinicopathologic, immunohistochemical, and molecular study of eight cases. Am J Surg Pathol 2010;34(1):44–52.
44. Amacher AM, Goyal B, Lewis JS, et al. Prevalence of a hobnail pattern in papillary, poorly differentiated, and anaplastic thyroid carcinoma: a possible manifestation of high-grade transformation. Am J Surg Pathol 2015;39(2):260–5.
45. Grogan RH, Kaplan SP, Cao H, et al. A study of recurrence and death from papillary thyroid cancer with 27 years of median follow-up. Surgery 2013; 154(6):1436–46, [discussion: 1446–7].
46. Ambrosi F, Righi A, Ricci C, et al. Hobnail variant of papillary thyroid carcinoma: a literature review. Endocr Pathol 2017;28(4):293–301.
47. Morandi L, Righi A, Maletta F, et al. Somatic mutation profiling of hobnail variant of papillary

thyroid carcinoma. Endocr Relat Cancer 2017;24: 107–17.
48. Teng L, Deng W, Lu J, et al. Hobnail variant of papillary thyroid carcinoma: molecular profiling and comparison to classical papillary thyroid carcinoma, poorly differentiated thyroid carcinoma and anaplastic thyroid carcinoma. Oncotarget 2017; 8(13):22023–33.
49. Watutantrige-Fernando S, Vianello F, Barollo S, et al. The hobnail variant of papillary thyroid carcinoma: clinical/molecular characteristics of a large monocentric series and comparison with conventional histotypes. Thyroid 2018;28(1):96–103.
50. Saltman B, Singh B, Hedvat CV, et al. Patterns of expression of cell cycle/apoptosis genes along the spectrum of thyroid carcinoma progression. Surgery 2006;140(6):899–905, [discussion: 905–6].
51. Evans HL. Columnar-cell carcinoma of the thyroid. A report of two cases of an aggressive variant of thyroid carcinoma. Am J Clin Pathol 1986;85(1): 77–80.
52. Ferreiro JA, Hay ID, Lloyd RV. Columnar cell carcinoma of the thyroid: report of three additional cases. Hum Pathol 1996;27(11):1156–60.
53. Wenig BM, Thompson LD, Adair CF, et al. Thyroid papillary carcinoma of columnar cell type: a clinicopathologic study of 16 cases. Cancer 1998;82(4): 740–53.
54. Evans HL. Encapsulated columnar-cell neoplasms of the thyroid. A report of four cases suggesting a favorable prognosis. Am J Surg Pathol 1996; 20(10):1205–11.
55. Haugen BR, Alexander EK, Bible KC, et al. 2015 American Thyroid Association Management Guidelines for Adult Patients with Thyroid Nodules and Differentiated Thyroid Cancer: The American Thyroid Association Guidelines Task Force on Thyroid Nodules and Differentiated Thyroid Cancer. Thyroid 2016;26:1–133.
56. Chen J-H, Faquin WC, Lloyd RV, et al. Clinicopathological and molecular characterization of nine cases of columnar cell variant of papillary thyroid carcinoma. Mod Pathol 2011;24(5):739–49.
57. Enriquez ML, Baloch ZW, Montone KT, et al. CDX2 expression in columnar cell variant of papillary thyroid carcinoma. Am J Clin Pathol 2012;137(5): 722–6.
58. Sujoy V, Pinto A, Nosé V. Columnar cell variant of papillary thyroid carcinoma: a study of 10 cases with emphasis on CDX2 expression. Thyroid 2013; 23(6):714–9.
59. Siami K, McCluggage WG, Ordonez NG, et al. Thyroid transcription factor-1 expression in endometrial and endocervical adenocarcinomas. Am J Surg Pathol 2007;31(11):1759–63.
60. Akaishi J, Kondo T, Sugino K, et al. Cribriform-morular variant of papillary thyroid carcinoma: clinical and pathological features of 30 cases. World J Surg 2018;42:3616–23.
61. Cetta F, Montalto G, Gori M, et al. Germline mutations of the APC gene in patients with familial adenomatous. Oncogene 2000;19:164–8.
62. Harach HR, Williams GT, Williams ED. Familial adenomatous polyposis associated thyroid carcinoma: a distinct type of follicular cell neoplasm. Histopathology 1994;25:549–61.
63. Hirokawa M, Maekawa M, Kuma S, et al. Cribriform-morular variant of papillary thyroid carcinoma—cytological and immunocytochemical findings of 18 cases. Diagn Cytopathol 2010;38:890–6.
64. Ito Y, Miyauchi A, Ishikawa H, et al. Our experience of treatment of cribriform morular variant of papillary thyroid carcinoma; difference in clinicopathological features of FAP-associated and sporadic patients. Endocr J 2011;58:685–9.
65. Jarrar AM, Milas M, Mitchell J, et al. Screening for thyroid cancer in patients with familial adenomatous polyposis. Ann Surg 2011;253:515–21.
66. Cameselle-Teijeiro JM, Peteiro-González D, Caneiro-Gómez J, et al. Cribriform-morular variant of thyroid carcinoma: a neoplasm with distinctive phenotype associated with the activation of the WNT/β-catenin pathway. Mod Pathol 2018;31:1168–79.
67. Cameselle-Teijeiro J, Menasce LP, Yap BK, et al. Cribriform-morular variant of papillary thyroid carcinoma molecular characterization of a case with neuroendocrine differentiation and aggressive behavior. Am J Clin Pathol 2009;131:134–42.
68. Cameselle-Teijeiro J, Ruiz-Ponte C, Loidi L, et al. Somatic but not germline mutation of the APC gene in a case of cribriform-morular variant of papillary thyroid carcinoma. Am J Clin Pathol 2001;115(4): 486–93.
69. Xu B, Yoshimoto K, Miyauchi A, et al. Cribriform-morular variant of papillary thyroid carcinoma: a pathological and molecular genetic study with evidence of frequent somatic mutations in exon 3 of the beta-catenin gene. J Pathol 2003;199(1):58–67.
70. Kurihara K, Shimizu S, Chong J, et al. Nuclear localization of immunoreactive beta-catenin is specific to familial adenomatous polyposis in papillary thyroid carcinoma. Jpn J Cancer Res 2000;91(11):1100–2.
71. Wells SA, Asa SL, Dralle H, et al. Revised American Thyroid Association guidelines for the management of medullary thyroid carcinoma. Thyroid 2015;25: 567–610.
72. Duan K, Mete O. Algorithmic approach to neuroendocrine tumors in targeted biopsies: practical applications of immunohistochemical markers. Cancer Cytopathol 2016;124(12):871–84.
73. Vahidi S, Stewart J, Amin K, et al. Metastatic medullary thyroid carcinoma or calcitonin-secreting carcinoid tumor of lung? A diagnostic dilemma in a

patient with lung mass and thyroid nodule. Diagn Cytopathol 2018;46(4):345–8.
74. Nikiforov YE, Seethala RR, Tallini G, et al. Nomenclature revision for encapsulated follicular variant of papillary thyroid carcinoma a paradigm shift to reduce overtreatment of indolent tumors. JAMA Oncol 2016;2:1023–9.
75. Zhao L, Dias-Santagata D, Sadow PM, et al. Cytological, molecular, and clinical features of noninvasive follicular thyroid neoplasm with papillary-like nuclear features versus invasive forms of follicular variant of papillary thyroid carcinoma. Cancer Cytopathol 2017;125:323–31.
76. Lloyd RV, Asa SL, LiVolsi VA, et al. The evolving diagnosis of noninvasive follicular thyroid neoplasm with papillary-like nuclear features (NIFTP). Hum Pathol 2018;74:1–4.
77. Howitt BE, Paulson VA, Barletta JA. Absence of BRAF V600E in non-infiltrative, non-invasive follicular variant of papillary thyroid carcinoma. Histopathology 2015;67:579–82.
78. Johnson DN, Sadow PM. Exploration of BRAFV600E as a diagnostic adjuvant in the non-invasive follicular thyroid neoplasm with papillary-like nuclear features (NIFTP). Hum Pathol 2018;82:32–8.
79. Pilarski R, Burt R, Kohlman W, et al. Cowden syndrome and the PTEN hamartoma tumor syndrome: systematic review and revised diagnostic criteria. J Natl Cancer Inst 2013;105:1607–16.
80. Pilarski R, Stephens JA, Noss R, et al. Predicting PTEN mutations: an evaluation of Cowden syndrome and Bannayan-Riley-Ruvalcaba syndrome clinical features. J Med Genet 2011;48:505–12.
81. Tan MH, Mester J, Peterson C, et al. A clinical scoring system for selection of patients for PTEN mutation testing is proposed on the basis of a prospective study of 3042 probands. Am J Hum Genet 2011;88:42–56.
82. Harach HR, Soubeyran I, Brown A, et al. Thyroid pathologic findings in patients with Cowden disease. Ann Diagn Pathol 1999;3:331–40.
83. Laury AR, Bongiovanni M, Tille J-C, et al. Thyroid Pathology in *PTEN*-hamartoma tumor syndrome: characteristic findings of a distinct entity. Thyroid 2011;21:135–44.
84. Pilarski R. Cowden syndrome: a critical review of the clinical literature. J Genet Couns 2009;18:13–27.
85. Ngeow J, Mester J, Rybicki LA, et al. Incidence and clinical characteristics of thyroid cancer in prospective series of individuals with Cowden and Cowden-like syndrome characterized by germline PTEN, SDH, or KLLN alterations. J Clin Endocrinol Metab 2011;96:2063–71.
86. Barletta JA, Bellizzi AM, Hornick JL. Immunohistochemical staining of thyroidectomy specimens for PTEN can aid in the identification of patients with Cowden syndrome. Am J Surg Pathol 2011;35:1505–11.

Molecular Alterations in Thyroid Carcinoma

Mohamed Rizwan Haroon Al Rasheed, MD, Bin Xu, MD, PhD*

KEYWORDS

• Thyroid carcinoma • Papillary thyroid carcinoma • Poorly differentiated thyroid carcinoma • Anaplastic thyroid carcinoma • *RAS* • *BRAF* • *TERT* promoter mutation

Key points

- ***BRAF***^{V600E} **mutation is frequent in classic and tall cell variants of papillary thyroid carcinoma.**
- **Follicular-patterned carcinoma (ie, follicular carcinoma and follicular variant of papillary thyroid carcinoma) is characterized by *RAS* mutation and *PAX8-PPAR*γ fusion.**
- **Thyroid carcinoma has stepwise molecular tumorigenesis from well-differentiated to poorly differentiated to anaplastic carcinoma in which *BRAF* and *RAS* mutations remain the main driver events.**
- ***TERT* promoter mutation, *TP53* mutation, and mutations in the PIK3CA (phosphatidylinositol-4,5-bisphosphate 3-kinase catalytic subunit alpha) pathway are associated with tumor aggressiveness and are common in poorly differentiated and anaplastic thyroid carcinoma.**
- **Novel tyrosine kinase inhibitor therapy targeting the mitogen-activated protein kinase pathway shows promising results in treating advanced thyroid carcinoma.**

ABSTRACT

Thyroid carcinoma is the most common cancer in the endocrine system. Recent advances, using next-generation sequencing, have shed light on the molecular pathogenesis of thyroid cancer. Constitutional activation of the mitogen-activated protein kinase pathway through *RAS* mutation, *BRAF* mutation, and/or fusions involving receptor tyrosine kinase (eg, (REarranged during Transfection) *RET-PTC*) plays a central role in tumorigenesis and opens doors to promising tyrosine kinase inhibitor therapy. Several molecular signatures, such as *TERT* promoter mutation and *TP53* mutation, are associated with tumor progression. This article provides a concise and updated summary of the main genetic alterations in thyroid carcinoma.

OVERVIEW

Most thyroid carcinomas can be divided into 2 broad categories based on their cell of origin: most (>95%) are of follicular cell origin, whereas the remaining 3% to 5% are medullary thyroid carcinomas (MTCs) arising from C cells. Follicular cell–derived carcinomas can be further divided into papillary thyroid carcinoma (PTC), follicular thyroid carcinoma (FTC), Hürthle cell carcinoma (HCC), poorly differentiated thyroid carcinoma (PDTC), and anaplastic thyroid carcinoma (ATC).[1] PTC, FTC, and HCC are considered well-differentiated thyroid carcinomas. PTC, the most common type of thyroid carcinoma, is composed of a heterogeneous group with more than 10

Conflicts of Interest and Sources of Funding: The authors have no significant relationships with, or financial interest in, any commercial companies pertaining to this article. Research reported in this publication was supported in part by the Cancer Center Support Grant of the National Institutes of Health/National Cancer Institute under award number P30CA008748. The content of this article is solely the responsibility of the authors and does not necessarily represent the official views of the National Institutes of Health.
Department of Pathology, Memorial Sloan Kettering Cancer Center, 1275 York Avenue, New York, NY 10065, USA
* Corresponding author.
E-mail address: xub@mskcc.org

Surgical Pathology 12 (2019) 921–930
https://doi.org/10.1016/j.path.2019.08.002
1875-9181/19/

phenotypes (ie, variants). Of them, classic variant PTC (CVPTC), follicular variant PTC (FVPTC), and papillary microcarcinoma are the most common variants.[1]

The past decade has witnessed significant progress in the understanding of the molecular pathogenesis of thyroid carcinoma, based on studies using next-generation sequencing (NGS) platforms.[2–8] In 2014, The Cancer Genome Atlas (TCGA) reported the comprehensive genomic characteristics of PTC[5]; 97% of PTCs have unique molecular alterations. This finding includes 74% with single nucleotide variants (eg, *BRAF* or *RAS* mutation), 15% with fusions, 7% with arm-level copy number alterations, and 1% with deletions. Merely 3% of PTC is characterized as dark matter; cases in which the molecular events underpinning the tumorigenesis remain to be discovered. Subsequently, the genomic characteristics of HCC, PDTC, and ATC have also been reported.[2–4] This article provides a concise summary of the molecular pathogenesis of thyroid carcinoma, focusing primarily on recent advances.

STEPWISE TUMORIGENESIS IN FOLLICULAR CELL-DERIVED THYROID CARCINOMA

EARLY MOLECULAR EVENTS: DRIVER MUTATIONS IN THE MITOGEN-ACTIVATED PROTEIN KINASE PATHWAY

The key molecular alterations in various types of thyroid carcinoma are summarized in **Table 1**. Constitutive activation of the mitogen-activated protein kinase (MAPK) signaling pathway plays a central role in the carcinogenesis of thyroid carcinoma. The essential proteins in this pathway are receptor tyrosine kinases (RTKs; including vascular endothelial growth factor receptor [VEGFR], RET, anaplastic lymphoma kinase (ALK), and neurotrophic receptor tyrosine kinase (NTRK)), RAS, Rapidly accelerated fibrosarcoma (RAF), mitogen-activated protein kinase (MEK), and extracellular signal–regulated kinase (ERK) (**Fig. 1**). RAS is a small G protein that is recruited on binding of growth factors to RTK and it, in turn, activates downstream pathways via

Table 1
Key molecular alterations in thyroid carcinoma

Tumor Types	Common Molecular Alterations	Uncommon Molecular Alterations
PTC	*BRAF* (62%), predominantly *BRAF*^{V600E} *RAS* (13%) *RET-PTC* (7%) *TERT* promoter mutation (9%)	*E1F1AX* *ALK* fusion *NTRK1* or *NTRK3* fusion
Encapsulated FVPTC and NIFTP	*RAS* (30%–52%) *PAX8-PPAR*γ (0%–38%) *THADA* fusion (0%–22%)	*BRAF*^{K601E} (3%–7%) Absence of *BRAF*^{V600E}
FTC	*RAS* (49%) *PAX8-PPAR*γ (30%–58%) *TERT* promoter mutation 17%	*TSHR* mutations *BRAF*^{K601E} *E1F1AX*
HCC	Widespread chromosomal losses Alteration of mitochondrial genome *RAS* (9%–15%) *TERT* promoter mutation (22%–27%) *TP53* mutation (7%–12%)	*CHCHD10-VPREB3* *HEPHL1-PANX1* *TMEM233-PRKAB1*
PDTC	*BRAF* 33% *RAS* 45% *TERT* promoter mutation (40%) *TP53* mutation (10%)	—
ATC	*BRAF* 29% *RAS* 23% *TERT* promoter mutation (73%) *TP53* mutation (59%)	Tumor suppressors: ATM, RB1, MEN1, NF1, and NF2 Mutation affecting PIK3CA-AKT-mTOR pathway, mismatch repair genes, SWI-SNF complex, and histone methyltransferase pathway
MTC	*RET* (40%–60%) *RAS* (up to 20%)	*MET* *ALK* fusion

Abbreviation: NIFTP, noninvasive follicular thyroid neoplasm with papillarylike nuclear features.

serine/threonine kinase BRAF. The cascade of downstream events in this pathway ultimately leads to altered cell proliferation, differentiation, and survival, resulting in various forms of thyroid carcinoma. In thyroid cancer, genetic alterations in the MAPK pathway are highly prevalent and mutually exclusive. Based on the cBioPortal data from the TCGA PTC cohort, alteration of the MAPK pathway is detected in 83% of all PTCs tested.[5,9] The common alterations are *BRAF* mutation (predominantly V600E) in 62%; *RAS* (including *HRAS*, *NRAS*, and *KRAS*) mutation in 13%; *RET-PTC* rearrangement in 6%; and, less frequently, *NTRK3* fusion in 1.5%, *NTRK1* fusion in 1.3%, and *ALK* fusion in 0.8%.

Key Points

1. Thyroid carcinoma is characterized by molecular alterations in the MAPK pathway.
2. $BRAF^{V600E}$ mutation is the most common mutation in papillary thyroid carcinoma.

GENOTYPE-PHENOTYPE CORRELATION

The TCGA study has shown that there is a strong correlation between histologic phenotypes and underlying genotypes. A review of cBioPortal TCGA data shows that the $BRAF^{V600E}$ mutation is highly prevalent in tall cell variant (TCV) and CVPTC with a frequency of 89% and 67% respectively. Meanwhile, a *RAS* mutation was detected in only 6% of CVPTCs and in none of the TCVs tested. In contrast, FVPTC has a high frequency of *RAS* mutations (38%), and infrequent $BRAF^{V600E}$ mutation (13%).[5,9] Two distinct molecular groups have emerged based on the mutation status of $BRAF^{V600E}$ and *RAS*: the $BRAF^{V600E}$-like and the RAS-like groups. The $BRAF^{V600E}$-like group, characterized by robust MAPK pathway activation, less differentiation, and dampened response to radioactive iodine (RAI), is enriched with tall cell and classic variants, whereas the RAS-like group shows activation of both MAPK and PI3K/AKT signaling pathways, is highly differentiated, and contains mostly FVPTC.[5] This genotype-phenotype correlation has been confirmed by multiple additional studies.[10–15] *PAX8-PPAR*γ rearrangement, a common

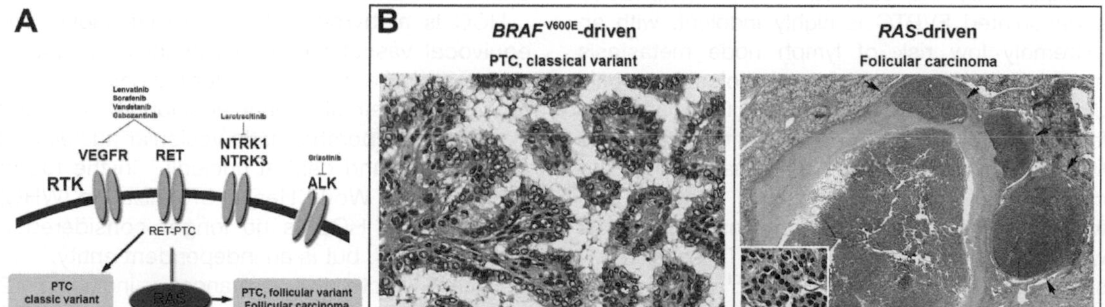

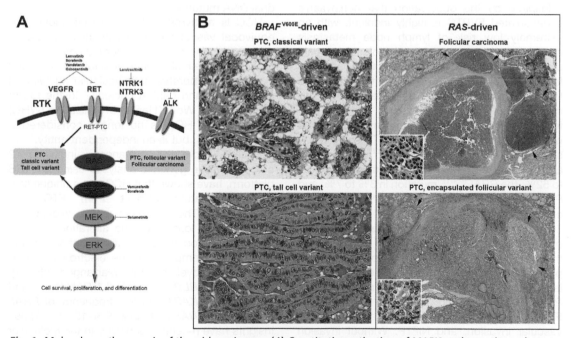

Fig. 1. Molecular pathogenesis of thyroid carcinoma. (*A*) Constitutive activation of MAPK pathway through mutations or fusions of its key components, including RTK (eg, RET, NTRK1, NTRK3, and ALK), RAS, and BRAF, plays a central role in tumorigenesis of thyroid carcinoma. Various tyrosine kinase inhibitors (eg, multiple kinase inhibitors sorafenib and lenvatinib and BRAF inhibitors vemurafenib and dabrafenib) have been investigated in treating advanced thyroid carcinoma. (*B*) There is a strong genotype-phenotype correlation, in which PTC classic variant and tall cell variant typically harbor $BRAF^{V600E}$ hotspot mutation, whereas follicular-patterned carcinomas (ie, follicular carcinoma and encapsulated follicular variant of PTC) are usually *RAS* mutated. Inserts show nuclear features of follicular carcinoma and follicular variant of PTC. Hematoxylin and eosin stain. Arrows indicate capsular invasion.

molecular event in thyroid carcinoma, is detected predominantly in follicular-patterned carcinoma, including 30% to 58% of FTC and 38% of FVPTC, whereas it is rare in CVPTC and TCV, accounting for less than 1% of all CVPTC and none of the TCV tested in the TCGA PTC cohort.[16–18] Therefore, it is now clear that TCV and CVPTCs are enriched with *BRAF*^{V600E} mutation and/or *RET-PTC* fusion, whereas the FVPTC is associated with a high frequency of *RAS* mutations and the *PAX8-PPAR*γ rearrangement, a low frequency of *BRAF*^{V600E} mutation, and a pattern of chromosomal gains/losses as well as a protein expression profile akin to FTC and follicular adenoma.

FVPTC can be further classified into infiltrative and encapsulated forms based on the absence or presence of a complete tumor capsule or well-circumscribed tumor border. The molecular profile and clinical behavior of infiltrative FVPTC resemble those of CVPTC, characterized by a 36% rate of *BRAF*^{V600E} mutation or *RET-PTC* fusion and 65% risk of nodal metastasis. Meanwhile, the encapsulated FVPTCs, especially those that show no evidence of invasion, are enriched in *RAS* mutations, lack *BRAF*^{V600E} mutations, and have a negligible risk of lymph node metastasis and recurrence.[19,20]

Inspired by the observation that noninvasive encapsulated FVPTC is highly indolent, with an extremely low risk of lymph node metastasis and/or recurrence, and has a molecular profile distinct from CVPTC, in 2016 Nikiforov and colleagues[21] revised the terminology to noninvasive follicular thyroid neoplasm with papillarylike nuclear features (NIFTP). Molecular profiling performed in a subset of the consensus cohort as well as subsequent studies on NIFTP consistently show that NIFTP lack the *BRAF*^{V600E} mutation and are instead associated with *RAS* mutations in 30% to 52%, the *BRAF*^{K601E} mutation in 3% to 7%, and *PPAR*γ and *THADA* fusions in 0% to 22% of cases.[22,23]

It is now clear that encapsulated follicular-patterned neoplasms, a group of encapsulated thyroid neoplasms with exclusive follicular growth pattern and absence of true papillae, are molecularly similar, and enriched in *RAS* mutations and *PAX8-PPAR*γ fusion. This group includes FA, FTC, encapsulated FVPTC with capsular and/or vascular invasion, and NIFTP. Without invasion (ie, FA and NIFTP), they follow a highly indolent course with negligible risk of regional spread and recurrence. With invasion (ie, FTC and encapsulated FVPTC), they have a propensity to spread distantly rather than to regional lymph nodes.

Before the birth of NIFTP, multiple studies, including a large meta-analysis of 5655 patients with PTC, showed that *BRAF* mutation is an adverse molecular signature in PTC, associated with advanced stage, high frequency of nodal metastasis, and increased risk of extrathyroidal extension and recurrence.[24,25] Because the implementation of NIFTP nomenclature exempts a proportion of *RAS*-related highly indolent tumors from a frank diagnosis of carcinoma, the prognostic significance of *BRAF* mutation in PTC needs to be reevaluated in the post-NIFTP era.

FOLLICULAR THYROID CARCINOMA

Given the preceding discussion on follicular-patterned carcinoma, it is no surprise that FTC is characterized by *RAS* point mutations and *PAX8-PPAR*γ fusion, detected in 49% and 30% to 58% of cases, respectively.[18,26–29] *TERT* (telomerase reverse transcriptase) promoter mutation has been detected in 17% of FTCs, a frequency that is higher than that seen in PTC (9%).[5,30] *TERT* promoter mutation is generally considered an aggressive molecular signature in thyroid carcinoma, and its significance is further elaborated later.

HCC is a unique thyroid cancer characterized by widespread chromosomal losses and mitochondrial DNA mutations.

HCC is a thyroid carcinoma that shows unequivocal vascular or capsular invasion and is composed of at least 75% Hürthle cells; characterized by their abundant eosinophilic granular cytoplasm, hyperchromatic/vesicular nuclei, and prominent round central nucleoli.[1] In the fourth edition of the World Health Organization (WHO) classification, HCC is no longer considered a variant of FTC, but is an independent entity.[1]

Recent molecular advances, including 2 comprehensive genomic analyses using an NGS platform, have shown that HCC has a unique molecular signature distinct from FTC and PTC.[2,3,31–33] These tumors show widespread chromosomal losses, unique alteration of mitochondrial genomes(especially mutations in the subunits of complex I in the electron transport chain), and novel recurrent rearrangements (eg, *CHCHD10-VPREB3*, *HEPHL1-PANX1*, and *TMEM233-PRKAB1*) but low frequency of *BRAF* (0%–5%) and *RAS* mutations (9%–15%).[2,3] These insights have recently been used in the molecular testing for thyroid fine-needle aspiration (FNA) to enhance its performance of these platforms in detecting HCC.[28,34] For example, Thyroseq version 3 has added a molecular group with copy number alterations. Not surprisingly, most nodules harboring copy number alterations are diagnosed as HCCs given the widespread chromosomal loss reported in these lesions.[28] Compared with PTC, which has a low frequency of *TERT* promoter mutation (9%) and *TP53* mutation (0.8%), *TERT* promoter mutation and *TP53* mutation are common in HCC, with a reported frequency of 22% to 27% and 7% to 12% respectively, suggesting that HCC has a more aggressive molecular signature compared with PTC.[2,3,5] The significance of *TERT* promoter mutation and *TP53* mutation is discussed in more detail later.

It is postulated that mitochondrial DNA mutations lead to an impaired electron transport chain and disruption of the oxidative phosphorylation system. Subsequent aberrant compensatory accumulation of mitochondria in tumor cells results in a Hürthle cell (oncocytic) phenotype histologically. It has recently been shown that oncocytic FVPTC, a tumor that shares the oncocytic cytomorphology, also commonly harbors nonsilent mitochondrial DNA mutations.[23]

Key Points

1. HCC is enriched with mitochondrial DNA mutations, which lead to aberrant mitochondria accumulation and Hürthle cell phenotype.
2. HCC shows widespread chromosomal losses.
3. HCC has low frequency of *BRAF* and *RAS* mutations.

TUMOR PROGRESSION AND DEDIFFERENTIATION: LATE MOLECULAR EVENTS OCCURRING IN POORLY DIFFERENTIATED THYROID CARCINOMA AND ANAPLASTIC THYROID CARCINOMA

Compared with well-differentiated thyroid carcinoma, PDTC and ATC are associated with a dismal clinic outcome. ATC, in particular, is nearly always fatal, with a median survival of 3–6 months after diagnosis.[1] The mortality for well-differentiated thyroid carcinoma, PDTC, and ATC is 3% to 10%, 38% to 57%, and approximately 100% respectively.[35–37] Considerable efforts have been undertaken in recent years to understand the molecular events that may predict tumor aggressiveness and may serve as treatment targets in advanced thyroid cancer.[6–8,38]

Similar to their well-differentiated counterparts, *BRAF* and *RAS* mutations remain the main drivers in PDTC and ATC, occurring in 33% and 45% of PDTC, and 29% and 23% of ATC, respectively.[4,6–8,39] The frequency of *BRAF* and *RAS* mutations in PDTC varies according to the definition of PDTC. When PDTCs are defined using the Turin proposal encompassing the following 3 criteria: (1) solid growth pattern; (2) absence of nuclear features of PTC; and (3) necrosis, mitotic index greater than or equal to 3 out of 10 high power fields (HPFs), or convoluted nuclei, they contain a high frequency (42%–64%) of *RAS* mutations and rare (6%–9%) *BRAF*^{V600E} mutations.[39,40] In contrast, when PDTCs are classified based solely on necrosis or a mitotic index of greater than or equal to 5 out of 10 HPFs regardless of architectural pattern and nuclear features (Memorial Sloan Kettering Cancer Center [MSKCC] criteria), they contain both tumors fulfilling Turin proposal and an additional set of tumors that fulfill MSKCC but not the Turin proposal. This subset of tumors has high frequency (67%–78%) of *BRAF* mutations and low rate (6%–13%) of *RAS* mutations.[39,40]

TERT promoter mutations, which activate telomerase and contribute to tumorigenesis, are detected at a low frequency in well-differentiated thyroid carcinoma: 10% of PTC, 17% of FTC, and 22% to 27% HCC.[30,41–45] In contrast, PDTC and ATC are characterized by high rates of *TERT* promoter mutation, occurring in 40% and 73%, respectively.[46] Furthermore, *TERT* promoter mutations are subclonal in PTC and clonal in PDTC and ATC, indicating that they are a vital event in tumor progression and evolution. In PTC, *TERT* promoter mutations seem to be an adverse prognostic factor associated with aggressive histology (TCV), high tumor stage, regional and distant metastases, and increased mortality.[25,41–45]

Inactivating *TP53* mutations, a genetic hallmark of ATC,[47] are infrequent in well-differentiated thyroid carcinoma, being detected in merely 0.8% of PTC in the TCGA cohort.[5] In contrast, they are highly prevalent in ATC, detected in up to 73% of tested ATC.[4,6–8,39] Similarly, *TP53* mutation also distinguishes ATC from PDTC, which has a lower frequency (10%) of *TP53* mutation. PDTC and ATC also have mutations in other tumor suppressor genes, such as *ATM*, *RB1*, *MEN1*, *NF1*, and *NF2* at a rate of 0% to 9%.[4]

In addition, mutations encoding components of PIK3CA (phosphatidylinositol-4,5-bisphosphate 3-kinase catalytic subunit alpha)-AKT (protein kinase B)-mTOR (mammalian target of rapamycin) pathway, SWI/SNF (switch/sucrose nonfermentable) nucleosome remodeling complex, mismatch repair genes, and histone methyltransferase are exceedingly rare in PTC but occur in 2% to 11% of PDTCs and 12% to 39% of ATCs.[4,39]

A recent study has identified a distinct subgroup of ATC with mutation in mismatch repair genes but with intact *BRAF*, *RAS*, and *RET* oncogenes.[29] Such findings indicate that a subset of ATC may arise through *BRAF/RAS*-independent mechanisms; for example, microsatellite instability.

In summary, the persistence of *BRAF* and *RAS* mutations throughout thyroid cancer development and the acquisition of additional mutations in PDTC and ATC indicate a stepwise tumor progression from well-differentiated carcinoma to PDTC and ATC in most PDTC and ATC. *BRAF* and *RAS* mutations are the driver mutations that occur early in the tumorigenesis and are present at a comparable rate throughout tumor progression, whereas mutations in *TERT* promoter, *TP53*, *PIK3CA*, SWI/SNF complex, mismatch repair genes, and histone methyltransferase pathway accumulate in the process of dedifferentiation and tumor progression, leading to the development of PDTC and ATC.[4,6–8,39]

GENETICS OF MEDULLARY THYROID CARCINOMA: THE *RET* PROTO-ONCOGENE

MTC is a neuroendocrine carcinoma originating from C cells.[5] Approximately 75% of MTCs are sporadic, whereas the remaining 25% arise in the setting of multiple endocrine neoplasm (MEN) type 2 with germline gain-of-function mutations in *RET*.[5,48] Three subtypes of MEN2 have been recognized by the WHO: MEN2A, MEN2B, and familial MTC.[5] The involved *RET* codons in each subtype are different; in MEN2A, C634R on codon 634 in exon 11 is most commonly altered, affecting approximately 85% of patients with MEN2A,[5,48,49] whereas patients with MEN2B have unique germline M918T and A883F mutations.[5,48,49]

RET point mutation is also the most common driver molecular event in sporadic MTCs, reported in 40% to 60% of cases.[5,48,49] A small percentage of sporadic MTCs may have a *RAS* mutation[49,50] or *ALK* fusion.[49]

NOVEL TARGETED THERAPIES IN THYROID CARCINOMA: TARGETING THE MITOGEN-ACTIVATED PROTEIN KINASE PATHWAY

The growing knowledge of MAPK alterations in thyroid carcinoma has led to multiple clinical trials of tyrosine kinase inhibitors (TKIs), with the ability to block the MAPK pathway, for the treatment of advanced thyroid cancer (see **Fig. 1**; **Table 2**). The presence of unique molecular alterations may drive decisions related to targeted therapy for advanced or metastatic thyroid carcinoma.[51,52] Recently, 4 multitargeted TKIs have been approved by the Food and Drug Administration (FDA): sorafenib and lenvatinib for RAI-refractory differentiated thyroid carcinoma, and cabozantinib and vandetanib for MTC based on results of phase III clinical trials.[53–55] **Table 2** provides a brief summary of selective TKIs in thyroid carcinoma. Lenvatinib targets VEGFR, FGFR, PDGFR, RET, and C-KIT; sorafenib has its effects on VEGFR, RET, and RAF; cabozantinib inhibits MET, VGEFR, and RET.[53–55] Vemurafenib and dabrafenib, 2 selective BRAF inhibitors, can restore RAI uptakes and efficacy, showing a partial response in 38% of patients with metastatic or unresectable RAI-resistant *BRAF*^{V600E}-mutated PTC.[56–58] Similarly, selumetinib, an inhibitor for MEK1/2, has also been shown to reverse the RAI refractoriness in metastatic thyroid carcinoma.[59] In response to these promising results of targeted therapy, the National Comprehensive Cancer Network (NCCN) guidelines have recently recommended molecular testing in patients with advanced thyroid carcinoma to identify actionable targets and to select patients that are eligible for clinical trials.[51]

Table 2
Molecular therapeutic targets in advanced thyroid carcinoma: selective tyrosine kinase inhibitors and their effects in thyroid carcinoma

Drugs	Targets	Cancers Treated
Sorafenib[53]	VEGFR, PDGFR, RET/PTC, BRAF, C-KIT	RAI-refractory DTC, ATC MTC
Lenvatinib[53]	VEGFR, PDGFR, FGFR, RET/PTC, C-KIT	RAI-refractory DTC ATC MTC
Cabozantinib[54]	VEGFR, RET, MET	MTC
Vandetanib[55]	VEGFR, EGFR, RET	MTC
Vemurafenib[56]	BRAF	RAI-refractory *BRAF*^{V600E}-mutated PTC
Debrafenib[58]	BRAF	RAI-refractory *BRAF*^{V600E}-mutated PTC
Selumetinib[59]	MEK1, MEK2	RAI-refractory DTC

Abbreviation: DTC, differentiated thyroid carcinoma.

TECHNIQUES

In the past decade, several ancillary molecular techniques have been developed to improve the diagnostic accuracy of thyroid FNA and are commercially available in the United States.[60] A brief summary of these platforms is provided in **Table 3**. According to the second edition of The Bethesda System for Reporting Thyroid Cytopathology, the current American Thyroid Association (ATA) guidelines, and the current NCCN guidelines, these molecular platforms may be considered as possible ancillary tests following thyroid FNA to further stratify the risk of malignancy in cases with indeterminate cytology, which in turn comprises 2 categories: atypia of undetermined significance (Bethesda category III), and follicular neoplasm/suspicious for follicular neoplasm (Bethesda category IV).[51,52,60,61]

Thyroseq version 3 is an NGS panel that detects mutations, fusions, copy number alterations, and gene expressions of 112 thyroid cancer–related genes, including commonly altered genes such as *BRAF*, *RAS*, and *RET-PTC*. In a multicenter prospective study of 257 FNA samples with an indeterminate diagnosis, it showed a high negative predictive value (NPV) of 97% and reasonable positive predictive value (PPV) of 68%.[28] ThyGenX/ThyraMIR is a combined stepwise platform. All samples are initially subjected to ThyGenX, an NGS mutation panel, and those with negative ThyGenX results then undergo ThyraMIR, a microRNA classifier.[34,62] Afirma gene expression classifier is a microarray assay of messenger RNA expression,[34,60,62] whereas RosettaGX is a microRNA classifier.[34,62] Tests with high NPVs (Afirma, ThyGenX/ThyraMIR, and RosettaGX) are considered rule-out tests, meaning a negative test result can be used to rule out a malignant diagnosis. In contrast, tests with a high PPV (Thyroseq version 3 and ThyGenX/ThyraMIR) are rule-in tests, meaning a positive result is associated with a high probability of malignant diagnosis, with the risk of malignancy depending on the mutation that is detected. These molecular testing platforms have been shown to reduce diagnostic uncertainty and assist clinical decision making in managing indeterminate thyroid nodules.

These molecular results should be interpreted in their appropriate context. First, the calculation of sensitivity, specificity, NPV, and PPV of the platforms mentioned earlier include NIFTP as one of the positive diagnoses. Because NIFTP has recently been reclassified as a nonmalignant tumor,[21] the sensitivity and PPV would decrease if NIFTP is removed from the calculation.[63–66] Second, detection of a molecular alteration using the Thyroseq platform or a suspicious result using the Afirma platform does not warrant a total thyroidectomy. The reported malignant rate of an RAS-mutated nodule detected by Thyroseq varies from as low as 10% to 62%.[28,67] Similarly, most thyroid nodules with indeterminate cytology and suspicious Afirma results have a surgical diagnosis of benign nodules or NIFTP.[68] Hence, a conservative surgical approach, such as lobectomy or hemithyroidectomy, may be more appropriate as the initial management for these patients. In addition, the PPV of these platforms can vary significantly based on characteristics of the population and incidence of thyroid cancer.[67] Therefore, it may

Table 3
Common commercially available molecular testing platforms for thyroid fine-needle aspiration

Platforms	Testing Methods	PPV (%)[a]	NPV (%)	Rule-in Test	Rule-out Test
Thyroseq genomic classifier version 3[28]	NGS platform of 112 genes: mutations, fusions, copy number alterations and gene expression	66	97	Yes	Yes
Afirma gene expression classifier[34,60,62]	Microarray essay of mRNA expression of 142 genes	42	93–97	No	Yes
ThyGenX/ThyraMIR[34,62]	Combined test of NGS mutation detection and miRNA classifier	74–82	92–94	Yes	Yes
RosettaGX[34,62]	miRNA classifier	42	92	No	Yes

Abbreviations: miRNA, microRNA; mRNA, messenger RNA; NPV, negative predictive value; PPV, positive predictive value.
[a] The PPV is calculated using a surgical diagnosis of carcinoma or NIFTP.

be prudent to determine the PPV of these platform at the institutional level.

SUMMARY

This article summarizes the recent genomic advances, prognostic molecular signatures, promising targeted therapies, and commercially available molecular platforms in thyroid carcinoma. Constitutive activation of the MAPK pathway is crucial for the pathogenesis and targeted therapy for thyroid cancer. A strong genotype-phenotype correlation exists in follicular cell–derived carcinoma. *RAS* mutations are commonly seen in follicular-patterned carcinoma, whereas the $BRAF^{V600E}$ mutation is the most prevalent event in classic and TCVs PTC.

REFERENCES

1. Lloyd RV, Osamura RY, Kloppel G, et al. WHO classification of tumours of endocrine organs. Lyon (France): International Agency for Research on Cancer (IARC); 2017.
2. Gopal RK, Kubler K, Calvo SE, et al. Widespread chromosomal losses and mitochondrial DNA alterations as genetic drivers in hurthle cell carcinoma. Cancer Cell 2018;34(2):242–55.e5.
3. Ganly I, Makarov V, Deraje S, et al. Integrated genomic analysis of hurthle cell cancer reveals oncogenic drivers, recurrent mitochondrial mutations, and unique chromosomal landscapes. Cancer Cell 2018;34(2):256–70.e5.
4. Landa I, Ibrahimpasic T, Boucai L, et al. Genomic and transcriptomic hallmarks of poorly differentiated and anaplastic thyroid cancers. J Clin Invest 2016; 126(3):1052–66.
5. Cancer Genome Atlas Research N. Integrated genomic characterization of papillary thyroid carcinoma. Cell 2014;159(3):676–90.
6. Jeon M, Chun SM, Kim D, et al. Genomic alterations of anaplastic thyroid carcinoma detected by targeted massive parallel sequencing in a BRAFV600E mutation-prevalent area. Thyroid 2016;26(5):683–90.
7. Sykorova V, Dvorakova S, Vcelak J, et al. Search for new genetic biomarkers in poorly differentiated and anaplastic thyroid carcinomas using next generation sequencing. Anticancer Res 2015;35(4):2029–36.
8. Kunstman JW, Juhlin CC, Goh G, et al. Characterization of the mutational landscape of anaplastic thyroid cancer via whole-exome sequencing. Hum Mol Genet 2015;24(8):2318–29.
9. Gao J, Aksoy BA, Dogrusoz U, et al. Integrative analysis of complex cancer genomics and clinical profiles using the cBioPortal. Sci Signal 2013; 6(269):pl1.
10. Viglietto G, Chiappetta G, Martinez-Tello FJ, et al. RET/PTC oncogene activation is an early event in thyroid carcinogenesis. Oncogene 1995;11(6): 1207–10.
11. Cohen Y, Xing M, Mambo E, et al. BRAF mutation in papillary thyroid carcinoma. J Natl Cancer Inst 2003; 95(8):625–7.
12. Kimura ET, Nikiforova MN, Zhu Z, et al. High prevalence of BRAF mutations in thyroid cancer: genetic evidence for constitutive activation of the RET/PTC-RAS-BRAF signaling pathway in papillary thyroid carcinoma. Cancer Res 2003;63(7):1454–7.
13. Yip L, Nikiforova MN, Yoo JY, et al. Tumor genotype determines phenotype and disease-related outcomes in thyroid cancer: a study of 1510 patients. Ann Surg 2015;262(3):519–25, [discussion: 524–5].
14. Rivera M, Ricarte-Filho J, Knauf J, et al. Molecular genotyping of papillary thyroid carcinoma follicular variant according to its histological subtypes (encapsulated vs infiltrative) reveals distinct BRAF and RAS mutation patterns. Mod Pathol 2010; 23(9):1191–200.
15. Howitt BE, Jia Y, Sholl LM, et al. Molecular alterations in partially-encapsulated or well-circumscribed follicular variant of papillary thyroid carcinoma. Thyroid 2013;23(10):1256–62.
16. Armstrong MJ, Yang H, Yip L, et al. PAX8/PPAR-gamma rearrangement in thyroid nodules predicts follicular-pattern carcinomas, in particular the encapsulated follicular variant of papillary carcinoma. Thyroid 2014;24(9):1369–74.
17. D'Cruz AK, Vaish R, Vaidya A, et al. Molecular markers in well-differentiated thyroid cancer. Eur Arch Otorhinolaryngol 2018;275(6):1375–84.
18. Acquaviva G, Visani M, Repaci A, et al. Molecular pathology of thyroid tumours of follicular cells: a review of genetic alterations and their clinicopathological relevance. Histopathology 2018;72(1):6–31.
19. Liu J, Singh B, Tallini G, et al. Follicular variant of papillary thyroid carcinoma: a clinicopathologic study of a problematic entity. Cancer 2006;107(6): 1255–64.
20. Zhu Z, Gandhi M, Nikiforova MN, et al. Molecular profile and clinical-pathologic features of the follicular variant of papillary thyroid carcinoma. An unusually high prevalence of ras mutations. Am J Clin Pathol 2003;120(1):71–7.
21. Nikiforov YE, Seethala RR, Tallini G, et al. Nomenclature revision for encapsulated follicular variant of papillary thyroid carcinoma: a paradigm shift to reduce overtreatment of indolent tumors. JAMA Oncol 2016;2(8):1023–9.
22. Johnson DN, Furtado LV, Long BC, et al. Noninvasive follicular thyroid neoplasms with papillary-like nuclear features are genetically and biologically similar to adenomatous nodules and distinct from

papillary thyroid carcinomas with extensive follicular growth. Arch Pathol Lab Med 2018;142(7):838–50.
23. Xu B, Reznik E, Tuttle RM, et al. Outcome and molecular characteristics of non-invasive encapsulated follicular variant of papillary thyroid carcinoma with oncocytic features. Endocrine 2019; 64(1):97–108.
24. Kim TH, Park YJ, Lim JA, et al. The association of the BRAF(V600E) mutation with prognostic factors and poor clinical outcome in papillary thyroid cancer: a meta-analysis. Cancer 2012;118(7):1764–73.
25. Vuong HG, Duong UN, Altibi AM, et al. A meta-analysis of prognostic roles of molecular markers in papillary thyroid carcinoma. Endocr Connect 2017; 6(3):R8–17.
26. Nikiforova MN, Lynch RA, Biddinger PW, et al. RAS point mutations and PAX8-PPAR gamma rearrangement in thyroid tumors: evidence for distinct molecular pathways in thyroid follicular carcinoma. J Clin Endocrinol Metab 2003;88(5):2318–26.
27. Nikiforova MN, Biddinger PW, Caudill CM, et al. PAX8-PPARgamma rearrangement in thyroid tumors: RT-PCR and immunohistochemical analyses. The Am J Surg Pathol 2002;26(8):1016–23.
28. Steward DL, Carty SE, Sippel RS, et al. Performance of a multigene genomic classifier in thyroid nodules with indeterminate cytology: a prospective blinded multicenter study. JAMA Oncol 2018;5(2):204–12.
29. Pozdeyev N, Gay LM, Sokol ES, et al. Genetic analysis of 779 advanced differentiated and anaplastic thyroid cancers. Clin Cancer Res 2018;24(13): 3059–68.
30. Liu R, Xing M. TERT promoter mutations in thyroid cancer. Endocr Relat cancer 2016;23(3):R143–55.
31. Tallini G, Hsueh A, Liu S, et al. Frequent chromosomal DNA unbalance in thyroid oncocytic (Hurthle cell) neoplasms detected by comparative genomic hybridization. Lab Invest 1999;79(5):547–55.
32. Dettori T, Frau DV, Lai ML, et al. Aneuploidy in oncocytic lesions of the thyroid gland: diffuse accumulation of mitochondria within the cell is associated with trisomy 7 and progressive numerical chromosomal alterations. Genes Chromosomes Cancer 2003; 38(1):22–31.
33. Ganly I, Ricarte Filho J, Eng S, et al. Genomic dissection of Hurthle cell carcinoma reveals a unique class of thyroid malignancy. J Clin Endocrinol Metab 2013;98(5):E962–72.
34. Rossi ED, Larocca LM, Pantanowitz L. Ancillary molecular testing of indeterminate thyroid nodules. Cancer Cytopathol 2018;126(Suppl 8):654–71.
35. Siegel R, Ma J, Zou Z, et al. Cancer statistics, 2014. CA Cancer J Clin 2014;64(1):9–29.
36. Hiltzik D, Carlson DL, Tuttle RM, et al. Poorly differentiated thyroid carcinomas defined on the basis of mitosis and necrosis: a clinicopathologic study of 58 patients. Cancer 2006;106(6):1286–95.
37. Volante M, Collini P, Nikiforov YE, et al. Poorly differentiated thyroid carcinoma: the Turin proposal for the use of uniform diagnostic criteria and an algorithmic diagnostic approach. Am J Surg Pathol 2007;31(8):1256–64.
38. Chen H, Luthra R, Routbort MJ, et al. Molecular profile of advanced thyroid carcinomas by next-generation sequencing: characterizing tumors beyond diagnosis for targeted therapy. Mol Cancer Ther 2018;17(7):1575–84.
39. Xu B, Ghossein R. Genomic landscape of poorly differentiated and anaplastic thyroid carcinoma. Endocr Pathol 2016;27(3):205–12.
40. Ibrahimpasic T, Xu B, Landa I, et al. Genomic alterations in fatal forms of non-anaplastic thyroid cancer: identification of MED12 and RBM10 as novel thyroid cancer genes associated with tumor virulence. Clin Cancer Res 2017;23(19):5970–80.
41. Melo M, da Rocha AG, Vinagre J, et al. TERT promoter mutations are a major indicator of poor outcome in differentiated thyroid carcinomas. J Clin Endocrinol Metab 2014;99(5):E754–65.
42. De-Tao Y, Kun Y, Run-Qing L, et al. Clinicopathological significance of TERT promoter mutation in papillary thyroid carcinomas: a systematic review and meta-analysis. Clin Endocrinol (Oxf). 2016;85(2): 299–305.
43. Song YS, Lim JA, Choi H, et al. Prognostic effects of TERT promoter mutations are enhanced by coexistence with BRAF or RAS mutations and strengthen the risk prediction by the ATA or TNM staging system in differentiated thyroid cancer patients. Cancer Endocrinol (Oxf) 2016;85(2):299–305.
44. Xing M, Liu R, Liu X, et al. BRAF V600E and TERT promoter mutations cooperatively identify the most aggressive papillary thyroid cancer with highest recurrence. J Clin Oncol 2014;32(25):2718–26.
45. Liu X, Bishop J, Shan Y, et al. Highly prevalent TERT promoter mutations in aggressive thyroid cancers. Endocr Relat Cancer 2013;20(4):603–10.
46. Landa I, Ganly I, Chan TA, et al. Frequent somatic TERT promoter mutations in thyroid cancer: higher prevalence in advanced forms of the disease. J Clin Endocrinol Metab 2013;98(9):E1562–6.
47. Fagin JA, Matsuo K, Karmakar A, et al. High prevalence of mutations of the p53 gene in poorly differentiated human thyroid carcinomas. J Clin Invest 1993; 91(1):179–84.
48. Accardo G, Conzo G, Esposito D, et al. Genetics of medullary thyroid cancer: An overview. Int J Surg 2017;41(Suppl 1):S2–6.
49. Ji JH, Oh YL, Hong M, et al. Identification of driving ALK fusion genes and genomic landscape of medullary thyroid cancer. PLoS Genet 2015;11(8): e1005467.
50. Vuong HG, Odate T, Ngo HTT, et al. Clinical significance of RET and RAS mutations in sporadic

medullary thyroid carcinoma: a meta-analysis. Endocrine-related cancer 2018;25(6):633–41.
51. Haddad RI, Nasr C, Bischoff L, et al. NCCN guidelines insights: thyroid carcinoma, version 2.2018. J Natl Compr Cancer Netw 2018;16(12):1429–40.
52. Haugen BRM, Alexander EK, Bible KC, et al. 2015 American Thyroid Association Management Guidelines for adult patients with thyroid nodules and differentiated thyroid cancer. Thyroid 2016;26: 1–133.
53. Lorusso L, Pieruzzi L, Biagini A, et al. Lenvatinib and other tyrosine kinase inhibitors for the treatment of radioiodine refractory, advanced, and progressive thyroid cancer. OncoTargets Ther 2016;9:6467–77.
54. Elisei R, Schlumberger MJ, Muller SP, et al. Cabozantinib in progressive medullary thyroid cancer. J Clin Oncol 2013;31(29):3639–46.
55. Trimboli P, Castellana M, Virili C, et al. Efficacy of vandetanib in treating locally advanced or metastatic medullary thyroid carcinoma according to RECIST criteria: a systematic review and meta-analysis. Front Endocrinol (Lausanne) 2018;9:224.
56. Brose MS, Cabanillas ME, Cohen EE, et al. Vemurafenib in patients with BRAF(V600E)-positive metastatic or unresectable papillary thyroid cancer refractory to radioactive iodine: a non-randomised, multicentre, open-label, phase 2 trial. Lancet Oncol 2016;17(9):1272–82.
57. Dunn LA, Sherman EJ, Baxi SS, et al. Vemurafenib redifferentiation of BRAF mutant, RAI-refractory thyroid cancers. J Clin Endocrinol Metab 2018;104(5): 1417–28.
58. Rothenberg SM, McFadden DG, Palmer EL, et al. Redifferentiation of iodine-refractory BRAF V600E-mutant metastatic papillary thyroid cancer with dabrafenib. Clin Cancer Res 2015;21(5):1028–35.
59. Ho AL, Grewal RK, Leboeuf R, et al. Selumetinib-enhanced radioiodine uptake in advanced thyroid cancer. N Engl J Med 2013;368(7):623–32.
60. Ferris RL, Baloch Z, Bernet V, et al. American Thyroid Association Statement on surgical application of molecular profiling for thyroid nodules: current impact on perioperative decision making. Thyroid 2015;25(7):760–8.
61. Ali SZ, Cibas ES. The Bethesda system for reporting thyroid Cytopathology: definitions, criteria, and explanatory notes. 2nd edition. Cham (Switzerland): Springer International; 2018.
62. Zhang M, Lin O. Molecular testing of thyroid nodules: a review of current available tests for fine-needle aspiration specimens. Arch Pathol Lab Med 2016;140(12):1338–44.
63. Lloyd RV, Asa SL, LiVolsi VA, et al. The evolving diagnosis of noninvasive follicular thyroid neoplasm with papillary-like nuclear features (NIFTP). Hum Pathol 2018;74:1–4.
64. Hung YP, Barletta JA. A user's guide to non-invasive follicular thyroid neoplasm with papillary-like nuclear features (NIFTP). Histopathology 2018;72(1):53–69.
65. Krane JF, Alexander EK, Cibas ES, et al. Coming to terms with NIFTP: a provisional approach for cytologists. Cancer 2016;124(11):767–72.
66. Strickland KC, Howitt BE, Barletta JA, et al. Suggesting the cytologic diagnosis of noninvasive follicular thyroid neoplasm with papillary-like nuclear features (NIFTP): a retrospective analysis of atypical and suspicious nodules. Cancer Cytopathol 2018;126(2): 86–93.
67. Marcadis AR, Valderrabano P, Ho AS, et al. Interinstitutional variation in predictive value of the ThyroSeq v2 genomic classifier for cytologically indeterminate thyroid nodules. Surgery 2019; 165(1):17–24.
68. Wong KS, Angell TE, Strickland KC, et al. Noninvasive follicular variant of papillary thyroid carcinoma and the afirma gene-expression classifier. Thyroid 2016;26(7):911–5.

Treatment of Differentiated Thyroid Carcinomas

Melissa G. Lechner, MD, PhD[a],
Stephanie Smooke Praw, MD[b], Trevor E. Angell, MD[c,*]

KEYWORDS

• Differentiated thyroid cancer • Dynamic risk stratification • Treatment • Active surveillance
• Surgery • Radioactive iodine • Tyrosine kinase inhibitor • BRAF

Key points

- Differentiated thyroid cancer is the most common endocrine malignancy, and its growing incidence and generally indolent course demand a careful approach to treatment.
- Initial management typically involves surgical resection of the primary tumor and regional lymph node metastases, but active surveillance may be considered in appropriately selected low-risk patients.
- After surgery, further management is guided predominantly by surgical pathology, which informs staging and risk of future disease recurrence, and thus guides the decision to perform further treatment.
- New therapies for progressive radioactive iodine–refractory metastatic differentiated thyroid cancer have emerged and are revolutionizing the approach to such patients.

ABSTRACT

Differentiated thyroid cancer (DTC) is the most common thyroid cancer and is frequently encountered in clinical practice. The incidence of DTC has increased significantly over the past three decades. Surgical resection, radioactive iodine (RAI), and levothyroxine suppression therapy remain the primary modalities for DTC treatment. Active surveillance for low-risk thyroid cancer may be an alternative to immediate surgery for appropriately selected patients. Patient characteristics influence treatment selection and intensity. In the subset of patients with progressive distant metastatic disease, not amenable to treatment with surgery or RAI, novel agents, including targeted therapies and immunotherapy, should be considered.

BACKGROUND

Thyroid cancer is the most common endocrine malignancy, accounting for 3.1% of all new cancers, and there were more than 750,000 people living with thyroid cancer in 2018 in the United States.[1] In the general population, the peak occurrence is between ages 51 and 60 years.[2] Thyroid cancer is more common in women and in those with radiation exposure or a family history of thyroid cancer.[1]

Disclosure: The authors have nothing to disclose.
[a] Division of Endocrinology, Diabetes, and Metabolism, David Geffen School of Medicine, University of California Los Angeles, 10833 Le Conte Avenue, CHS 57-145, Los Angeles, CA 90095, USA; [b] Division of Endocrinology, Diabetes, and Metabolism, David Geffen School of Medicine, University of California, Los Angeles, 10833 Le Conte Avenue, CHS 57-145, Los Angeles, CA 90095, USA; [c] Division of Endocrinology, Diabetes, and Metabolism, Keck School of Medicine, University of Southern California, 1333 San Pablo Avenue, BMT-B11, Los Angeles, CA 90033, USA
* Corresponding author.
E-mail address: Trevor.angell@med.usc.edu

Surgical Pathology 12 (2019) 931–942
https://doi.org/10.1016/j.path.2019.08.003

Most thyroid malignancies are well-differentiated thyroid follicular cell–derived cancers (differentiated thyroid cancer [DTC]), subdivided into several histopathologic types: papillary thyroid carcinoma (PTC, 80%–85% of cases), follicular thyroid carcinoma (FTC, 10%–15% of cases), and Hürthle cell carcinoma (HCC, 5% of cases). This article reviews DTC and does not cover other less common subtypes of thyroid cancer, such as medullary thyroid cancer, anaplastic thyroid cancer, or thyroid lymphoma.

The incidence of DTC has tripled over the past three decades, predominantly attributable to the increased diagnosis of small (<2 cm), indolent PTCs.[3,4] The observed increase seems related to the increased detection of subclinical cancers by the growing use of diagnostic imaging, such as ultrasonography, computed tomography (CT), magnetic resonance (MR), or positron emission tomography [PET] studies, and fine-needle aspiration biopsy (FNAB).[5,6] Some data suggest that there also may be a true increase in new cancers, perhaps caused by environmental factors, aging populations, and increasing obesity rates.[3,4,7,8]

DTC is most commonly detected as a thyroid nodule incidentally found on imaging, whereas some patients present with a palpable neck mass, or, rarely, with compressive neck symptoms or voice changes. A diagnosis of malignancy is usually made by FNAB of a thyroid nodule. Cytology specimens collected by FNAB are classified by the Bethesda System for Reporting Thyroid Cytopathology[9] across 6 categories to stratify the risk of malignancy and guide decisions about continued clinical observation or treatment with surgical resection.[9] Those categories (along with corresponding estimate of cancer risk) are (I) nondiagnostic or unsatisfactory (5%–10%); (II) benign (0%–3%); (III) atypia of undetermined significance or follicular lesion of undetermined significance (AUS/FLUS) (6%–30%); (IV) follicular neoplasm or suspicious for a follicular neoplasm (10%–40%); (V) suspicious for malignancy (45%–75%); and (VI) malignant (94%–99%).[9]

In the so-called indeterminate categories, particularly Bethesda categories III and IV, the diagnosis or exclusion of cancer preoperatively is more challenging and often requires additional studies. In some cases, diagnostic lobectomy is required to obtain histopathology confirmation of the diagnosis. More recently, improved cancer risk stratification before surgery has been facilitated by molecular diagnostic tests performed on preserved FNAB material. Commercially available molecular tests use different strategies, including detection of high-risk cancer variants and fusions (ThyroSeq, University of Pittsburgh Medical Center and CBL PATH, Pittsburgh, PA), messenger RNA expression classification (Genomic Sequencing Classifier, Veracyte, San Francisco, CA), and combined analysis of genetic variants/fusions and microRNA expression (ThyGeNEXT + ThyraMIR, Interpace Diagnostics, Parsippany, NJ).[10–12] A current limitation to such molecular tests for thyroid nodule diagnosis is that only a few mutations (eg, v-raf murine sarcoma viral oncogene homolog B [BRAF]V600E, rearranged during transfection [RET]/PTC fusions) are specific for malignancy, and most genomic alterations associated with DTC are also seen in some benign lesions. Therefore, although high sensitivity and negative predictive values of 94% to 97% have been reported for the best-studied molecular tests (ThyroSeq and Afirma), the specificity and positive predictive values for these assays are only moderate (47% and 66%, respectively).[10,11] The predictive values of these tests are also influenced by the institution-specific true prevalence of malignancy within Bethesda III to IV nodules. As molecular testing continues to evolve, clinicians and patients will have additional tools to aid in diagnosis and treatment decisions for indeterminate nodules.

MANAGEMENT OF DIFFERENTIATED THYROID CANCER

Treatment outcomes for DTC are generally excellent, with 98% disease-specific survival at 10 years and variable rates of recurrence depending on disease characteristics.[13,14] A general approach to the management of DTC is presented in **Fig. 1**. The cornerstone of therapy is a combination of surgery, with or without radioactive iodine (RAI) therapy, and levothyroxine (LT4)-induced suppression of thyroid-stimulating hormone (TSH). Serum thyroglobulin (Tg) trends and postoperative neck ultrasonography imaging are used to monitor patients over time. Patients with progressive or metastatic disease may benefit from additional surgery, RAI, local therapies (eg, external beam radiation), or systemic therapies. Historically, effective systemic therapy for unresectable or distantly metastatic disease was lacking, but recently targeted small molecule inhibitors and immunotherapy have changed the approach to such patients.

SURGICAL TREATMENT

Surgery is almost universally the initial treatment of DTC. Usual management includes lobectomy or total thyroidectomy and resection of lymph node metastases identified preoperatively or found to

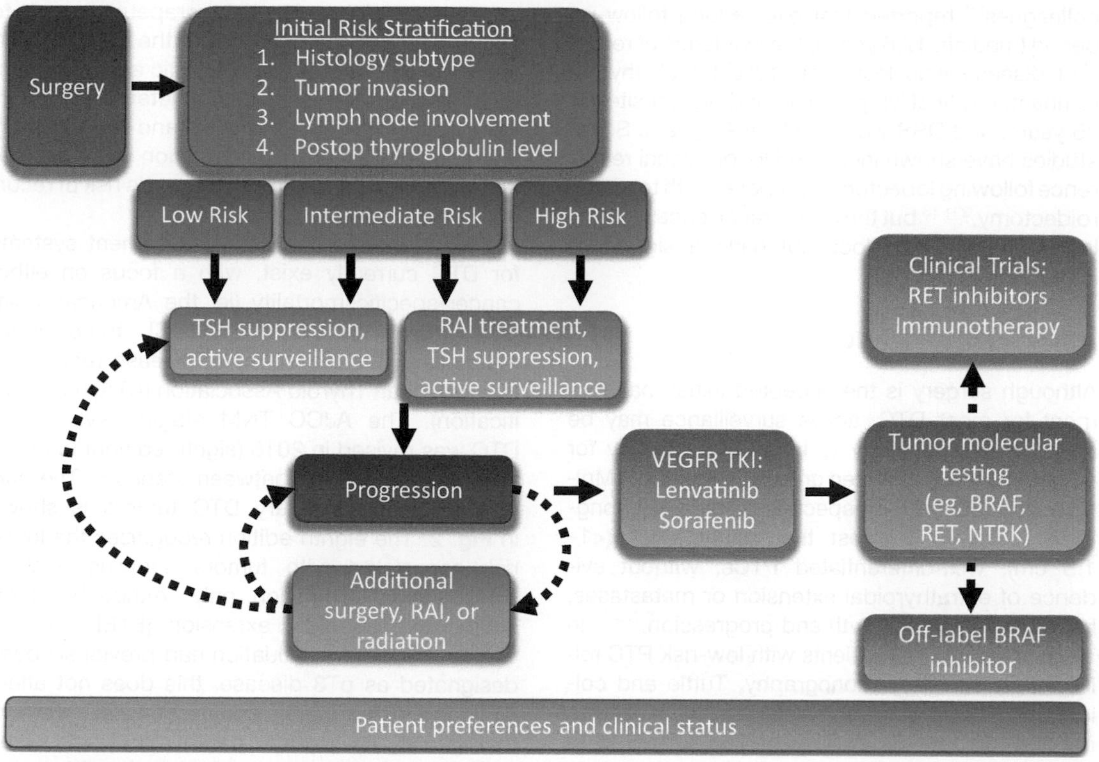

Fig. 1. General approach to the treatment of differentiated thyroid cancer. Following surgery, treatment with radioactive iodine (RAI) therapy and levothyroxine-induced suppression of thyroid-stimulating hormone (TSH) is determined by initial risk stratification. For progressive disease, additional surgery, local therapies, RAI, or systemic therapies may be considered. NTRK, neurotrophic receptor tyrosine kinase; Postop, postoperative; TKI, tyrosine kinase inhibitor; VEGFR, vascular endothelial growth factor receptor.

be grossly involved during surgery.[13] The most common complications of thyroidectomy include hypoparathyroidism, recurrent laryngeal nerve injury, hematoma, and wound infection. The risk of surgical complications is inversely associated with surgeon volume,[13,15] although most thyroid resections for cancer continue to be performed by low-volume surgeons.[16] In one recent study of US surgeons, the complication rates for patients who underwent total thyroidectomy for cancer ranged from 7.5% with the highest-volume surgeons (>100 cases/y), to 13.4% with intermediate-volume surgeons (10–100 cases/y) and 18.9% with low-volume surgeons (<10 cases/y).[16]

For select patients who have unifocal DTC greater than 1 cm and less than 4 cm, without extrathyroidal extension or lymph node metastases, thyroid lobectomy may be considered for the initial surgical procedure.[13] Increasing evidence from long-term population and retrospective studies suggest that, for such low-risk patients, lobectomy offers noninferior disease-specific survival outcomes and decreased surgical complications, and may obviate lifelong thyroid hormone replacement. Barney and colleagues,[17] in a study of 23,605 patients with DTC from the Surveillance, Epidemiology, and End Result (SEER) database, compared those treated with total thyroidectomy (12,598) versus lobectomy (3,266) and found no difference in 10-year overall survival (OS) (90.4% vs 90.8%) or 10-year disease-specific survival (DSS) (96.8% vs 98.6%). Furthermore, in a multivariate analysis that included age, tumor stage, nodal status, distant metastasis status, sex, year of diagnosis, extent of surgery, and RAI use, no difference in OS or DSS was seen with respect to the extent of initial surgery. These data were corroborated by Adam and colleagues[18] in a study of 61,775 patients with DTC in the National Cancer Database, which found no survival difference between patients treated with lobectomy compared with total thyroidectomy, after adjustment for initial extent and severity of disease. Mendelsohn and colleagues[19] similarly found no differences in OS or DSS in a comparison between total thyroidectomy and lobectomy for 22,274 patients with low-risk PTC. In addition, in a Japanese cohort of 1088 patients with PTC, confined to low-risk disease treated with lobectomy, Matsuzu and colleagues[20] reported that over a long follow-up period (median, 17.6 years), the incidence of recurrent disease was less than 10% for all thyroid remnant, regional lymph node, and distant sites at 25 years, and DSS was 95.2% at 25 years. Some studies have shown increased locoregional recurrence following lobectomy compared with total thyroidectomy,[21–23] but the rate of recurrence remains low (1%–4%) and does not have a significant impact on DSS.[20,24–26]

ACTIVE SURVEILLANCE

Although surgery is the accepted initial management for most DTC, active surveillance may be an alternative strategy to immediate surgery for an appropriately selected group of patients.[27] Multiple international retrospective studies with long-term follow-up suggest that many small (<1–1.5 cm), well-differentiated PTCs, without evidence of extrathyroidal extension or metastases, have low rates of growth and progression.[28–30] In a cohort of 291 US patients with low-risk PTC followed by serial ultrasonography, Tuttle and colleagues[29] showed significant growth in only a minority of patients over a median follow-up of 25 months: volume increase of greater than 50% in only 36 (12%) patients and size increase greater than 3 mm in 11 (3.8%) patients. Ito and colleagues[30] similarly showed in a cohort of 1235 Japanese patients with small PTCs followed with active ultrasonographic surveillance for a median of 75 months that, by 5 and 10 years, only 4.9% and 8% of patients experienced tumor growth of more than 3 mm, and 1.7% and 3.8% of patients experienced new lymph node metastases, respectively. Importantly, in a subset of patients who ultimately underwent thyroid surgery in this study, none were found to have distant metastases and no patient died of PTC, suggesting that delaying intervention until the time of growth or detection of lymph node spread did not adversely affect mortality. Active surveillance for low-risk PTC may avoid unwarranted surgery, surgical complications, RAI administration, and lifelong thyroid hormone replacement therapy and should be considered for appropriate patients, particularly those with reliable follow-up, high surgical risk, shorter life expectancy, or with concomitant medical issues that need to be addressed before surgery.[27,31]

RISK STRATIFICATION AND DETERMINATION OF POSTOPERATIVE THERAPY

Following surgery, patients may be treated with RAI and TSH suppression depending on an overall assessment of the potential therapeutic benefit to patient outcome compared with the risks of treatment. Surgical and histopathologic assessment of tumor aggressiveness and completeness of resection, postoperative serum Tg and Tg antibody (TgAb) measurement, and detection of distant metastases primarily inform the patient's risk of recurrence and/or death from DTC.

Several staging and risk assessment systems for DTC currently exist, with a focus on either cancer-specific mortality (ie, the American Joint Committee on Cancer [AJCC] tumor-node-metastasis [TNM] system) or disease recurrence (eg, American Thyroid Association [ATA] risk stratification). The AJCC TNM staging system for DTC was revised in 2016 (eighth edition) to better stratify mortality risk between stages.[32] The current staging of primary DTC tumors is shown in **Fig. 2**. The eighth edition recognizes the lower risk associated with tumors showing minimal extrathyroidal extension only. Although microscopic extrathyroidal extension [ETE] detected only on histologic evaluation had previously been designated as pT3 disease, this does not affect pT stage in the eighth edition of AJCC. Tumors that grossly invade into perithyroidal soft tissue structures (ie, sternohyoid, sternothyroid, thyrohyoid, omohyoid muscles) are now categorized as pT3b. Designation of pT4 disease is limited to tumors with gross ETE, regardless of tumor size, involving the larynx, trachea, esophagus, recurrent laryngeal nerve, subcutaneous soft tissue (T4a) or the perivertebral fascia, carotid, or mediastinal vasculature (T4b) (see **Fig. 2**).

In the AJCC eighth edition, the age threshold for increased risk also was increased from 45 to 55 years, based on reports suggesting that this improved staging prediction.[33,34] Other data indicate that thyroid cancer mortality and recurrence prediction is more robust when age is modeled as a continuous variable, leading some experts to argue for the elimination of a specific age cutoff from staging completely.[35] In a study of 3664 patients with DTC, Ganly and colleagues[36] found that disease-specific mortality increased progressively with advancing age, without a threshold age. Similarly, evaluation of more than 30,000 patients in the SEER database by Orosco and colleagues[37] showed a linear association with age and thyroid cancer death.

Overall the revised eighth edition AJCC staging for thyroid cancer resulted in many patients being downstaged and greater distinction in the disease-specific mortality among stages of disease.[14,38,39] In patients <55 years old, Stage I includes all disease without distant metastases (M0) and any disease with distant metastases

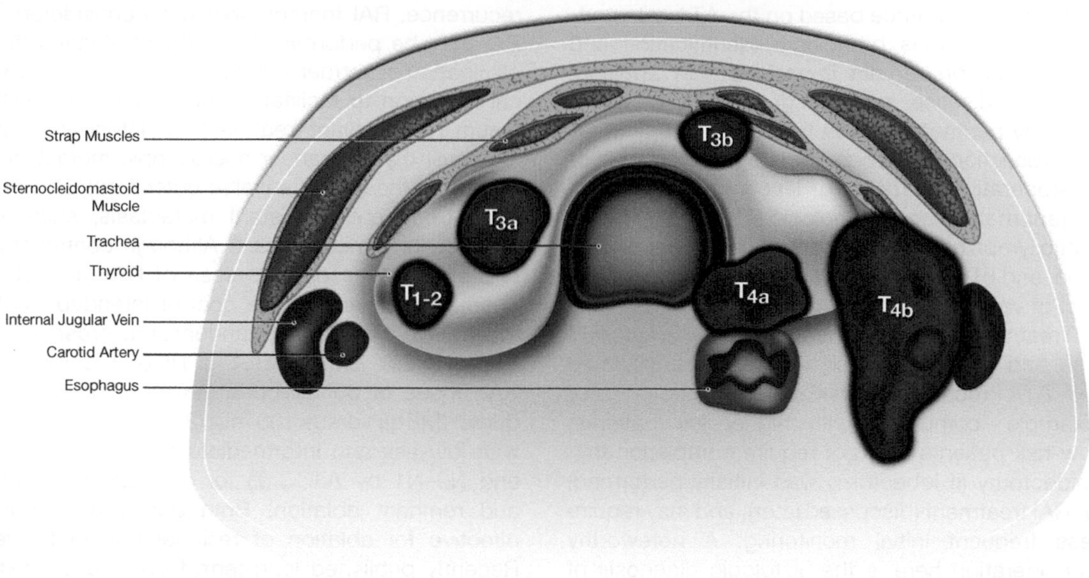

Fig. 2. Tumor staging of differentiated thyroid cancer by AJCC eighth edition. T1, intrathyroidal less than 2 cm; T2, intrathyroidal less than 2 to 4 cm; T3a, intrathyroidal greater than 4 cm; T3b, gross extrathyroidal extension invading only strap muscles (sternohyoid, sternothyroid, thyrohyoid, or omohyoid muscles) from a tumor of any size; T4a, gross extrathyroidal extension invading subcutaneous soft tissues, larynx, trachea, esophagus, or recurrent laryngeal nerve from a tumor of any size; T4b, gross extrathyroidal extension invading prevertebral fascia or encasing carotid artery or mediastinal vessels from a tumor of any size.

(M1) is considered Stage II. For patients ≥55 years who are M0, Stage I includes intrathyroidal tumors no more than 4cm without lymph node metastases (N0), and Stage II includes intrathyroidal tumors no more than 4cm with lymph node metastases, as well as intrathyroidal tumors >4cm and tumors that are pT3b. Compared to the previous edition, pT4a was downgraded and defines Stage III, with only pT4b included as Stage IVA. Patients ≥55 years with distant metastases are Stage IVB. Using the revised AJCC eighth edition, several recent retrospective cohort studies report 10-year DSS across DTC: 98.9% to 99.8% for stage I, 85.2% to 95.4% for stage II, 45.6% to 80.4% for stage III, and 27.6% to 71.9% for stage IV.[14,38–41] These rates compare with 10-year DSS across AJCC seventh edition staging: 99.1% to 100% for stage I, 92.5% to 100% for stage II, 94.3% to 98.8% for stage III, and 59% to 83.2% for stage IV.[14,38–41]

Although the AJCC TNM system provides useful estimates of mortality, the risk of cancer-specific mortality for most DTC is very low and treatment is often directed toward disease recurrence or persistence. Therefore, alternative prognostic systems that seek to more accurately predict disease recurrence in DTC have been developed, such as the ATA Risk Stratification System.[13] The ATA Risk Stratification System defines patients as having low, intermediate, or high risk of disease recurrence,[13] with estimated recurrence rates of 9% to 14% for ATA low-risk, 37% to 48% for intermediate-risk, and 69% to 86% for high-risk disease over a median follow-up time of 4 to 10 years.[13,42–45]

Briefly, ATA low-risk disease includes PTC (excluding aggressive histologic variants) without local or distant metastasis; complete macroscopic surgical resection; and no evidence of capsular, vascular, or surrounding structure invasion. Lymph node metastases must be absent or limited (≤5 pathologic N1 micrometastases, <0.2 cm in largest dimension). FTC tumors can be classified as low risk if surgical pathology shows an intrathyroidal, well-differentiated lesion with only capsular or minimal vascular (<4 foci) invasion. Intermediate-risk DTC includes cancers with microscopic invasion of tumor into the perithyroidal soft tissues (including multifocal papillary microcarcinoma with ETE), PTC with aggressive histology subtypes (eg, tall cell, hobnail variant, columnar cell carcinoma) and/or vascular invasion, lymph node metastasis involving more than 5 nodes but with disease limited to less than 3 cm in largest dimension, and RAI-avid metastatic foci in the neck on the first posttreatment whole-body RAI scan. Of note, although microscopic ETE no longer influences staging in the eighth edition of AJCC based on the absence of significant impact on patient survival, it is relevant to predicting recurrence based on the ATA risk stratification and thus pathologic identification and documentation remain important.[13] In addition, high-risk disease includes gross ETE of tumor into any perithyroidal soft tissues, incomplete tumor resection, presence of distant metastases or postoperative serum Tg levels suggestive of distant metastases, pathologic N1 with any metastatic lymph node 3 cm or greater in largest dimension, and FTC with extensive vascular invasion ($\geq$4 foci of vascular invasion).

Treatment recommendations for initial RAI use and TSH suppression targets are informed by ATA recurrence risk categorization.[13] For example, compared with higher-risk patients, low-risk patients may not require completion thyroidectomy (if lobectomy was initially performed) or RAI treatment (discussed later), and may require less frequent initial monitoring. A noteworthy consideration here is the histologic diagnosis of noninvasive follicular thyroid neoplasm with papillarylike nuclear features (NIFTP), the criteria of which were defined in 2016.[46] These tumors previously represented a subset of noninvasive follicular variant of PTC with particularly indolent features and clinical course. NIFTP are predominantly found within the indeterminate Bethesda cytology categories and most frequently harbor a mutation in one of the *RAS* genes.[47] Although not definitively considered benign, metastatic behavior is not observed, so they are perhaps best considered a premalignant lesion.[48] Importantly, because of the very indolent behavior of these tumors, more conservative treatment is recommended, including foregoing completion thyroidectomy and RAI therapy.[46]

The assessment of DTC risk and the decision to pursue further treatment remains complex and increasingly incorporates not only intraoperative and pathology findings but also mutational information and postoperative measurement of Tg and TgAb levels. In the future, prognostic systems may incorporate additional information to further refine the estimation of mortality or recurrence risk.

RADIOACTIVE IODINE THERAPY

DTCs are well-differentiated tumors that often retain functions of normal thyroid follicular tissue, including the ability to concentrate iodine through expression of the sodium-iodine symporter, allowing successful targeted therapy with I^{131}. Treatment with RAI should not be universally given, because data indicate that many patients at low risk of thyroid cancer death or recurrence do not benefit from this additional treatment.[13] For patients with ATA intermediate and high risk of recurrence, RAI therapy should be considered.[13] RAI may be performed for remnant ablation (the elimination of normal thyroid tissue following surgical resection to facilitate cancer monitoring with serum Tg); adjuvant treatment (the intended elimination of thyroid cancer microscopic metastases to reduce the risk of adverse outcomes); and primary treatment of distant metastasis, such as bone or lung metastasis.[49] Although controversy exists about the optimal dose of RAI, accepted dose ranges vary by the goal of intended treatment. Two multicenter, randomized, prospective clinical trials (ESTIMABL1[50]; HiLo[51]) compared RAI doses of 30 millicurie (mCi) (1.1 megabecquerel (MBq)) versus 100 mCi (3.7 MBq) in patients with low-risk and intermediate-risk DTC (pT1–T3 and N0–N1 by AJCC 7) for adjuvant treatment and remnant ablation. Both doses were 90% effective for ablation of residual thyroid tissue. Recently published long-term follow-up of these study cohorts showed that the RAI dose did not affect recurrence rates of DTC, with a median 5-year follow-up in the ESTIMABL1 trial[52] and a 6.5-year follow-up in the HiLo trial.[53] Higher doses of RAI (eg, 100–200 mCi) are often used for adjuvant and distant metastatic disease treatment, without high-quality evidence to support a specific dose recommendation at this time.[13] Adverse effects of RAI include transient neck pain and swelling, sialadenitis, xerostomia, and secondary malignancy, and correlate positively with higher doses.[54]

THYROID HORMONE REPLACEMENT AND THYROID-STIMULATING HORMONE SUPPRESSION

Following surgery, and irrespective of RAI treatment, patients may be treated with thyroid hormone to provide physiologic hormone replacement and to sufficiently suppress pituitary secretion of TSH, which is a growth-promoting factor for follicular cell–derived thyroid cancers. The revised guidelines from the American Thyroid Association[13] suggest individualized goals for TSH suppression in DTC that generally target the low-normal range of TSH (0.5–2.0 mIU/L) for low-risk DTC and greater TSH suppression (0.1–0.5 mIU/L) for those at increased risk for recurrence. More excessive TSH suppression (<0.1 mIU/L) should be reserved for those at the highest risk,[13] and be balanced against increased cardiac and bone complications.

A population-based study of patients taking levothyroxine for any cause found a significantly higher risk of cardiac arrhythmias (hazard ratio [HR] 1.6 [1.10–2.33]) and cardiovascular admission or death (1.37 [1.17–1.60]) in those with suppressed serum TSH (≤0.03 mU/L) compared with those with TSH level in the reference range.[55] Specifically, in patients with thyroid cancer treated with levothyroxine with modestly suppressed TSH (mean TSH level, <0.35 mU/L), atrial fibrillation was common (17.5% prevalence) in those patients greater than or equal to 60 years old.[55]

Long-standing hyperthyroidism is associated with osteoporotic fractures and loss of bone mineral density. Postmenopausal women greater than or equal to 65 year old with suppressed TSH levels (0.1 mU/L) caused by endogenous or exogenous thyroid hormone have significantly higher rates of new hip (OR, 3.6; 95% confidence interval [CI], 1.0–12.9) and vertebral (OR, 4.5; 95% CI, 1.3–15.6) fractures compared with similar women with normal TSH levels over 3.7 years of follow-up.[56] In adult patients on levothyroxine therapy, a suppressed TSH level (≤0.03 mU/L) was associated with a 2-fold increase in risk of new osteoporotic fracture compared with similar levothyroxine-treated patients who had TSH levels within the reference interval (HR, 2.02 [1.55–2.62]).[55] Studies evaluating patients with thyroid cancer are limited by evaluation of bone mineral density (BMD) rather than fracture incidence but generally support similar conclusions regarding lower BMD with suppressive-dose levothyroxine therapy.[57–59]

TSH goals in DTC should be individualized and reevaluated over time. Dynamic risk stratification, with continued reassessment of treatment response to therapy using serum tumor markers and imaging, should guide selection of the TSH suppression target based on low (TSH, 0.5–2 mIU/L), intermediate (0.1–0.5 mIU/L), or high risk (<0.1 mIU/L) of disease recurrence or progression.[13] Particularly in older patients and in those with comorbid cardiac disease and/or osteoporosis, the goal for TSH suppression may be more conservative to balance the risks of thyroid hormone excess with the possible benefit they may derive from therapy.

POSTOPERATIVE SURVEILLANCE AND DYNAMIC RISK STRATIFICATION

Recommended follow-up of DTC includes biochemical surveillance with measurement of serum Tg and TgAb concentrations and structural surveillance with neck ultrasonography at clinically appropriate intervals.[13]

Serum Tg and TgAb, in conjunction with TSH, may be assessed initially at 4 to 6 weeks postoperatively to stratify the risk of persistent disease.[13] After initial treatment, Tg and TgAb measurement should be performed at an interval appropriate to the clinical risk of detecting disease recurrence or progression. This interval may be 3 to 4 months in high-risk patients, whereas annual assessment is appropriate for many lower-risk patients and those with a more distant history of DTC without evidence of recurrence. Complete thyroid removal with or without RAI ablation facilitates Tg use as a tumor marker because Tg is also produced by residual normal thyroid tissue. In patients who underwent near-total thyroidectomy and RAI, a serum Tg level greater than 0.2 ng/mL with concurrent TSH suppression, a TSH-stimulated Tg level greater than 2 to 5 ng/mL, an increasing Tg level, or the persistence of TgAb warrant further evaluation for persistent or recurrent disease.[13,60] The optimal use of Tg in patients not treated with RAI or treated with thyroid lobectomy alone remains uncertain.[61]

Measurement of serum Tg is confounded by the presence of TgAb, which occurs in approximately 20% of patients with DTC and can mask recurrent or persistent disease by causing falsely low or undetectable serum Tg levels.[61,62] Evidence from retrospective studies suggests that increasing TgAb levels (measured using validated assays), compared with stable or decreasing titers, can be used as a surrogate tumor marker in these patients.[60,62,63]

Previously, nearly all patients with DTC received RAI and lifelong levothyroxine suppression therapy. This strategy has since evolved to current recommendations for treatment guided by dynamic risk stratification. Dynamic risk stratification involves the continued reassessment of serum Tg and TgAb and imaging for the detection of recurrence or persistent disease over time at regular intervals and with changes in clinical symptoms. At each juncture, the estimated risk of recurrence or disease progression is determined, and treatment is continued or changed accordingly, as outlined in **Fig. 3**. Tuttle and colleagues[64] and the ATA guidelines[13] outline four categories of disease response, defined by the presence or absence of biochemical and structural disease as detected by clinically available modalities.[64] An excellent response implies no clinical, biochemical, or structural evidence of disease. A biochemical incomplete response indicates persistent abnormal Tg values or increasing TgAb levels in the absence of localizable disease. Structural incomplete response indicates persistent or newly identified locoregional or distant metastases. In addition, an indeterminate response is defined as nonspecific biochemical or structural findings that cannot be confidently classified as representing malignant disease.

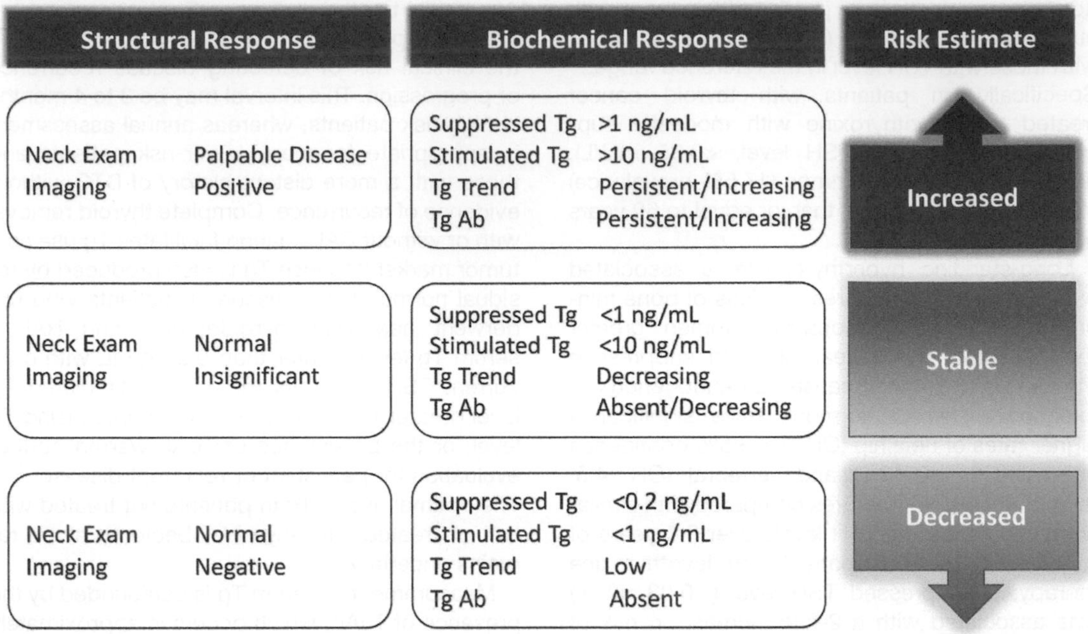

Fig. 3. Dynamic risk stratification approach to treatment. Dynamic risk stratification includes ongoing reevaluation using serum Tg levels, TgAb levels, and imaging to determine the patient's response to treatment. This approach helps to distinguish those patients, throughout the course of their disease, requiring more aggressive treatment from those in whom additional treatment may be safely postponed or attenuated.

When the risk estimate for recurrent disease increases, additional evaluation, such as neck ultrasonography, whole-body RAI scanning, and/or PET/CT depending on level of clinical suspicion, should be performed to locate residual thyroid tissue/cancer. Identification of abnormal lymph nodes or tumor mass can then be evaluated for possible further treatment with RAI, surgery, or targeted therapy. In addition, the TSH suppression target is modified as the patient's risk of recurrence changes over time to optimize disease control while minimizing adverse effects of levothyroxine therapy, as discussed earlier.

TREATMENT OF RECURRENT, PERSISTENT, AND METASTATIC DISEASE

For DTC that persists or recurs after surgery, RAI, and TSH suppression, additional therapies may be required. If a metastatic lesion is identified, it may be amenable to repeat surgery or external beam radiation. Risks of repeat surgery in the neck, such as recurrent laryngeal nerve injury and hypoparathyroidism, are increased compared with initial thyroid surgery. External radiation to the neck region is appropriate for local control and preservation of vital structures in patients with aggressive cancers that cannot be completely resected surgically, but has not been shown to convey survival benefit.[13]

SYSTEMIC THERAPY

For multifocal disease, not amenable to surgery or external radiation, systemic therapies may be used. Older cytotoxic drugs (eg, doxorubicin) have shown little benefit for progressive or metastatic DTC and cause significant side effects. Improved understanding of the pathogenesis of these cancers is leading to the development of new agents targeting specific oncogenic mechanisms. Mitogen-activated protein kinase (MAPK) signaling is a major driver of PTC through BRAFV600E and mutated RAS proteins. RET/PTC fusions also are seen in a minority of PTC tumors. Mutations in *RAS*, *PAX8-PPAR*γ translocations, and activation of the phosphatidylinositol 3 kinase (PI3K)/ protein kinase B (AKT) pathway are frequently seen in FTC.[46,65] Multiple clinical trials targeting these pathways are ongoing for the treatment of advanced DTC.[65] At present, two tyrosine kinase inhibitors are US Food and Drug Administration (FDA) approved for the treatment of metastatic, RAI-resistant DTC: sorafenib and lenvatinib. Sorafenib, an oral multikinase inhibitor, inhibits vascular endothelial growth factor receptors (VEGFRs: VEGFR-1, VEGFR-2, and VEGFR-

3), RET kinase (including RET/PTC), BRAFV600E, and platelet-derived growth factor receptor (PDGFR) beta. In the DECISION phase 3 trial, patients randomly assigned to sorafenib treatment showed improved progression-free survival compared with placebo.[66] Lenvatinib is a tyrosine kinase inhibitor of VEGFR-1, VEGFR-2, and VEGFR-3; fibroblast-derived growth factor receptors 1 through 4; PDGFRα; RET; and KIT signaling pathways. Longer progression-free survival in subjects receiving lenvatinib versus placebo was shown in the randomized phase 3 SELECT trial.[67] For patients who progress despite these treatments, off-label use of BRAF or multiple kinase inhibitors is sometimes considered. Selective BRAF inhibitors (eg, dabrafenib, vemurafenib) are approved for use in melanoma and have been tested for efficacy in BRAF-mutated PTC. Falchook and colleagues[68] have reported partial response and stable disease with dabrafenib in a subset of patients with metastatic BRAF-mutated thyroid cancer. Brose and colleagues[69] reported efficacy of vemurafenib in a phase II open-label trial of patients with BRAFV600E-mutated recurrent or metastatic, RAI-refractory PTC. Additional clinical trials of dabrafenib and vemurafenib are ongoing for the treatment of advanced and radioresistant BRAF-mutated thyroid cancer, including NCT03244956, NCT01723202, NCT01947023, NCT01534897, and NCT02145143. Treatment with multiple kinase inhibitors is another therapy option. Some phase II clinical trials evaluating multiple kinase inhibitors, including with axitinib, motesanib, sunitinib, pazopanib, dovitinib, and selumetinib, for the treatment of advanced, RAI-resistant DTC have shown modest benefit as measured by partial treatment response and progression-free survival, although phase III clinical trials and FDA approval have not been completed. In addition, immunotherapy may be considered in some patients. Checkpoint inhibitors are a kind of immunotherapy that blocks immune regulatory pathways with the goal of increasing antitumor immune responses and producing tumor killing by host leukocytes. Two primary classes of immunotherapy being evaluated for advanced thyroid cancer are inhibitors of cytotoxic T lymphocyte A (CTLA) 4 (eg, ipilimumab) and inhibitors of programmed cell death (PD) receptor/ligand interactions (eg, nivolumab, pembrolizumab, atezolizumab). At present, immune checkpoint inhibitors are being evaluated alone and in combination with targeted therapies for metastatic DTC in clinical trials[70] (for more information on the treatment of RAI-refractory DTC, see Julian Huang's article, "Treatment of Aggressive Thyroid Cancer," in this issue).

SUMMARY

Differentiated thyroid cancer is a frequent diagnosis and includes malignancies with diverse clinical behavior. Although overall prognosis is excellent, treatment carries substantial morbidity risks. Stratification of risk, based on pathology, tumor biology, ongoing biochemical and imaging assessments, and patient comorbidities, now forms the essential basis of DTC management with an imperative to provide care that is individualized and disease appropriate.

REFERENCES

1. Noone AM, Howlader N, Krapcho M, et al. SEER cancer statistics review, 1975-2015. Bethesda (MD): National Cancer Institute; 2018. Available at: https://seer.cancer.gov/csr/1975_2015/, based on November 2017 SEER data submission, posted to the SEER web site, April.
2. Girardi FM. Thyroid carcinoma pattern presentation according to age. Int Arch Otorhinolaryngol 2017; 21(1):38–41.
3. Kitahara CM, Sosa JA. The changing incidence of thyroid cancer. Nat Rev Endocrinol 2016;12(11):646–53.
4. Lim H, Devesa SS, Sosa JA, et al. Trends in thyroid cancer incidence and mortality in the United States, 1974-2013. JAMA 2017;317(13):1338–48.
5. Guth S, Theune U, Aberle J, et al. Very high prevalence of thyroid nodules detected by high frequency (13 MHz) ultrasound examination. Eur J Clin Invest 2009;39:699–706.
6. Ezzat S, Sarti DA, Cain DR, et al. Thyroid incidentalomas prevalence by palpation and ultrasonography. Arch Intern Med 1994;154:1838–40.
7. Kwong N, Medici M, Angell TE, et al. The influence of patient age on thyroid nodule formation, multinodularity, and thyroid cancer risk. J Clin Endocrinol Metab 2015;100(12):4434–40.
8. Dauksiene D, Petkeviciene J, Klumbiene J, et al. Factors associated with the prevalence of thyroid nodules and goiter in middle-aged euthyroid subjects. Int J Endocrinol 2017;2017:8401518.
9. Cibas ES, Ali SZ. The 2017 Bethesda system for reporting thyroid cytopathology. Thyroid 2017;27(11): 1341–6.
10. Patel KN, Angell TE, Babiarz J, et al. Performance of a genomic sequencing classifier for the preoperative diagnosis of cytologically indeterminate thyroid nodules. JAMA Surg 2018;153(9):817–24.
11. Steward DL, Carty SE, Sippel RS, et al. Performance of a multigene genomic classifier in thyroid nodules with indeterminate cytology: a prospective blinded multicenter study. JAMA Oncol 2019;5(2):204–12.
12. Labourier E, Shifrin A, Busseniers AE, et al. Molecular testing for miRNA, mRNA, and DNA on fine-

needle aspiration improves the preoperative diagnosis of thyroid nodules with indeterminate cytology. J Clin Endocrinol Metab 2015;100(7):2743–50.
13. Haugen BR, Alexander EK, Bible KC, et al. 2015 American Thyroid Association management guidelines for adult patients with thyroid nodules and differentiated thyroid cancer: the American Thyroid Association guidelines task force on thyroid nodules and differentiated thyroid cancer. Thyroid 2016; 26(1):1–133.
14. van Velsen EFS, Stegenga MT, van Kemenade FJ, et al. Comparing the prognostic value of the eighth edition of the American Joint Committee on cancer/tumor node metastasis staging system between papillary and follicular thyroid cancer. Thyroid 2018; 28(8):976–81.
15. Sosa JA, Bowman HM, Tielsch JM, et al. The importance of surgeon experience for clinical and economic outcomes from thyroidectomy. Ann Surg 1998;228:320–30.
16. Kandil E, Noureldine SI, Abbas A, et al. The impact of surgical volume on patient outcomes following thyroid surgery. Surgery 2013;154: 1346–52.
17. Barney BM, Hitchcock YJ, Sharma P, et al. Overall and cause-specific survival for patients undergoing lobectomy, near-total, or total thyroidectomy for differentiated thyroid cancer. Head Neck 2011;33: 645–9.
18. Brauer VF, Eder P, Miehle K, et al. Interobserver variation for ultrasound determination of thyroid nodule volumes. Thyroid 2005;15:1169–75.
19. Mendelsohn AH, Elashoff DA, Abemayor E, et al. Surgery for papillary thyroid carcinoma: is lobectomy enough? Arch Otolaryngol Head Neck Surg 2010;136:1055–61.
20. Matsuzu K, Sugino K, Masudo K, et al. Thyroid lobectomy for papillary thyroid cancer: long-term follow-up study of 1,088 cases. World J Surg 2014; 38:68–79.
21. Grant CS, Hay ID, Gough IR, et al. Local recurrence in papillary thyroid carcinoma: is extent of surgical resection important? Surgery 1988;104: 954–62.
22. Hay ID, Grant CS, Bergstralh EJ, et al. Unilateral total lobectomy: is it sufficient surgical treatment for patients with AMES low-risk papillary thyroid carcinoma? Surgery 1998;124:958–64.
23. Mazzaferri EL, Kloos RT. Clinical review 128: current approaches to primary therapy for papillary and follicular thyroid cancer. J Clin Endocrinol Metab 2001;86:1447–63.
24. Nixon IJ, Ganly I, Patel SG, et al. Thyroid lobectomy for treatment of well differentiated intrathyroid malignancy. Surgery 2012;151:571–9.
25. Adam MA, Pura J, Gu L, et al. Extent of surgery for papillary thyroid cancer is not associated with survival: an analysis of 61,775 patients. Ann Surg 2014;260:601–5.
26. Vaisman F, Shaha A, Fish S, et al. Initial therapy with either thyroid lobectomy or total thyroidectomy without radioactive iodine remnant ablation is associated with very low rates of structural disease recurrence in properly selected patients with differentiated thyroid cancer. Clin Endocrinol (Oxf) 2011; 75:112–9.
27. Tuttle RM, Zhang L, Shaha A. A clinical framework to facilitate selection of patients with differentiated thyroid cancer for active surveillance or less aggressive initial surgical management. Expert Rev Endocrinol Metab 2018;13(2):77–85.
28. Sugitani I, Fujimoto Y, Yamada K. Association between serum thyrotropin concentration and growth of asymptomatic papillary thyroid microcarcinoma. World J Surg 2014;38(3):673–8.
29. Tuttle RM, Fagin JA, Minkowitz G, et al. Natural history and tumor volume kinetics of papillary thyroid cancers during active surveillance. JAMA Otolaryngol Head Neck Surg 2017;143(10): 1015–20.
30. Ito Y, Miyauchi A, Kihara M, et al. Patient age is significantly related to the progression of papillary microcarcinoma of the thyroid under observation. Thyroid 2014;24(1):27–34.
31. Tufano RP, Shindo M, Shaha AR. New recommendations for extent of thyroidectomy and active surveillance for the treatment of differentiated thyroid cancer. JAMA Otolaryngol Head Neck Surg 2016; 142(7):625–6.
32. Brierley JD, Gospodarowicz MK, Wittekind C. TNM classification of malignant tumours. 8th edition. Weinheim (Germany): John Wiley & Sons; 2017. p. 69–71.
33. Nixon IJ, Wang LY, Migliacci JC, et al. An international multi-institutional validation of age 55 years as a cutoff for risk stratification in the AJCC/UICC staging system for well-differentiated thyroid cancer. Thyroid 2016;26(3):373–80.
34. Nixon IJ, Kuk D, Wreesmann V, et al. Defining a valid age cutoff in staging of well-differentiated thyroid cancer. Ann Surg Oncol 2016;23(2):410–5.
35. Ylli D, Burman KD, Van Nostrand D, et al. Eliminating the age cutoff in staging of differentiated thyroid cancer: the safest road? J Clin Endocrinol Metab 2018;103(5):1813–7.
36. Ganly I, Nixon IJ, Wang LY, et al. Survival from differentiated thyroid cancer: what has age got to do with it? Thyroid 2015;25(10):1106–14.
37. Orosco RK, Hussain T, Brumund KT, et al. Analysis of age and disease status as predictors of thyroid cancer-specific mortality using the surveillance, epidemiology, and end results database. Thyroid 2015;25(1):125–32.

38. Kim M, Kim WG, Oh HS, et al. Comparison of the seventh and eighth editions of the American Joint Committee on cancer/union for international cancer control tumor-node-metastasis staging system for differentiated thyroid cancer. Thyroid 2017;27(9): 1149–55.
39. Tam S, Boonsripitayanon M, Amit M, et al. Survival in differentiated thyroid cancer: comparing the AJCC cancer staging seventh and eighth editions. Thyroid 2018;28(10):1301–10.
40. Verburg FA, Mäder U, Luster M, et al. The effects of the Union for International Cancer Control/American Joint Committee on Cancer Tumour, Node, Metastasis system version 8 on staging of differentiated thyroid cancer: a comparison to version 7. Clin Endocrinol (Oxf) 2018;88(6):950–6.
41. Kim TH, Kim YN, Kim HI, et al. Prognostic value of the eighth edition AJCC TNM classification for differentiated thyroid carcinoma. Oral Oncol 2017;71: 81–6.
42. Tuttle RM, Tala H, Shah J, et al. Estimating risk of recurrence in differentiated thyroid cancer after total thyroidectomy and radioactive iodine remnant ablation: using response to therapy variables to modify the initial risk estimates predicted by the new American Thyroid Association staging system. Thyroid 2010;20:1341–9.
43. Vaisman F, Momesso D, Bulzico DA, et al. Spontaneous remission in thyroid cancer patients after biochemical incomplete response to initial therapy. Clin Endocrinol (Oxf) 2012;77:132–8.
44. Castagna MG, Maino F, Cipri C, et al. Delayed risk stratification, to include the response to initial treatment (surgery and radioiodine ablation), has better outcome predictivity in differentiated thyroid cancer patients. Eur J Endocrinol 2011;165:441–6.
45. Pitoia F, Bueno F, Urciuoli C, et al. Outcomes of patients with differentiated thyroid cancer risk-stratified according to the American Thyroid Association and Latin American Thyroid Society risk of recurrence classification systems. Thyroid 2013;23:1401–7.
46. Nikiforov YE, Seethala RR, Tallini G, et al. Nomenclature revision for encapsulated follicular variant of papillary thyroid carcinoma: a paradigm shift to reduce overtreatment of indolent tumors. JAMA Oncol 2016;2(8):1023–9.
47. Fagin JA, Wells SA Jr. Biologic and clinical perspectives on thyroid cancer. N Engl J Med 2016;375(11): 1054–67.
48. Sahli ZT, Umbricht CB, Schneider EB, et al. Thyroid nodule diagnostic markers in the face of the new NIFTP category: time for a reset? Thyroid 2017; 27(11):1393–9.
49. Tuttle MR. Differentiated thyroid cancer: radioiodine treatment. Ross DS, editor. UpToDate. UpToDate Inc: Waltham, (MA): 2018. Available at: https://www.uptodate.com. Accessed February 1, 2019.
50. Schlumberger M, Catargi B, Borget I, et al. Strategies of radioiodine ablation in patients with low-risk thyroid cancer. N Engl J Med 2012;366:1663–73.
51. Mallick U, Harmer C, Yap B, et al. Ablation with low-dose radioiodine and thyrotropin alfa in thyroid cancer. N Engl J Med 2012;366:1674–85.
52. Schlumberger M, Leboulleux S, Catargi B, et al. Outcome after ablation in patients with low-risk thyroid cancer (ESTIMABL1): 5-year follow-up results of a randomised, phase 3, equivalence trial. Lancet Diabetes Endocrinol 2018;6:618–26.
53. Dehbi HM, Mallick U, Wadsley J, et al. Recurrence after low-dose radioiodine ablation and recombinant human thyroid-stimulating hormone for differentiated thyroid cancer (HiLo): long-term results of an open-label, non-inferiority randomised controlled trial. Lancet Diabetes Endocrinol 2019; 7(1):44–51.
54. Andresen NS, Buatti JM, Tewfik HH, et al. Radioiodine ablation following thyroidectomy for differentiated thyroid cancer: literature review of utility, dose, and toxicity. Eur Thyroid J 2017;6(4):187–96.
55. Flynn RW, Bonellie SR, Jung RT, et al. Serum thyroid stimulating hormone concentration and morbidity from cardiovascular disease and fractures in patients on long-term thyroxine therapy. J Clin Endocrinol Metab 2010;95:186–93.
56. Bauer DC, Ettinger B, Nevitt MC, et al. Risk for fracture in women with low serum levels of thyroid-stimulating hormone. Ann Intern Med 2001;134: 561–8.
57. Kung AW, Yeung SS. Prevention of bone loss induced by thyroxine suppressive therapy in postmenopausal women: the effect of calcium and calcitonin. J Clin Endocrinol Metab 1996;81:1232–6.
58. Sugitani I, Fujimoto Y. Effect of postoperative thyrotropin suppressive therapy on bone mineral density in patients with papillary thyroid carcinoma: a prospective controlled study. Surgery 2011;150:1250–7.
59. Wang LY, Smith AW, Palmer FL, et al. Thyrotropin suppression increases the risk of osteoporosis without decreasing recurrence in ATA low- and intermediate-risk patients with differentiated thyroid carcinoma. Thyroid 2015;25(3):300–7.
60. Spencer C, Fatemi S. Thyroglobulin antibody (TgAb) methods - Strengths, pitfalls and clinical utility for monitoring TgAb-positive patients with differentiated thyroid cancer. Best Pract Res Clin Endocrinol Metab 2013;27(5):701–12.
61. Momesso DP, Vaisman F, Yang SP, et al. Dynamic risk stratification in patients with differentiated thyroid cancer treated without radioactive iodine. J Clin Endocrinol Metab 2016;101(7):2692–700.
62. Chung JK, Park YJ, Kim TY, et al. Clinical significance of elevated level of serum antithyroglobulin antibody in patients with differentiated thyroid

cancer after thyroid ablation. Clin Endocrinol (Oxf) 2002;57(2):215–21.
63. Pedrazzini L, Baroli A, Lomuscio G, et al. Prevalence, clinical significance and prognostic value of anti-thyroglobulin antibodies in the follow-up of patients with differentiated thyroid carcinoma: a retrospective study. Minerva Endocrinol 2009;34(3):195–203.
64. Tarasova VD, Tuttle RM. A risk-adapted approach to follow-up in differentiated thyroid cancer. Rambam Maimonides Med J 2016;7(1):1–10.
65. Naoum GE, Morkos M, Kim B, et al. Novel targeted therapies and immunotherapy for advanced thyroid cancers. Mol Cancer 2018;17(1):51.
66. Brose MS, Nutting CM, Jarzab B, et al. Sorafenib in radioactive iodine-refractory, locally advanced or metastatic differentiated thyroid cancer: a randomised, double-blind, phase 3 trial. Lancet 2014;384:319–28.
67. Schlumberger M, Tahara M, Wirth LJ, et al. Lenvatinib versus placebo in radioiodine-refractory thyroid cancer. N Engl J Med 2015;372:621–30.
68. Falchook GS, Millward M, Hong D, et al. BRAF inhibitor dabrafenib in patients with metastatic BRAF-mutant thyroid cancer. Thyroid 2015;25(1): 71–7.
69. Brose MS, Cabanillas ME, Cohen EE, et al. Vemurafenib in patients with BRAF(V600E)-positive metastatic or unresectable papillary thyroid cancer refractory to radioactive iodine: a non-randomised, multicentre, open-label, phase 2 trial. Lancet Oncol 2016;17(9):1272–82.
70. Rao SN, Cabanillas ME. Navigating systemic therapy in advanced thyroid carcinoma: From standard care to personalized therapy and beyond. J Endocr Soc 2018;2(10):1109–30.

Treatment of Aggressive Thyroid Cancer

Julian Huang, AB[a], Ethan James Harris, BS[b], Jochen H. Lorch, MD, MS[c,*]

KEYWORDS

• Differentiated thyroid cancer • Medullary thyroid cancer • Anaplastic thyroid cancer • Aggressive • Therapeutics

Key points

- Most cases of thyroid cancer have a good prognosis with standard-of-care treatment.
- Patients with radioactive iodine-refractory differentiated thyroid cancer, anaplastic thyroid cancer, and progressive medullary thyroid cancer have a much poorer prognosis, with limited treatment options available.
- Major classes of treatments in clinical development for these aggressive cases of thyroid cancer include tyrosine kinase inhibitors, mammalian target of rapamycin inhibitors, and mitogen-activated protein kinase kinase inhibitors.

ABSTRACT

Although thyroid cancer generally has a good prognosis, there is a subset of patients for whom standard care (ie, treatment limited to surgery or surgery plus radioactive iodine) is either not appropriate because of the aggressive nature of their disease or not sufficient because of disease progression through standard treatment. Most of these tumors are in 3 groups: radioactive iodine–refractory differentiated thyroid carcinoma including poorly differentiated thyroid carcinoma anaplastic thyroid carcinoma, and progressive medullary thyroid carcinoma. Major classes of treatments in clinical development for these aggressive thyroid tumors include tyrosine kinase inhibitors, mammalian target of rapamycin inhibitors, and mitogen-activated protein kinase kinase inhibitors.

OVERVIEW

The American Cancer Society estimates that there were approximately 53,990 new cases of thyroid cancer and 2060 deaths from thyroid cancer in 2018.[1] Relative 5-year survival rates for thyroid cancer as a whole have been among the highest of all cancers, ranging from 92% in 1975 to 1977 to 94% in 1987 to 89, and 98% in 2007 to 2013, but there is still a subset of patients who are not responsive to the typically curative standard of care.[2] For these patients, treatment options are limited, and outcomes are sobering. For instance, patients with differentiated thyroid carcinoma (DTC) with distant metastases diagnosed during the course of their disease have a 35% 5-year survival rate,[3] and patients with medullary thyroid cancer (MTC) with distant metastases at diagnosis have been reported to have a 5-year survival rate as low as 28%.[4] Meanwhile, patients with anaplastic thyroid cancer (ATC) have an even more dismal 5-year survival rate of 7%.[4] Patients with these tumors have the highest unmet need for effective treatments among patients with thyroid cancer, and thus the bulk of research on thyroid cancer treatment is focused on strategies to improve outcomes for these patients.

Disclosure: JH Lorch: Receives Research Funding from Novartis, Bristol-Myers-Squibb, Millennium and Bayer Consulting honoraria Genentech, Bayer. J Huang and E Harris have no disclosures.
[a] Yale University School of Medicine, 123 York Street, 15A, New Haven, CT 06511, USA; [b] University of Illinois College of Medicine, 901 South Ashland Avenue, 01-715, Chicago, IL 60602, USA; [c] Department of Medical Oncology, Dana-Farber Cancer Institute, 450 Brookline Avenue, D2136, Boston, MA 02115, USA
* Corresponding author.
E-mail address: jochen_lorch@dfci.harvard.edu

Surgical Pathology 12 (2019) 943–950
https://doi.org/10.1016/j.path.2019.08.004

This article discusses advances in the treatment of aggressive thyroid carcinomas, including treatment of radioactive iodine (RAI)–refractory DTC, ATC, and MTC. For each of these thyroid cancer subtypes, a brief background is provided on the disease and current standard of care, as well as a glimpse into the many therapeutic candidates currently in clinical development. This article is specifically written for pathologists interested in how aggressive thyroid carcinomas are treated. Therefore, the aim is to emphasize key points rather than providing an exhaustive review of therapeutic candidates in clinical development.

DIFFERENTIATED THYROID CARCINOMA

> ***Key Points***
> **DIFFERENTIATED THYROID CANCER**
>
> - DTC generally has a very good prognosis with surgery and RAI as standard of care, but options for patients with distant metastases or RAI-refractory disease are limited.
> - Sorafenib and lenvatinib are tyrosine kinase inhibitors (TKIs) approved for RAI-refractory DTC, but many patients still do not respond to these drugs.
> - Drugs in development for this population of DTC include other TKIs, mitogen-activated protein kinase kinase (MEK) inhibitors, mammalian target of rapamycin (mTOR) inhibitors, histone deacetylase (HDAC) inhibitors, tropomyosin receptor kinase (TRK) inhibitors, gene therapy, RET inhibitors, and immunotherapy

RADIOACTIVE IODINE–REFRACTORY DIFFERENTIATED THYROID CARCINOMA BACKGROUND

DTC comprises about 92% of all thyroid carcinomas. DTC originates from the thyroid follicular cells, and includes papillary, follicular, and Hürthle cell thyroid carcinomas.[5] These cancers are typically treated with surgery and RAI as standard of care, which generally produces excellent survival rates of more than 90%.[6] However, there are patients x for whom this standard of care is not sufficient or effective, such as patients that develop distant metastases (10%–15% of patients)[7] or those with tumors that become refractory to RAI (5%–15% of patients).[8–10] Distant metastatic and RAI-refractory DTC have 5-year survival rates of 35%[3] and 66%,[11] respectively.

CURRENT TREATMENT OPTIONS FOR RADIOACTIVE IODINE–REFRACTORY DIFFERENTIATED THYROID CARCINOMA

Although RAI may still be effective against metastatic disease that is RAI avid, once the disease progresses through RAI or becomes nonavid to RAI, alternative systemic therapies should be explored. In the past, doxorubicin was used, but it showed poor response rates with limited improvement in progression-free survival (PFS); moreover, it has numerous side effects.[12–15] By far the most well-researched class of agents for treating RAI-refractory DTC are tyrosine kinase inhibitors (TKIs) targeting the mitogen-activated protein kinase (MAPK) pathway.[16] Sorafenib and lenvatinib, both TKIs, are US Food and Drug Administration (FDA) approved for RAI-refractory DTC. Sorafenib is a multikinase inhibitor of vascular endothelial growth factor receptor (VEGFR), platelet-derived growth factor receptor (PDGFR), c-Kit, and Rapidly Accelerated Fibrosarcoma (Raf) family kinases such as B-Rapidly Accelerated Fibrosarcoma (B-RAF) and C-Rapidly Accelerated Fibrosarcoma (C-Raf), whereas lenvatinib is a multikinase inhibitor of VEGFR, Fibroblast growth factor receptor (FGFR), PDGFR, c-Kit, and RET. Several of the kinases that are inhibited by sorafenib and lenvatinib have been suggested to have roles in cancer progression.

FDA approval was based on studies showing treatment response to these therapies. For example, sorafenib showed a response rate of 12.2% and a PFS of 10.8 months versus 5.7 months with placebo in a randomized phase 3 study (DECIDE).[17] In a similarly designed trial (SELECT), lenvatinib elicited a 64.8% response rate, with a PFS of 15.2 months versus 3.6 months on placebo.[18] For both trials, response rate was defined as either a complete or partial response per Response evaluation criteria in solid tumors (RECIST) criteria. These treatments represent the current standard of care in patients with RAI-refractory DTC. However, side effects can be severe, and include catastrophic vascular effects, including stroke and heart attacks.[19] Approximately 75% of patients in the pivotal randomized phase 3 trials required dose interruptions or dose reductions.[17,18] Fatigue and lack of appetite are also frequently observed, and in numerous cases lead to interruptions or discontinuation of therapy. Furthermore, none of these treatments are curative and resistance eventually develops, highlighting the need for treatment options beyond first-line therapy.

THERAPEUTIC CANDIDATES IN CLINICAL DEVELOPMENT FOR RADIOACTIVE IODINE–REFRACTORY DIFFERENTIATED THYROID CARCINOMA

Numerous drugs are in development for patients with DTC for whom surgery and RAI are not effective. Many of these drugs, such as sorafenib and lenvatinib, are TKIs.[16] TKIs that have been tested include cabozantinib, cediranib, vemurafenib, and dabrafenib. Vemurafenib and dabrafenib are TKIs that specifically inhibit BRAF and have shown some efficacy in patients with RAI-refractory DTC. For example, a response rate of 38.5% was reported in an open-label phase II trial conducted by Brose and colleagues[20] evaluating the efficacy of vemurafenib in patients with RAI-refractory papillary thyroid carcinoma harboring the BRAF V600E mutation. The BRAF V600E mutation has been shown to reduce RAI uptake in tumor cells because of suppression of the sodium iodide symporter.[21] Based on this finding, studies have evaluated whether vemurafenib and dabrafenib are able to increase RAI uptake in RAI-refractory DTC. Dunn and colleagues[22] showed that, of 9 evaluable patients treated with vemurafenib, 4 became appropriate candidates for RAI, and 3 of those experienced tumor regression after RAI. In addition, Rothenberg and colleagues[23] showed that 6 of 10 patients had RAI uptake after dabrafenib, with 2 of these patients showing partial responses. Although early data with vemurafenib and dabrafenib suggested that BRAF inhibition may have a role in improving RAI refractoriness, data with pazopanib (another inhibitor of BRAF) seem to suggest the contrary.[22–24] Further studies are needed to explore their utility in the modulation of RAI uptake.

TKIs have found success in terms of the FDA approval of sorafenib and lenvatinib for DTC and have produced encouraging results in select studies of drug candidates still in clinical development. As a whole, however, even in complete responders, resistance eventually develops and the disease returns if treatment is discontinued. As such, researchers have been exploring other treatment targets and modalities. Selumetinib is a MEK inhibitor that inhibits the enzyme MEK, which is directly downstream of BRAF. In 2013, Ho and colleagues[25] published a study evaluating selumetinib in 20 patients with RAI-refractory metastatic thyroid cancer. The study reported that 12 of these 20 patients experienced increased iodine uptake, and 8 of those patients became appropriate candidates for RAI. Five of the 8 patients treated had partial responses. AstraZeneca followed up these promising midstage results by conducting a larger randomized phase III trial: the ASTRA study. This study recruited 233 patients with nonmetastatic DTC after thyroidectomy, but before receipt of RAI, in order to assess whether selumetinib improved the complete remission rate for patients at high risk of failing standard of care. However, recent announcement of study results confirmed no significant difference in complete response rate between the selumetinib and placebo arms.[26]

The PI3K-AKT-mTOR pathway is another signaling pathway that has been implicated in thyroid cancer.[27] Specifically, inhibition of mTOR has been proposed as an emerging strategy for thyroid cancer because of existing development of rapamycin analogs, antiproliferative action of mTOR inhibition, and potential stimulation of thyroid iodide uptake.[28] In 2013, Lim and colleagues[29] published a phase II study of everolimus (an mTOR inhibitor) in 24 patients with DTC. Two partial responses were observed, and median PFS was 43 weeks. In 2017, Schneider and colleagues[30] reported on a phase II study of everolimus in 28 patients with DTC, this time observing no responses; median PFS was 9 months. Most recently, Hanna and colleagues[31] reported on 33 patients with DTC treated with everolimus, observing 1 partial response and a median PFS of 12.9 months. In particular, Hürthle cell carcinoma seems to be susceptible to mTOR inhibition.[31] Based on these data, everolimus is now listed in the National Comprehensive Cancer Network (NCCN) guidelines for treatment of RAI-refractory disease if clinical trials are not available or applicable.[32] mTOR inhibitors have also been studied in combination with other agents, namely TKIs. For example, in 2015, combination therapy with everolimus and sorafenib was assessed via a phase II study in 28 patients with DTC, eliciting an encouraging 61% response rate, with only 1 patient progressing at the time of the published update.[33] Overall, results from mTOR inhibitors in combination with TKIs seem to be more encouraging than those of mTOR inhibitors alone, and larger trials are needed to confirm the positive findings observed in these midstage studies.

Aside from TKIs and mTOR inhibitors, there have been numerous other classes of targeted agents and treatment modalities in active clinical development. These agents include HDAC inhibitors, VB-111 (a gene therapy that targets the tumor vasculature to induce cell death in angiogenic endothelial cells in the tumor microenvironment), and larotrectinib (LOXO-101; a potent inhibitor of TRK), a gene seen mutated in papillary thyroid cancer.[34] In addition, the advent of immunotherapy has redefined cancer treatment, and this emerging strategy has permeated into thyroid cancer as well. Although there are many trials currently ongoing involving immunotherapeutic agents in thyroid cancer, they have not yet produced data. Of note, Mehnert and colleagues[35] reported preliminary results at American Society Of Clinical Oncology (ASCO) in 2016 of a phase II trial with pembrolizumab in 22 patients with thyroid cancer. Two patients had partial responses for a response rate of 9.1%, and the 6-month PFS rate was 58.7%.

ANAPLASTIC THYROID CANCER

> ***Key Points***
> **ANAPLASTIC THYROID CANCER**
>
> - The prognosis for ATC is one of the worst among all cancers, with limited treatment options and a 5-year survival rate of 7%.
> - Combination treatment with dabrafenib, a TKI inhibiting BRAF, and trametinib, a MEK inhibitor, became the first targeted treatment approved for ATC.
> - Drugs in development for ATC include TKIs such as lenvatinib; mTOR inhibitors such as everolimus; crolibulin, a microtubule destabilizing agent; and anti–PD-1 immunotherapies.

BACKGROUND ON ANAPLASTIC THYROID CANCER

ATC, also known as undifferentiated thyroid cancer, is the rarest subtype of thyroid cancer but also the most lethal. Comprising 1.6% to 1.7% of all thyroid cancers in the United States,[36] ATC nevertheless is responsible for up to 14% to 50% of annual mortality for thyroid cancer.[37] In addition, the prognosis for ATC is one of the worst among all cancers, with a 5-year survival rate of 7%.[4] Because nearly half of all patients with ATC are diagnosed with metastatic disease,[38] and ATC does not take up radioactive iodine,[39] treatment options are limited. Thus, management of ATC often involves surgery (if possible), chemotherapy, and radiation.[40] Nevertheless, disease progression is rapid, and the unmet need in this small population is large.

In May of 2018, the FDA approved the first targeted treatment of patients with ATC with a BRAFV600E mutation: dabrafenib, a TKI that inhibits BRAF, in combination with trametinib, a MEK inhibitor. The data on which the approval was granted included 16 patients with ATC, for whom the combination therapy elicited a 61% response rate, with a duration of response greater than or equal to 6 months in 64% of responders.[41]

THERAPEUTIC CANDIDATES IN CLINICAL DEVELOPMENT FOR ANAPLASTIC THYROID CANCER

Although the development pipeline for ATC is smaller than that for RAI-refractory DTC, many similar classes of drugs are in development for ATC. In 2017, Tahara and colleagues[42] reported on a phase II trial with lenvatinib in ATC, RAI-refractory DTC, and MTC. Lenvatinib was assessed in 17 patients with ATC, eliciting a response rate of 24%, and a median PFS of 7.4 months. Also in 2017, Ito and colleagues[43] published results of a phase II study with sorafenib in 10 patients with ATC, observing a median PFS of 2.8 months and no responses.

There have also been multiple trials evaluating mTOR inhibitors in ATC. In 2013, Lim and colleagues[29] observed that everolimus in 6 patients with ATC failed to elicit any responses, with a median PFS of 10 weeks. Schneider and colleagues[30] evaluated everolimus in 7 patients with ATC, similarly observing no responses and a median time to progressive disease of 9 weeks. In our phase II study with 7 patients with ATC, 1 had a partial response until 17.9 months after study entry. However, the median PFS of the ATC cohort as a whole was 2.2 months, similar to results of prior studies with everolimus.[31] Temsirolimus, another mTOR inhibitor, has been evaluated in combination with sorafenib in a phase II thyroid cancer study. Among the overall cohort, there were 2 patients with ATC, and 1 experienced an objective response.[44]

Gramza and colleagues[45] investigated the combination of crolibulin, a microtubule destabilizing agent, and cisplatin in a basket trial of solid tumors, including 16 patients with ATC. Of the 8 patients with ATC treated at the highest dose level, there was 1 who experienced a complete response and had been on the study for more than 12 months as of publication of the results. Most recently, Wirth and colleagues[46] reported on data from a basket trial of spartalizumab (PDR001), an anti–PD-1 immunotherapy agent, which included 37 patients with ATC. The study observed a 17% overall response rate by RECIST 1.1, and a 20% response rate by immune-related response criteria. This first glimpse into the potential for immunotherapy with several trials ongoing.

MEDULLARY THYROID CARCINOMA

Key Points
MEDULLARY THYROID CANCER

- For patients with MTC for whom surgical treatment is insufficient, systemic treatment options are limited
- Vandetanib and cabozantinib are two TKIs approved for refractory MTC, but there are still many patients who seek alternative treatments after exhausting these options
- Drugs in development for ATC include TKIs such as sulfatinib, anlotinib, and sorafenib; mTOR inhibitors such as everolimus; antibody-drug conjugates; and RET inhibitors

BACKGROUND ON MEDULLARY THYROID CARCINOMA

MTC, which originates from neural crest–derived parafollicular C cells of the thyroid gland, comprises approximately 2% of all thyroid cancers.[47] Approximately a quarter of MTC is associated with the inherited diseases multiple endocrine neoplasia 2A and 2B. At present, standard of care for MTC revolves around thyroidectomy and lymph node dissection. If surgical treatment is insufficient because of disease burden, there are limited systemic treatment options.[48,49] The 10-year survival rate for patients with localized disease is 95.6%, compared with 40% if there are distant metastases at diagnosis.[50]

Given that RET mutations are present in all heritable MTC and a significant percentage of sporadic tumors (especially MTC pursuing an aggressive clinical course), systemic therapies targeting RET have been developed to treat MTC.[51] So far, there have been 2 targeted therapies approved for MTC: vandetanib and cabozantinib, both TKIs. In 2011, vandetanib became the first FDA-approved agent for progressive MTC. The approval was based on data from a 331-patient phase III trial evaluating vandetanib in advanced MTC. The pivotal trial found significant prolongation of PFS on vandetanib compared with placebo (predicted median 30.5 months vs 19.3 months), as well as a higher response rate (45% vs 13%).[52] However, the long PFS in the control arm raises questions about the patient population studied, because there was no requirement for disease progression to enter the study. Cabozantinib was approved for advanced MTC in 2018. In a 330-patient randomized phase III trial with cabozantinib, study investigators estimated a median PFS of 11.2 months versus 4.0 months on placebo, and a response rate of 28% on cabozantinib versus 0% on placebo in patients with MTC and documented disease progression.[53] Vandetanib and cabozantinib changed the treatment landscape for patients with MTC after surgery, but there are still many patients for whom these approved agents do not work, emphasizing the need for alternative treatments.

THERAPEUTIC CANDIDATES IN CLINICAL DEVELOPMENT FOR MEDULLARY THYROID CANCER

Sulfatinib is a TKI targeting VEGR, FGFR1, and CSF1R. In a phase II study including 6 patients with advanced MTC, 1 partial response was confirmed, with manageable toxicities overall.[54] Anlotinib is another TKI inhibiting Vascular endothelial growth factor receptor 2 (VEGFR2)/Vascular endothelial growth factor receptor 3 (VEGFR3) and Fibroblast growth factor receptor 1 (FGFR1) to Fibroblast growth factor receptor 4 (FGFR4), as well as PDGFR, c-Kit, and RET. Sun and colleagues[55] evaluated anlotinib in 58 patients with advanced or metastatic MTC and found that the drug showed an impressive 56.9% response rate and 85.5% PFS rate at 48 weeks. Sorafenib has also been assessed in MTC. Ito and colleagues[43] conducted a phase II trial with 18 patients with thyroid cancer, 8 of whom had MTC. The response rate for the MTC cohort was 25%, with median PFS not yet reached at the time of publication.

mTOR inhibitors have also been tested in MTC. Lim and colleagues[29] reported on their experience with everolimus in 9 patients with MTC; however, the drug failed to elicit a treatment response. Our phase II study with everolimus included an exploratory cohort of 10 patients with MTC that had radiographic progression before enrollment. There was a median PFS of 13.1 months in the MTC cohort with 1 partial response.[31] In a phase II study open to all histologic subtypes of thyroid cancer, Sherman and colleagues[33] observed in 10 patients with MTC a 40% response rate, with a median 209 days on study. Everolimus has also been assessed in combination with pasireotide, a somatostatin analog, in a proof-of-concept study with 19 patients with MTC. Seven patients advanced on the trial to receive pasireotide in combination with everolimus, with response observed in 1 patient.[56] These results in MTC mirror the improved findings of the mTOR inhibitor/TKI combination compared with mTOR inhibitor monotherapy observed in DTC, described earlier.

Rovalpituzumab tesirine (Rova-T) is an antibody-drug conjugate targeting a DNA cross-linking agent to deltalike protein 3 (DLL3), which is expressed on certain tumor cells. Aggarwal and colleagues[57] reported an update on a phase I basket study with Rova-T, which included 2 patients with MTC. However, as of the trial update presented in October 2017, it does not seem that either of the patients with MTC responded.

In addition, LOXO-292 is a RET inhibitor that is being developed by Loxo Oncology for tumor types harboring RET mutations, such as MTC. In an October 2018 press release, the company presented impressive early-stage data for LOXO-292 in MTC. Of 29 patients with RET-mutant MTC, 17 patients showed an objective response (2 complete responses, 15 partial responses, and 2 unconfirmed partial responses) for an overall response rate of 59%. In addition, 7 other patients with MTC showed tumor regression. There were also 9 patients with RET fusion-positive papillary thyroid cancer, 7 of whom responded, with 1 additional patient showing tumor regression for an overall response rate of 78%. The drug has also shown durability, with 16 of 17 responding patients with MTC on therapy with a median follow-up of 8.4 months, and all responding patients with papillary thyroid cancer on therapy with a median follow-up of 8.5 months.[58,59]

SUMMARY

Improved understanding of molecular pathways driving thyroid cancer has accelerated development of targeted therapies for all histologic subtypes of thyroid cancer. Recent approvals of different systemic TKIs targeting the MAPK pathway for DTC, ATC, and MTC have fundamentally changed outcomes for patients who are not appropriate for, or progress through, standard-of-care treatment. Although TKIs comprise a substantial portion of drugs in clinical development for thyroid cancer, many other novel targets and treatment modalities, such as mTOR inhibitors and immunotherapy, have produced encouraging clinical data. Of particular interest is the potential for synergistic combinations with emerging treatments.

REFERENCES

1. American Cancer Society. Cancer facts & figures 2017. Atlanta (GA): American Cancer Society; 2017.
2. Noone AM, Howlader N, Krapcho M, et al, editors. SEER cancer statistics review, 1975-2015. Bethesda (MD): National Cancer Institute; 2018. Available at: https://seer.cancer.gov/csr/1975_2015/.
3. Ruegemer JJ, Hay ID, Bergstralh EJ, et al. Distant metastases in differentiated thyroid carcinoma: a multivariate analysis of prognostic variables. J Clin Endocrinol Metab 1988;67(3):501–8.
4. Edge SB, Compton CC. The American Joint Committee on Cancer: the 7th edition of the AJCC cancer staging manual and the future of TNM. Ann Surg Oncol 2010;17(6):1471–4.
5. Gilliland FD, Hunt WC, Morris DM, et al. Prognostic factors for thyroid carcinoma. A population-based study of 15,698 cases from the Surveillance, Epidemiology and End Results (SEER) program 1973-1991. Cancer 1997;79(3):564–73.
6. Lerch H, Schober O, Kuwert T, et al. Survival of differentiated thyroid carcinoma studied in 500 patients. J Clin Oncol 1997;15(5):2067–75.
7. O'Neill CJ, Oucharek J, Learoyd D, et al. Standard and emerging therapies for metastatic differentiated thyroid cancer. Oncologist 2010;15(2):146–56.
8. Pacini F, Castagna MG. Approach to and treatment of differentiated thyroid carcinoma. Med Clin North Am 2012;96(2):369–83.
9. Sciuto R, Romano L, Rea S, et al. Natural history and clinical outcome of differentiated thyroid carcinoma: a retrospective analysis of 1503 patients treated at a single institution. Ann Oncol 2009; 20(10):1728–35.
10. Amin A, Badwey A, El-Fatah S. Differentiated thyroid carcinoma: an analysis of 249 patients undergoing therapy and aftercare at a single institution. Clin Nucl Med 2014;39(2):142–6.
11. Nixon IJ, Whitcher MM, Palmer FL, et al. The impact of distant metastases at presentation on prognosis in patients with differentiated carcinoma of the thyroid gland. Thyroid 2012;22(9):884–9.
12. Williams SD, Birch R, Einhorn LH. Phase II evaluation of doxorubicin plus cisplatin in advanced thyroid cancer: a Southeastern Cancer Study Group Trial. Cancer Treat Rep 1986;70(3):405–7.
13. Gottlieb JA, Hill CS Jr, Ibanez ML, et al. Chemotherapy of thyroid cancer. An evaluation of experience with 37 patients. Cancer 1972;30(3):848–53.
14. Gottlieb JA, Hill CS Jr. Chemotherapy of thyroid cancer with adriamycin. Experience with 30 patients. N Engl J Med 1974;290(4):193–7.
15. Bukowski RM, Brown L, Weick JK, et al. Combination chemotherapy of metastatic thyroid cancer. Phase II study. Am J Clin Oncol 1983;6(5):579–81.
16. Donato S, Santos R, Simões H, et al. Novel therapies against aggressive differentiated thyroid carcinomas. Int J Endocr Oncol 2018;5(1):IJE05.
17. Brose MS, Nutting CM, Jarzab B, et al. Sorafenib in radioactive iodine-refractory, locally advanced or metastatic differentiated thyroid cancer: a randomised, double-blind, phase 3 trial. Lancet 2014; 384(9940):319–28.
18. Schlumberger M, Tahara M, Wirth LJ, et al. Lenvatinib versus placebo in radioiodine-refractory thyroid cancer. N Engl J Med 2015;372(7):621–30.

19. Groden PJ, Lee TC, Bhattacharyya S, et al. Lenvatinib-associated cervical artery dissections in a patient with radioiodine-refractory metastatic papillary thyroid carcinoma. Front Med (Lausanne) 2017;4:220.
20. Brose MS, Cabanillas ME, Cohen EE, et al. Vemurafenib in patients with BRAF(V600E)-positive metastatic or unresectable papillary thyroid cancer refractory to radioactive iodine: a non-randomised, multicentre, open-label, phase 2 trial. Lancet Oncol 2016;17(9):1272–82.
21. Riesco-Eizaguirre G, Rodriguez I, De la Vieja A, et al. The BRAFV600E oncogene induces transforming growth factor beta secretion leading to sodium iodide symporter repression and increased malignancy in thyroid cancer. Cancer Res 2009;69(21): 8317–25.
22. Dunn LA, Sherman EJ, Baxi SS, et al. Vemurafenib Redifferentiation of BRAF Mutant, RAI-Refractory Thyroid Cancers. J Clin Endocrinol Metab 2018; 104(5):1417–28.
23. Rothenberg SM, McFadden DG, Palmer EL, et al. Redifferentiation of iodine-refractory BRAF V600E-mutant metastatic papillary thyroid cancer with dabrafenib. Clin Cancer Res 2015;21(5): 1028–35.
24. Chow LQ, Santana-Davila R, Pantel A, et al. A phase I study of pazopanib in combination with escalating doses of 131I in patients with well-differentiated thyroid carcinoma borderline refractory to radioiodine. PLoS One 2017;12(6):e0178325.
25. Ho AL, Grewal RK, Leboeuf R, et al. Selumetinib-enhanced radioiodine uptake in advanced thyroid cancer. N Engl J Med 2013;368(7):623–32.
26. Ho A, Dedecjus M, Wirth LJ, et al. ASTRA: a phase III, randomized, placebo-controlled study evaluating complete remission rate (CRR) with short-course selumetinib plus adjuvant radioactive iodine (RAI) in patients (pts) with differentiated thyroid cancer (DTC). Presented at: the 88th Annual Meeting of the American Thyroid Association. Washington, DC, October 3–7, 2018. [Abstract short call oral 8].
27. Xing M. Recent advances in molecular biology of thyroid cancer and their clinical implications. Otolaryngol Clin North Am 2008;41(6):1135–46, ix.
28. Souza EC, Ferreira AC, Carvalho DP. The mTOR protein as a target in thyroid cancer. Expert Opin Ther Targets 2011;15(9):1099–112.
29. Lim SM, Chang H, Yoon MJ, et al. A multicenter, phase II trial of everolimus in locally advanced or metastatic thyroid cancer of all histologic subtypes. Ann Oncol 2013;24(12):3089–94.
30. Schneider TC, de Wit D, Links TP, et al. Everolimus in patients with advanced follicular-derived thyroid cancer: results of a phase II clinical trial. J Clin Endocrinol Metab 2017;102(2):698–707.
31. Hanna GJ, Busaidy NL, Chau NG, et al. Genomic correlates of response to everolimus in aggressive radioiodine-refractory thyroid cancer: a phase II study. Clin Cancer Res 2018;24(7):1546–53.
32. Haddad RI, Nasr C, Bischoff L, et al. NCCN guidelines insights: thyroid carcinoma, version 2.2018. J Natl Compr Cancer Netw 2018;16(12):1429–40.
33. Sherman EJ, Ho AL, Fury MG, et al. Combination of everolimus and sorafenib in the treatment of thyroid cancer: Update on phase II study. J Clin Oncol 2015;33(15_suppl):6069.
34. Greco A, Miranda C, Pierotti MA. Rearrangements of NTRK1 gene in papillary thyroid carcinoma. Mol Cell Endocrinol 2010;321(1):44–9.
35. Mehnert JM, Varga A, Brose M, et al. Pembrolizumab for advanced papillary or follicular thyroid cancer: preliminary results from the phase 1b KEYNOTE-028 study. J Clin Oncol 2016; 34(15_suppl):6091.
36. Hundahl SA, Fleming ID, Fremgen AM, et al. A National Cancer Data Base report on 53,856 cases of thyroid carcinoma treated in the U.S., 1985-1995 [see comments]. Cancer 1998;83(12): 2638–48.
37. Nagaiah G, Hossain A, Mooney CJ, et al. Anaplastic thyroid cancer: a review of epidemiology, pathogenesis, and treatment. J Oncol 2011;2011:542358.
38. McIver B, Hay ID, Giuffrida DF, et al. Anaplastic thyroid carcinoma: a 50-year experience at a single institution. Surgery 2001;130(6):1028–34.
39. Smallridge RC, Ain KB, Asa SL, et al. American Thyroid Association guidelines for management of patients with anaplastic thyroid cancer. Thyroid 2012; 22(11):1104–39.
40. Keutgen XM, Sadowski SM, Kebebew E. Management of anaplastic thyroid cancer. Gland Surg 2015;4(1):44–51.
41. FDA approves dabrafenib plus trametinib for anaplastic thyroid cancer with BRAFV600E mutation. Available at: https://www.fda.gov/drugs/informationondrugs/approveddrugs/ucm606708.htm. Accessed February 1, 2019.
42. Tahara M, Kiyota N, Yamazaki T, et al. Lenvatinib for anaplastic thyroid cancer. Front Oncol 2017;7:25.
43. Ito Y, Onoda N, Ito KI, et al. Sorafenib in Japanese patients with locally advanced or metastatic medullary thyroid carcinoma and anaplastic thyroid carcinoma. Thyroid 2017;27(9):1142–8.
44. Sherman EJ, Dunn LA, Ho AL, et al. Phase 2 study evaluating the combination of sorafenib and temsirolimus in the treatment of radioactive iodine-refractory thyroid cancer. Cancer 2017;123(21): 4114–21.
45. Gramza AW, Balasubramaniam S, Fojo AT, et al. Phase I/II trial of crolibulin and cisplatin in solid tumors with a focus on anaplastic thyroid cancer:

Phase I results. J Clin Oncol 2013;31(15_suppl): 6074.
46. Wirth LJ, Eigendorff E, Capdevila J, et al. Phase I/II study of spartalizumab (PDR001), an anti-PD1 mAb, in patients with anaplastic thyroid cancer. J Clin Oncol 2018;36(15_suppl):6024.
47. Wells SA Jr, Asa SL, Dralle H, et al. Revised American Thyroid Association guidelines for the management of medullary thyroid carcinoma. Thyroid 2015; 25(6):567–610.
48. Sippel RS, Kunnimalaiyaan M, Chen H. Current management of medullary thyroid cancer. Oncologist 2008;13(5):539–47.
49. Lai AZ, Gujral TS, Mulligan LM. RET signaling in endocrine tumors: delving deeper into molecular mechanisms. Endocr Pathol 2007;18(2):57–67.
50. Roman S, Lin R, Sosa JA. Prognosis of medullary thyroid carcinoma: demographic, clinical, and pathologic predictors of survival in 1252 cases. Cancer 2006;107(9):2134–42.
51. Ernani V, Kumar M, Chen AY, et al. Systemic treatment and management approaches for medullary thyroid cancer. Cancer Treat Rev 2016;50: 89–98.
52. Wells SA Jr, Robinson BG, Gagel RF, et al. Vandetanib in patients with locally advanced or metastatic medullary thyroid cancer: a randomized, double-blind phase III trial. J Clin Oncol 2012; 30(2):134–41.
53. Elisei R, Schlumberger MJ, Muller SP, et al. Cabozantinib in progressive medullary thyroid cancer. J Clin Oncol 2013;31(29):3639–46.
54. Chen J, Ji Q, Cao J, et al. A phase II multicenter trial of the multitargeted kinase inhibitor sulfatinib in advanced medullary thyroid cancer (MTC) and radioiodine (RAI)-refractory differentiated thyroid cancer (DTC). J Clin Oncol 2017;35(15_suppl): 6037.
55. Sun Y, Du F, Gao M, et al. Anlotinib for the treatment of patients with locally advanced or metastatic medullary thyroid cancer. Thyroid 2018;28(11): 1455–61.
56. Faggiano A, Modica R, Severino R, et al. The antiproliferative effect of pasireotide LAR alone and in combination with everolimus in patients with medullary thyroid cancer: a single-center, open-label, phase II, proof-of-concept study. Endocrine 2018; 62(1):46–56.
57. Aggarwal R, Smith D, Soares HP, et al. 436PDPreliminary safety and efficacy of rovalpituzumab tesirine in patients with delta-like protein 3-expressing advanced solid tumors. Ann Oncol 2017; 28(suppl_5):145.
58. Drilon AE, Subbiah V, Oxnard GR, et al. A phase 1 study of LOXO-292, a potent and highly selective RET inhibitor, in patients with RET-altered cancers. J Clin Oncol 2018;36(15_suppl):102.
59. Loxo oncology announces LOXO-292 durability update in patients with RET-mutant medullary thyroid cancer and RET fusion-positive thyroid cancer from LIBRETTO-001 at the 88th Annual Meeting of the American Thyroid Association. 2018. Available at: https://ir.loxooncology.com/press-releases. Accessed February 1, 2019.

A Guide to Pheochromocytomas and Paragangliomas

Julie Guilmette, MD[b], Peter M. Sadow, MD, PhD[a,*]

KEYWORDS

• Pheochromocytoma • Paraganglioma • PASS • GAPP • Succinate dehydrogenase

Key points

- Pheochromocytomas and paragangliomas are uncommon chromaffin cell tumors estimated to occur in about 0.4 to 9.5 per 1 million individuals per year.
- Most pheochromocytomas and paragangliomas show the classic zellballen morphology characterized by nests of uniform polygonal chromaffin/chief cells surrounded by support sustentacular cells.
- Nine percent of pheochromocytomas present with a composite morphology made up of ganglioneuroma, ganglioneuroblastoma, neuroblastoma, or peripheral nerve sheath tumors.
- Current (controversial) grading systems include Pheochromocytoma of the Adrenal Gland Scaled Score and Grading System for the Adrenal Pheochromocytoma and Paraganglioma.
- As much as 24% of pheochromocytomas and paragangliomas are part of a hereditary syndrome.

ABSTRACT

Pheochromocytomas and extra-adrenal paragangliomas are rare neuroendocrine neoplasms with characteristic histologic and immunohistochemical features. These tumors can arise in several anatomic locations, necessitating that their diagnostic recognition extends beyond the realm of endocrine disorders. A practical and reproducible risk stratification system for these tumors is still in development. In this rapidly evolving era of molecular medicine, it is essential for pathologists to equip themselves with a framework for understanding the classification of paragangliomas and pheochromocytomas and be informed of how they might advise their colleagues with regard to prognostication and appropriate follow-up.

OVERVIEW

Pheochromocytomas and paragangliomas (PPGLs) are uncommon neural crest–derived tumors estimated to occur in about 0.4 to 9.5 per 1 million individuals per year and in about 0.1% of patients with hypertension.[1–3] Depending on location, they are diagnosed with variable ease and their biological and clinical behavior ranges from benign to potentially aggressive with a high risk of metastasis. Current scoring systems have been variably used in the assessment of risk of metastasis and overall survival, which have contributed to stratifying patient care and treatment. Although most of these tumors occur in isolation, they are clearly associated with several underlying familial/genetic disorders. Identifying the presence of an underlying hereditary cancer

Conflict of Interest: The authors have no conflicts of interest to report.
Ethical Approval: This article does not contain any studies with human participants performed by the authors.
[a] Department of Pathology, Massachusetts General Hospital, Harvard Medical School, 55 Fruit Street, Boston, MA 02114-2696, USA; [b] Department of Pathology, Charles-Lemoyne Hospital, Sherbrooke University Affiliated Health Care Center, 3120 Boulevard Taschereau, Greenfield Park, Quebec J4V 2H1, Canada
* Corresponding author.
E-mail address: psadow@mgh.harvard.edu

Surgical Pathology 12 (2019) 951–965
https://doi.org/10.1016/j.path.2019.08.009

syndrome is critical. Genetic testing and referral are necessary for patients diagnosed with PPGL.

ANATOMIC DISTRIBUTION AND MORPHOLOGY

Pheochromocytomas and extra-adrenal paragangliomas are tumors of neural crest–derived endocrine cells or organs known as paraganglia. The paraganglia occupy several anatomic locations within the body and are categorized as sympathetic or parasympathetic based on location and neural association. They are found in an asymmetric and axial distribution along the supradiaphragmatic branches of the parasympathetic system, including the head and neck and aorticopulmonary region, and interconnect with the sympathetic adrenal neuroendocrine system (**Table 1**).[4]

The largest collection of parasympathetic paraganglia are the carotid bodies in the head and neck region. These small, ovoid structures are located medially to the carotid bifurcation and, in a normal state, they weigh approximately 12 mg combined.[5,6] Other paraganglia are microscopic with variable weights.

Regardless of location, all paraganglia share nearly identical histomorphology. Their key functional units are chromaffin cells or chief cells, which are organized into lobules or nests, also known as zellballen. Supporting sustentacular cells help in maintaining the lobular structures, which are in turn surrounded by a prominent capillary network made up of pericytes, endothelial cells, and Schwann cells. The chromaffin/chief cells belong to the diffuse neuroendocrine system, discrete aggregates of neuroendocrine cells scattered throughout the body, and contain secretory granules and enzymes involved in catecholamine synthesis.[7]

Table 1
Anatomic distribution of paraganglia

System	Locations
Adrenal (sympathetic)	• Adrenal medulla
Extra-adrenal	
Parasympathetic	• Carotid bodies • Middle ear • Adventitia of the jugular bulb • Vagus nerve • Larynx • Aorticopulmonary region • Orbit • Nasal cavity • Nasopharynx • Cheek • Pineal gland • Sellar region • Thyroid gland • Lung
Sympathetic	• Aortic region/organs of Zuckerkandl • Gallbladder • Urinary bladder • Thorax/lung • Spermatic cord • Prostate gland and urethra • Pancreas • Uterus

Data from Sternberg SS, Mills SE, and Carter D. Paragangliomas. In: Mills SE editor. Sternberg's diagnostic surgical pathology, 6th edition (vol 1). Philadelphia: Wolters Kluwer Health/Lippincott Williams & Wilkins; 2015.

PHEOCHROMOCYTOMA AND EXTRA-ADRENAL PARAGANGLIOMA

The updated 2017 World Health Organization (WHO) Classification of Tumors of Endocrine Organs has incorporated new definitions, recent scientific advances, and novel genetic discoveries into the sections dedicated to PPGL. The term pheochromocytoma is now reserved for intra-adrenal tumors, whereas similar tumors arising outside the adrenal medulla are defined as extra-adrenal paragangliomas and further named according to their anatomic origin.[8] In addition, the well-established 10% rule (10% familial/hereditary, 10% malignant, and 10% extra-adrenal) for sympathetic paragangliomas is no longer considered applicable. Recently documented germline mutations characteristic of familial pheochromocytoma/paraganglioma syndromes have increased the percentage of heritable lesions to more than 30%.[9,10]

DIAGNOSIS

CLINICAL PRESENTATION

Clinical manifestations of PPGL diverge in several ways. Most pheochromocytomas are capable of catecholamine overproduction and release, which, in turn, is responsible for the clinical signs and symptoms associated with these tumors.[11,12] More than 95% of patients with functional pheochromocytomas present with variable signs of sustained or paroxysmal hypertension, whereas the remainder are normotensive.[13,14] The classic clinical triad characterized by headaches, tachycardia, and sweating occurs in approximately

25% of patients, with less than half of patients presenting with only 1 of these symptoms.[15] Other nonspecific findings include orthostatic hypotension, pallor, tremors, constipation, and psychological symptoms, including acute anxiety and panic attacks.[16] Functional pheochromocytomas may also cause endocrine paraneoplastic syndromes (PNSs) through the secretion of bioactive substances from tumor cells. The most commonly encountered PNS is Cushing syndrome driven by adrenocorticotropic hormone or corticotropin-releasing hormone secretion. Watery diarrhea, hypokalemia, and achlorhydria syndrome caused by vasoactive intestinal peptide production, and polycythemia arising from erythropoietin (EPO) oversecretion or oversensitivity of EPO receptors, can also occur.[17–21]

Unlike pheochromocytomas, many extra-adrenal paragangliomas are asymptomatic. Although sympathetic paragangliomas are often functional (and therefore may be symptomatic), less than 4% of head and neck paragangliomas are linked to catecholamine overproduction.[22] As a result, many of these parasympathetic paragangliomas are found incidentally by imaging or present as slow-growing painless masses.[23]

BIOCHEMICAL TESTING

When a pheochromocytoma or extra-adrenal paraganglioma is suspected, biochemical analysis can be helpful in making the diagnosis. The Endocrine Society Clinical Guidelines Subcommittee has established biochemical testing recommendations for the diagnosis of PPGL.[24] The initial investigation should include measurements of plasma free metanephrines or urinary fractionated metanephrines. For measurements of plasma free metanephrines, the patient should be in the supine position as the blood is drawn and reference intervals of the supine position should be used. Liquid chromatography with mass spectrometric or electrochemical detection methods are preferred to other laboratory techniques and algorithms to render a diagnosis of PPGL. Patients with positive laboratory results require appropriate clinical follow-up.

MACROSCOPY AND MICROSCOPY

PPGLs are well circumscribed but typically unencapsulated. On cross section, they have a firm, rubbery consistency and vary from pale pink to a dark reddish brown, likely secondary to their well-established vascular network (**Fig. 1**A). On occasion, they show degenerative cystic changes with associated fibrosis and/or hemorrhage. PPGLs are variably sized, but range, on average, between 3 and 6 cm, depending on the site of origin. Some pheochromocytomas have been reported to be more than 10 cm in largest diameter.[25]

Microscopically, PPGLs show mild histologic heterogeneity. Most have the classic zellballen pattern formed by nests of uniform, polygonal chromaffin/chief cells surrounded by sustentacular support cells and well-formed vascular cuffing (**Fig. 1**B). However, when these lesions present with nonclassic morphology, a PPGL diagnosis may be challenging with a broader differential diagnosis, especially in more compact sites, such as the middle ear, with specimens often showing crush artifact. Although unusual, other architectural configurations, such as trabecular, diffuse, and vessel-rich patterns, may be observed.[26] Cytologically, chromaffin/chief cells range from fairly monomorphic polygonal cells with granular basophilic to amphophilic cytoplasm and round vesicular nuclei to cells showing marked pleomorphism with nuclear pseudoinclusions or prominent nucleoli. Less commonly, spindled and oncocytic cells may be observed but generally comprise a small percentage of the tumor. Intracytoplasmic hyaline globules are often present. Necrosis and mitoses are rare and may cause suspicion for more biologically aggressive behavior, and atypical mitoses, under any circumstances, should be especially concerning.

Composite morphology can be found in more than 9% of all pheochromocytomas.[27,28] Composite pheochromocytomas are partly made up of neurogenic tumors such as ganglioneuroma (70%–80% of cases) (**Fig. 2**), ganglioneuroblastoma (10%–20% of cases), and rarely neuroblastoma or peripheral nerve sheath tumors.[29–31] These tumors can arise in either a sporadic setting or as part of a syndrome. About 17% of all documented composite pheochromocytomas are diagnosed in patients with neurofibromatosis type 1 (NF1), with more than half of them presenting as bilateral masses.[31]

IMMUNOHISTOCHEMISTRY

Immunohistochemical studies are usually not needed to confirm the diagnosis of PPGL. Nonetheless, in ambiguous cases, chromaffin/chief cells express neuroendocrine markers, such as synaptophysin, chromogranin A, and CD56 (cluster of differentiation 56) but do not express epithelial markers (**Fig. 1**C–E).[32] Other markers, such as catecholamines, neuron-specific enolase, and neurofilament, may be expressed. If cells fail to stain for chromogranin A, then the diagnosis of PPGL should be reconsidered. In addition, sustentacular cells are highlighted by S100 protein (see **Fig. 1**F), which

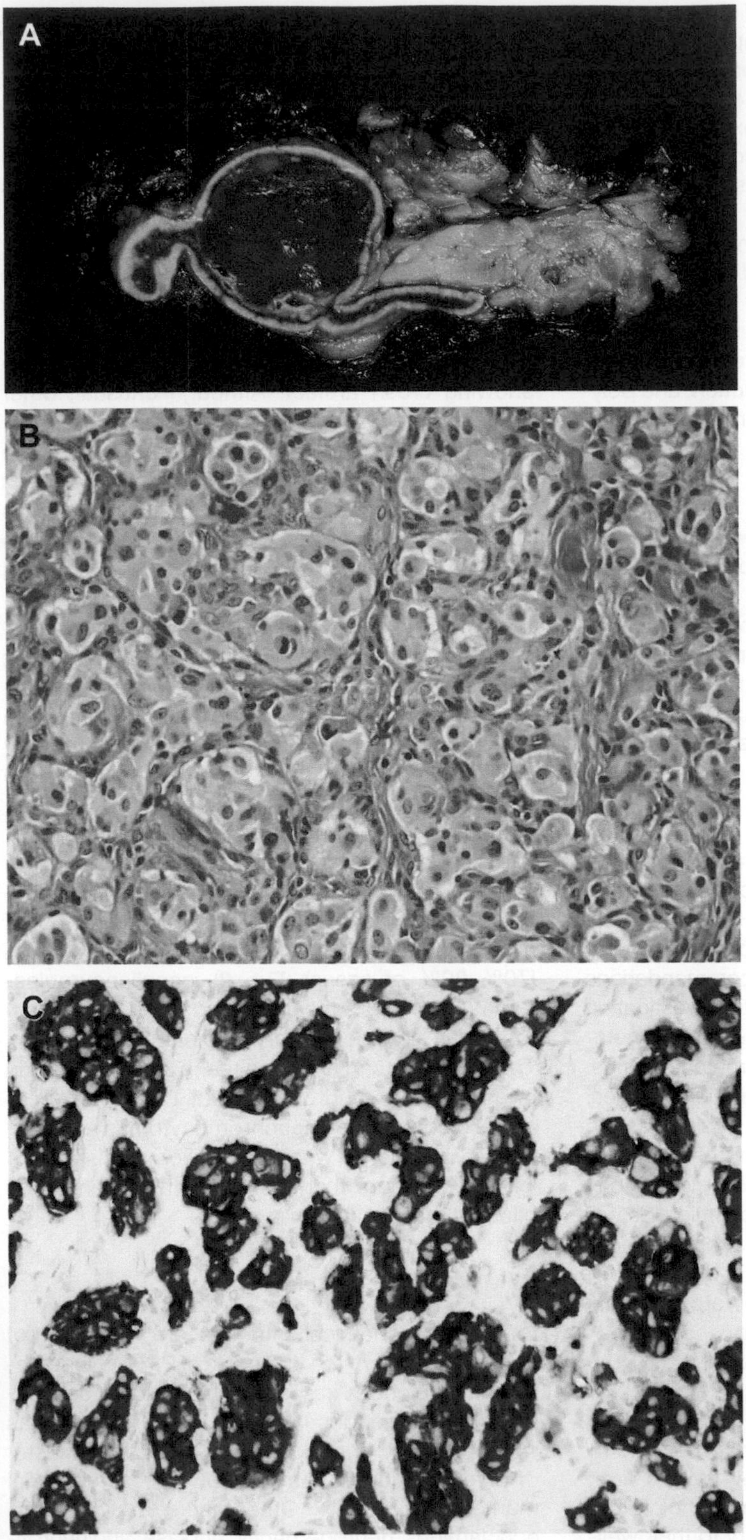

Fig. 1. Pheochromocytoma. (*A*) Gross resection specimen reveals a well-circumscribed tan-brown adrenal medullary mass. Histologic assessment (B-F, original magnification ×400). (*B*) shows the characteristic zellballen morphology with uniform chromaffin cell nests (hematoxylin-eosin). Immunohistochemistry shows the chromaffin cells are positive for. (*C*) synaptophysin.

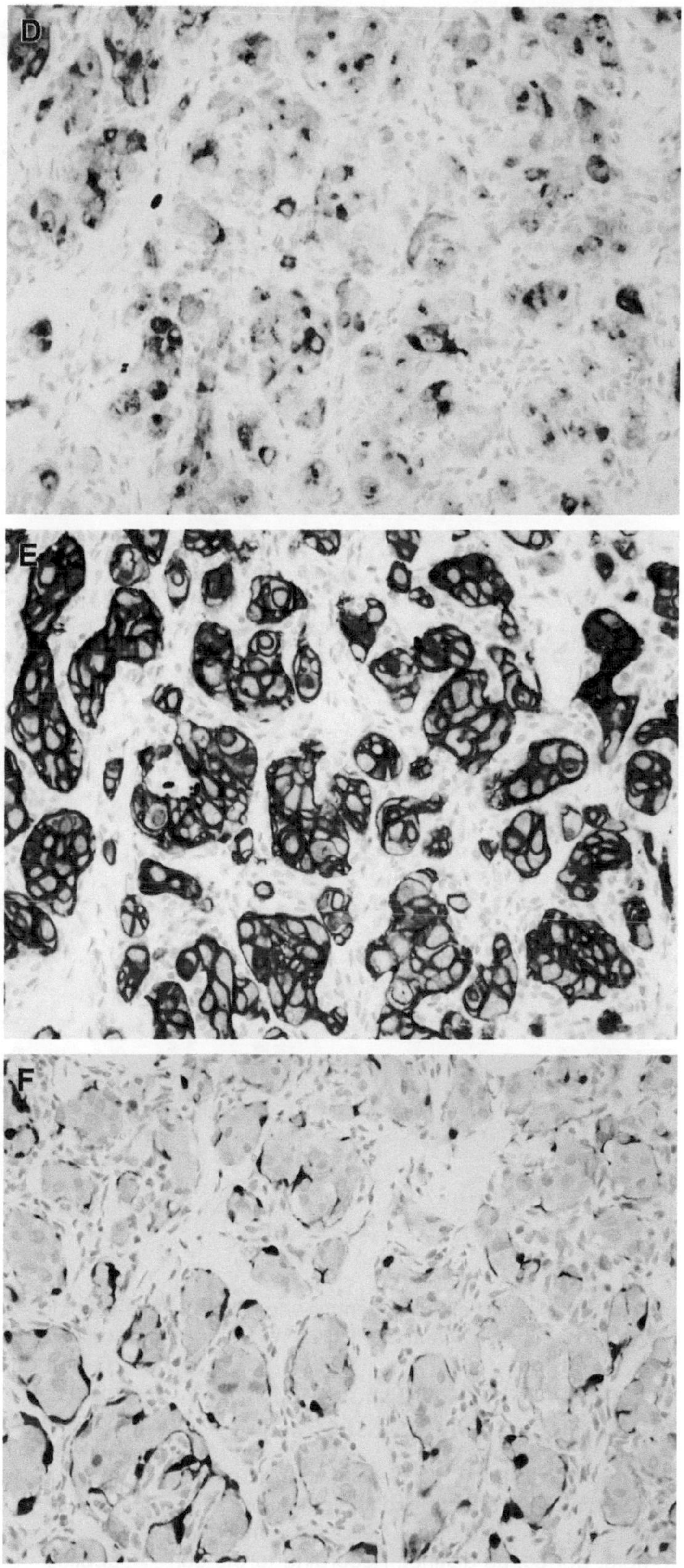

Fig. 1. (*continued*). (*D*) chromogranin A. (*E*) CD56 (cluster of differentiation 56), and (*F*) The sustentacular cells are highlighted by S100.

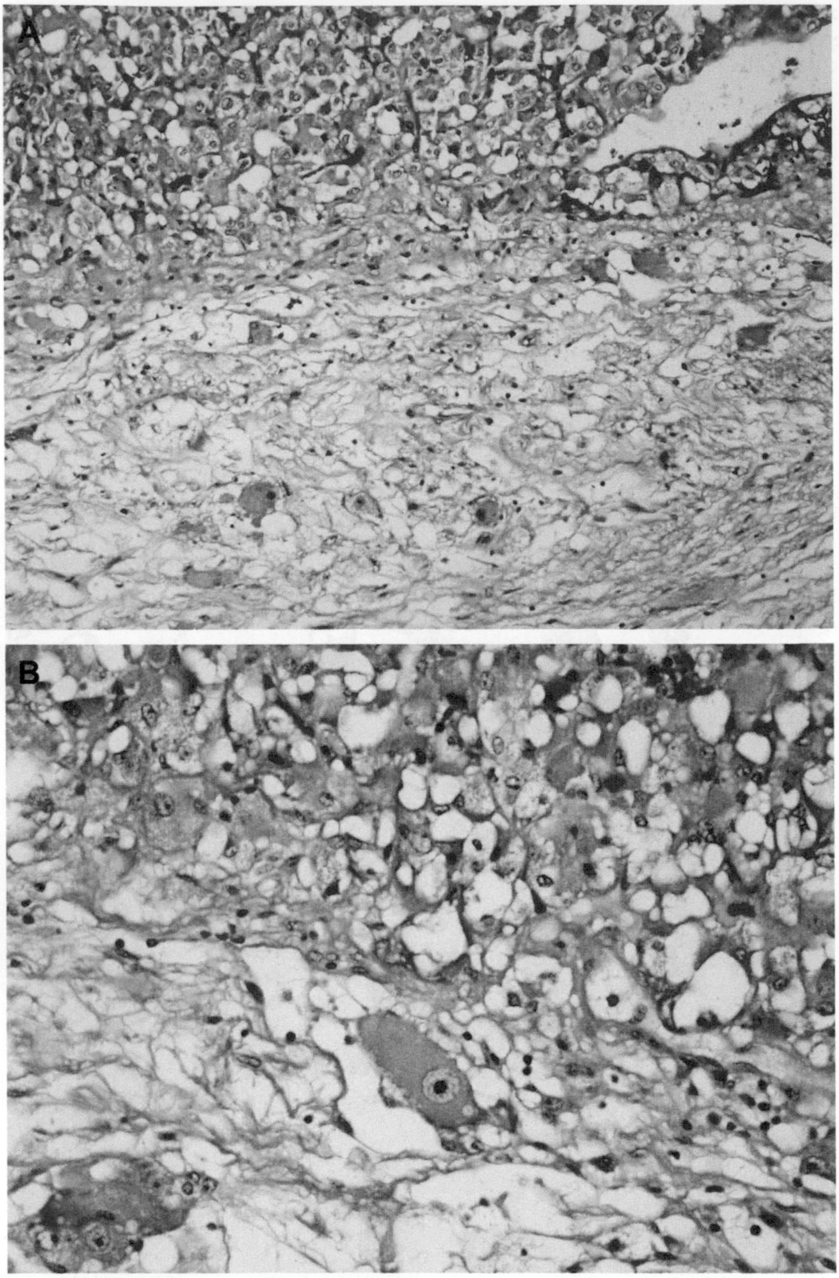

Fig. 2. Composite pheochromocytoma. (*A*, *B*) Typical pheochromocytoma is identified in the upper parts, whereas large ganglion cells compatible with a ganglioneuroma are observed in the lower parts (hematoxylin-eosin, original magnification ×200 [*A*] and ×400 [*B*]).

may be particularly helpful to identify when encountering architectural variants of PPGL.[33]

DETERMINATION OF BIOLOGICAL AGGRESSION AND RISK ASSESSMENT

The newly revised WHO classification considers PPGL to adopt a spectrum of biological behaviors and no longer distinguishes benign and malignant tumors, per se, as distinct. According to the current WHO classification, PPGL should all be considered to have some malignant potential (defined as a risk of metastasis). Determining the magnitude of that risk for individual PPGLs before metastasis is more challenging. At the current time, there is no well-established consensus that can definitively predict the malignant potential of these tumors. Among the most widely used grading systems are Pheochromocytoma of the Adrenal Gland Scaled Score (PASS), which applies solely to pheochromocytoma, and the Grading System for the Adrenal

Pheochromocytoma and Paraganglioma (GAPP), which, as its name implies, applies to both pheochromocytoma and paraganglioma.[34–37]

In 2002, the PASS system was developed to identify pheochromocytomas at risk for metastasis (**Table 2**). PASS evaluates 12 histopathologic parameters that are most commonly observed in metastatic pheochromocytomas and sums to a maximum score of 20 points. Neoplasms with a score greater than or equal to 4 are defined as having increased risk of metastatic potential; those with a score of less than 4 are considered biologically inert.[36] Eight histologic features (large nests, central or confluent tumor necrosis, hypercellularity, cellular spindling, monotonous growth pattern, increased mitotic activity, atypical mitoses, and invasion into surrounding periadrenal soft tissue) are each worth 2 points (**Fig. 3**). The remaining features of vascular invasion, capsular invasion, profound nuclear pleomorphism, and nuclear hyperchromasia score 1 point each. Although its usefulness in predicting metastatic potential has proved controversial and its utility is discounted by most endocrine pathologists, the PASS system is still recognized by clinical colleagues, even requested at some institutions, and therefore warrants presentation at the current time without a recommendation for usage (and is not used by the authors of this article).[38–40]

Recently validated, the GAPP is used for both pheochromocytoma and paraganglioma and incorporates both clinical and histologic parameters[41] (**Table 3**). GAPP provides a stepwise assessment of both metastatic risk and patient survival. Histologic grading is based on a scoring system made up of 6 parameters considered risk factors for metastasis. These parameters are histologic pattern, cellularity, comedo-type necrosis, capsular or vascular invasion, Ki67 proliferative index, and catecholamine phenotype, all summing up to a maximum of 10 possible points. A neoplasm with an overall score ranging from zero to 2 points is considered to be well differentiated. A tumor with an intermediate score ranging from 3 to 6 points is defined as moderately differentiated. A score greater than or equal to 7 is considered to be poorly differentiated.[25,34] Approximately 70% of tumors assessed by GAPP are well-differentiated PPGL and very rarely metastasize. Patients virtually never die of these biologically inert tumors. Moderately differentiated PPGL comprise 20% of PPGLs, with the remaining 10% characterized as poorly differentiated. Both moderately and poorly differentiated PPGLs are associated with an increased metastatic potential, estimated close to 60% and 88%, respectively. The 5-year survival rates of the patients with well-differentiated, moderately differentiated, and poorly differentiated PPGLs are 100%, 67%, and 22%, respectively.[37,41,42] Similar to PASS, because some of the parameters are subjective, reproducibility of GAPP is uncertain, and hence it has not been broadly adopted as a prognostic tool. However, because the validation study is recent, practitioners who treat patients with PPGL may request this evaluation.

Table 2
Grading system for Pheochromocytoma of the Adrenal Gland Scaled Score (PASS)

Histologic Parameters	Points Scored
(1) Large nest of diffuse growth (>10% of tumor volume)	2
(2) Central or confluent tumor necrosis	2
(3) High cellularity	2
(4) Cell spindling (even if focal)	2
(5) Mitotic figures (>3/HPF)	2
(6) Atypical mitotic figure	2
(7) Extension into periadrenal adipose tissue	2
(8) Cellular monotony	2
(9) Vascular invasion	1
(10) Capsular invasion	1
(11) Profound nuclear pleomorphism	1
(12) Nuclear hyperchromasia	1

Abbreviation: HPF, high-power field.

MOLECULAR INSIGHTS AND DISCOVERIES

Although most PPGLs arise sporadically, germline mutations in known susceptibility genes are identified in up to 24% of sporadic-appearing PPGL cases.[43–45] At least 19 hereditary susceptibility genes have been described, namely *NF1*, ATRX Chromatin Remodeler (*ATRX*), HRas Proto-Oncogene, GTPase (*HRAS*), VonHippel-Lindau (*VHL*), endothelial PAS domain-contain protein (*EPAS1*) or HIF2alpha, cyclin dependent kinase inhibitor 2A (*CDKN2A*), rearranged during transfection (RET), tumor protein p53 (*TP53*), hepatocyte growth factor precursor (*MET*), serine/threonine-protein kinase B-Raf (*BRAF*), myc associated facotr X (*MAX*), isocitrate dehydrogenase 1 (*IDH1*), kinesin-like protein KIF1B (*KIF1B*), and succinate dehydrogenase (*SDH*) subunits.[46–49] Somatic mutations of hereditary susceptibility genes can also occur. *NF1* mutations, the most commonly mutated gene, are present in more than 25% of sporadic PPGLs, followed by *VHL*

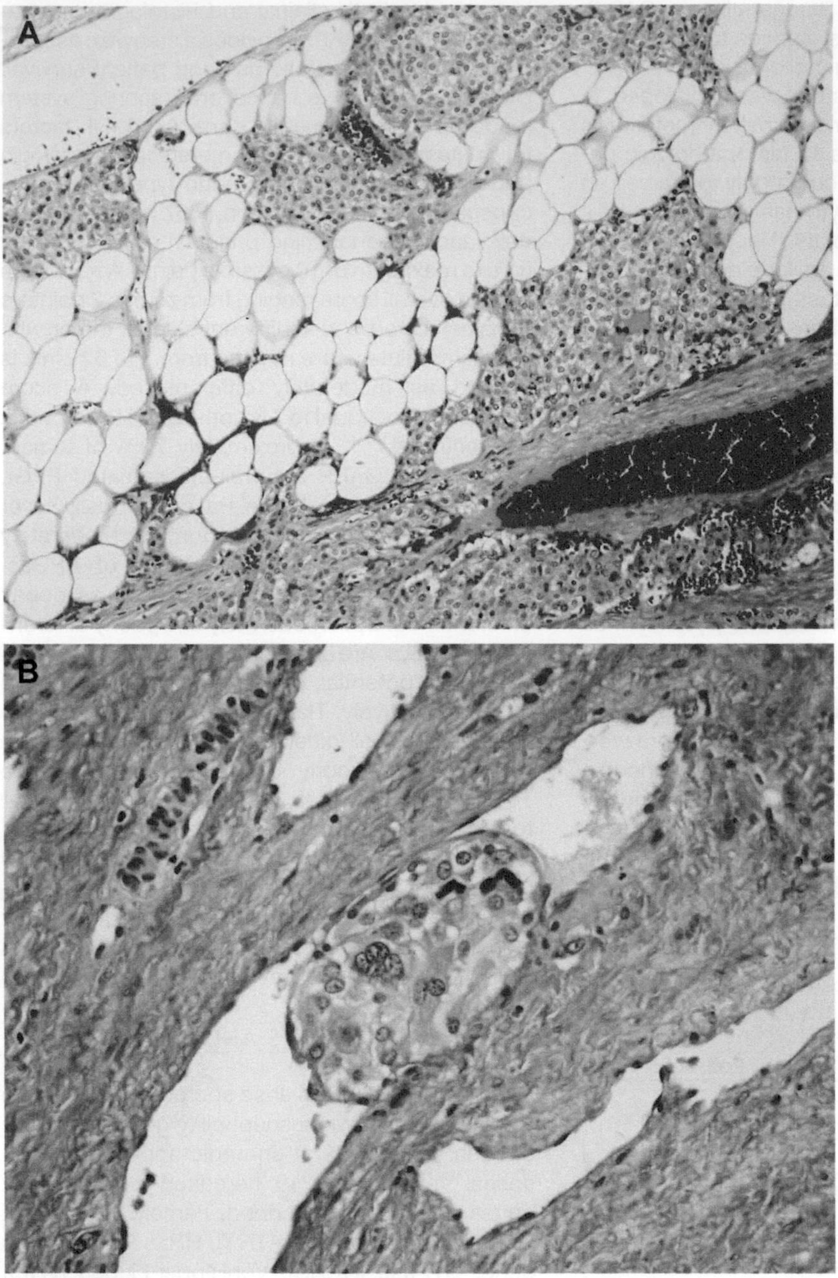

Fig. 3. Risk assessment for PPGL. (*A*) Pheochromocytoma infiltrating the periadrenal adipose tissue (hematoxylin-eosin, original magnification ×200). (*B*) Vascular invasion is also a feature associated with an increased risk of metastasis (hematoxylin-eosin, original magnification ×400).

(9%) and *RET* (5%). In addition, some tumors harbor gain-of-function *EPAS1* mutations.[50]

The 2017 Cancer Genome Atlas (TCGA) study has separated PPGL into 3 clusters or groups with distinct transcriptional and functional profiles.[48] Each cluster has a unique molecular-clinical-biochemical imaging phenotype that can be used for clinical prognostication and to identify biomarkers relevant for personalized care by targeted therapeutics. The first cluster is associated with pseudohypoxic signaling and is subdivided into 2 subgroups: tricarboxylic acid (TCA) cycle-related mutations, involving germline mutations in all 5 of the succinate dehydrogenase (*SDH*) subunits (*SDHA*, *SDHB*, *SDHC*, *SDHD*, and *SDHAF2*) and fumarate hydratase (*FH*), also an enzyme in the TCA cycle; and *VHL/EPAS1*-related mutations.[51] Cluster 1–related PPGLs cause fewer catecholamine-related symptoms than the other 2 clusters. In addition, they have a tendency to

Table 3
Grading system for the adrenal pheochromocytoma and paraganglioma (GAPP)

Parameters	Points Scored
(1) Histologic Pattern	
Classic zellballen	0
Large and irregular cell nest	1
Pseudorosette	1
(2) Cellularity	
Low (<150 cells/U)	0
Moderate (150–250 cells/U)	1
High (>250 cells/U)	2
(3) Comedo necrosis	
Absence	0
Presence	2
(4) Vascular or Capsular Invasion	
Absence	0
Presence	1
(5) Ki67 Proliferative Index (%)	
<1	0
1–3	1
>3	2
(6) Catecholamine Type	
Epinephrine	0
Norepinephrine	1
Nonfunctioning	0

Abbreviation: U, number of tumor cells in a square of a 10-mm micrometer observed under high-power magnification (×400).

grow larger and reach more advanced stages at the time of presentation.[52] The second group is characterized by *Wnt* signaling and includes newly recognized *CSDE1* somatic mutations as well as *MAML3* somatic gene fusion events. This category contains more aggressive PPGLs, with some patients presenting with metastatic disease. The last group consists of abnormalities of tyrosine kinase signaling pathways and encompass germline or somatic mutations in *RET*, *NF1*, *TMEM127*, *MAX*, and *HRAS* genes.[23,48,53] Because of the significant rate of identified susceptibility genes found in PPGL, genetic assessment for at least the most common ones is recommended in patients with or without known family history. Patients with known germline mutations should benefit from appropriate medical referral.[54]

HEREDITARY CANCER SYNDROMES

It was formerly thought that 10% of pheochromocytomas were associated with familial syndromes; however, it is now known that up to 24% of sporadic-appearing PPGLs harbor germline mutations.[43,44,55–59] Familial PPGLs are often multifocal or bilateral and often arise at an earlier age (often in the first 2 decades of life) than sporadic PPGLs, which typically occur following the fourth decade.[12,60] Hereditary PPGLs are often associated with the emergence of other neoplasms. Several hereditary disorders are well known to be associated with development of PPGL (**Table 4**). Among the most common ones are multiple endocrine neoplasia type 2 (MEN2), von Hippel-Lindau (VHL), NF1, and familial pheochromocytoma/paraganglioma syndromes.

MULTIPLE ENDOCRINE NEOPLASIA TYPE 2

MEN2 is a well-known autosomal dominant syndrome caused by activating germline mutations of the *RET* gene, located on chromosome 10q11.2.[61] MEN2 is subdivided into MEN2A and MEN2B. Although similar, MEN2A and MEN2B each have their own clinical features and associated neoplasms. MEN2A is associated with a classic tumor triad. Ninety percent of mutations with MEN2A develop medullary thyroid carcinoma, 50% develop pheochromocytomas, and 20% to 30% have hyperparathyroidism secondary to parathyroid hyperplasia.[62] Patients with MEN2B also present with a similar percentage of medullary thyroid carcinoma and pheochromocytoma but do not manifest parathyroid disease. Pheochromocytomas arising as part of MEN2 syndromes are often associated with adjacent hyperplasia of the adrenal medulla and are usually biologically low risk, with few rare cases reported to show malignant behavior.[63] Although paroxysms of life-threatening hypertension may occur as a result of pheochromocytoma, morbidity and mortality associated with MEN2 are most commonly attributed to medullary thyroid carcinoma.[64]

VON HIPPEL-LINDAU

VHL syndrome is a rare genetic disorder caused by germline mutations in the *VHL* tumor suppressor gene located on chromosome 3p25.3.[65] VHL is characterized by the occurrence of several neoplasms, such as retinal and central nervous system hemangioblastomas, clear cell renal cell carcinoma, various cysts, endolymphatic sac tumors, and neuroendocrine tumors (see **Table 4**). The incidence of this hereditary syndrome is estimated as close to 1 case per 36,000 individuals.[66] VHL is inherited in an autosomal dominant manner and shows a high penetrance rate. As consequence, more than 90% of gene-carrying patients manifest

Table 4
Hereditary syndromes associated with pheochromocytoma and paraganglioma

Syndrome	Inheritance	Chromosome	Genes	Frequency of Mutation (%)	Associated Tumors
MEN2a	Autosomal dominant	10q11.2	*RET*	3–5	MTC and C-cell hyperplasia, parathyroid hyperplasia
MEN2b	Autosomal dominant Sporadic	10q11.2	*RET*	3–5	MTC and C-cell hyperplasia, mucosal neuroma, ganglioneuroma, marfanoid body habitus
VHL	Autosomal dominant	3p25.5	*VHL*	2–9	Cysts of kidney, pancreas, liver, and epididymis; clear cell RCC; hemangioblastoma; pancreatic and other NETs; cerebellar hemangioblastoma; endolymphatic sac tumors; papillary cystadenoma of the epididymis
FPPGL	Autosomal				
PGL1	dominant	11q23	*SDHD*	6–8	RCC, GIST, pituitary adenoma
PGL2	Maternal	—	*SDHAF2*	Rare	None reported
PGL3	imprinting	1q21	*SDHC*	1–2	RCC, GIST
PGL4		1p36.13	*SDHB*	2–7	RCC, GIST, pituitary adenoma
PGL5		—	*SDHA*	1	RCC
NF1	Autosomal dominant	17q11.2	*NF1*	2–4	Neurofibroma, café-au-lait spots, Lisch nodules, GIST, schwannoma, meningioma, optic nerve glioma, MPNST, duodenal NET, juvenile xanthogranuloma
HLRCC	Autosomal dominant	1q42.1	*FH*	1	Leiomyomatosis, RCC
PZS	unknown	2p21	*EPAS1*	Rare	Polycythemia, somatostatinoma, retinal abnormalities, cysts
MAX	Autosomal dominant	14q23.3	*MAX*	1	Renal oncocytoma
TMEM127	Autosomal dominant	2q11.2	*TMEM127*	1	RCC
EGLN1	Unknown	1q42.1	*EGLN1*	Rare	Polycythemia
EGLN2	Unknown	19q13.2	*EGLN2*	Rare	Polycythemia
MDH2	Unknown	7q11.23	*MDH2*	Rare	None reported
KIF1B	Unknown	1p36.22	*KIF1B*	Rare	Ganglioneuroma, leiomyosarcoma, pulmonary adenocarcinoma, neuroblastoma

Abbreviations: FPPGL, familial pheochromocytoma/paraganglioma syndrome; GIST, gastrointestinal spindle cell tumor; HLRCC, hereditary leiomyomatosis and renal cell carcinoma syndrome; MEN2a, multiple endocrine neoplasia type 2a; MEN2b, multiple endocrine neoplasia type 2b; MPNST, malignant peripheral nerve sheath tumor; MTC, medullary thyroid carcinoma; NET, neuroendocrine tumor; PGL1, paraganglioma syndrome type 1; PGL2, paraganglioma syndrome type 2; PGL3, paraganglioma syndrome type 3; PGL4, paraganglioma syndrome type 4; PGL5, paraganglioma type 5; PZS, Pacak-Zhuang syndrome; RCC, renal cell carcinoma; VHL, von Hippel-Lindau.

1 or more of the clinical sequelae of the syndrome by age 65 years and up to 30% develop PPGL at a mean patient age of 30 years.[67–71] More than half of patients with VHL-related PPGLs present with minimal or even no symptoms of catecholamine excess.[12,72,73] Unlike nonhereditary PPGL, PPGLs associated with VHL often have a thick, vessel-rich capsule. The tumor's chromaffin cells frequently contain clear to slightly amphophilic cytoplasm. Hypoxia-inducible factor, a transcription factor linked to the development of VHL phenotypes, is responsible for clear cell changes through the accumulation of lipid and glycogen in tumor cells (**Fig. 4**). In less than 10% of cases, sporadic PPGL may also present with VHL germline mutation without being part of a hereditary syndrome.[43,74,75] Long-term morbidity and mortality associated with VHL are often related to complications from retinal and central nervous system hemangioblastomas and metastatic renal cell carcinoma.[70,71,76,77]

NEUROFIBROMATOSIS TYPE 1

NF1 is an autosomal dominant syndrome caused by mutations in the NF1 gene on chromosome 17q11.2.[78] NF1 is characterized by a constellation of lesions and tumors, especially neurofibromas, which develop in more than 90% of patients with NF1.[79] The occurrence of pheochromocytoma is uncommon, with an estimated lifetime incidence of less than 5% during the fourth or fifth decade.[68,80–83] On histology, NF1-related PPGLs are very similar to the sporadic ones, although NF1-related lesions include composite PPGLs.[84] Although rare, metastatic pheochromocytoma occur in less than 5% of cases.[12]

FAMILIAL PHEOCHROMOCYTOMA/ PARAGANGLIOMA SYNDROMES

Familial pheochromocytoma/paraganglioma syndromes are a group of inherited genetic disorders caused by mutations of the succinate dehydrogenase (*SDH*) gene complex.[43,59,65] Germline mutations in *SDH* genes are responsible for approximately 10% of sporadic PPGLs, 30% of pediatric cases, and more than 80% of familial collections of PPGLs.[85] These *SDH*-related syndromes are inherited in an autosomal dominant manner with a variable penetrance rate. So far, 5 familial PPGL syndromes have been described and are referred to as paraganglioma syndrome (PGL) 1 to 5, in addition to the Carney triad (see **Table 4**).[78,86] Among these, the major PGL syndromes are caused by mutations of the *SDHB* (PGL4), *SDHD* (PGL1) and *SDHC* (PGL3) subunits. PGL4 is characterized by an intermediate penetrance rate, with 40% of patients developing PPGL by the age of 40 years, whereas patients with PGL1 have a penetrance rate of at least 75% by the same age.[86] Both PGL1 and PGL3 are predominantly associated with PGL arising in the head and neck region, with PGL1 lesions often multifocal. PGL4 may also present with head and neck tumors; however, extra-adrenal abdominal and thoracic neoplasms are most frequent. The risk of malignancy varies significantly based on the mutated *SDH* subunit. In PGL4-related tumors, mutation in *SDHB* is associated with

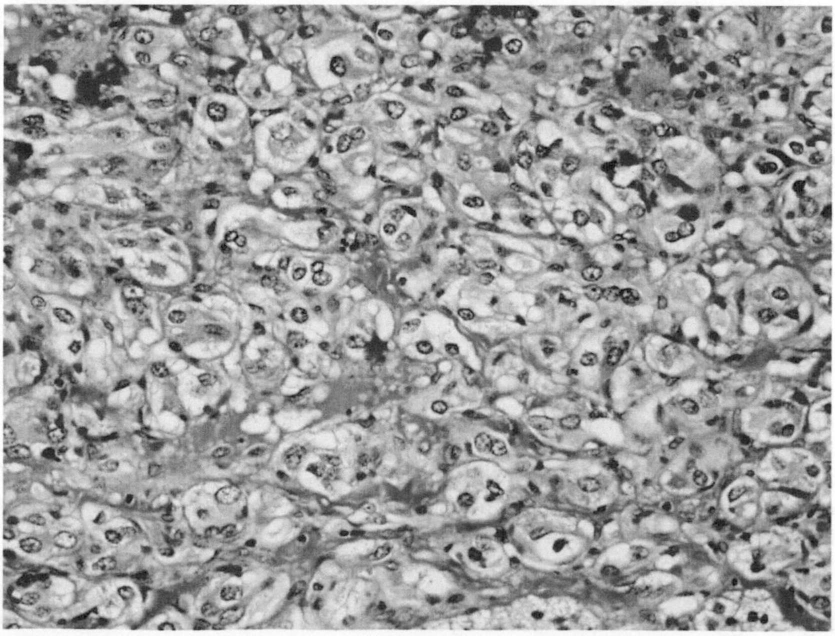

Fig. 4. PPGL in patient with von Hippel-Lindau syndrome. VHL-related paraganglioma shows clear cell changes and mild nuclear atypia (hematoxylin-eosin, original magnification ×400).

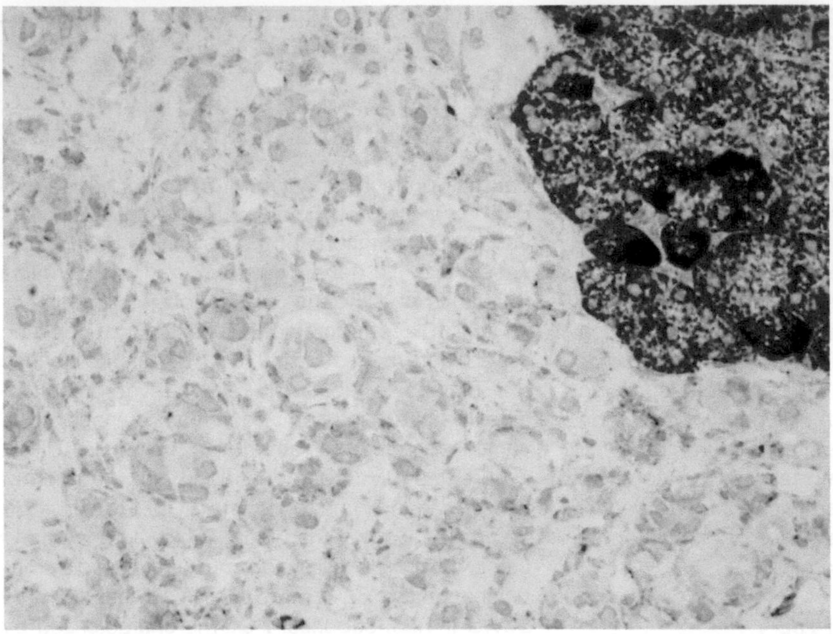

Fig. **5.** Familial pheochromocytoma/paraganglioma syndrome caused by SDH subunit mutation. SDHB immunohistochemistry shows loss of cytoplasmic expression in an SDHB-deficient tumor. Internal positive SDHB control is seen in residual normal chromaffin cells, upper right corner (SDHB, original magnification ×400).

the worst prognosis because at least 30% of these neoplasms metastasize or show extensive multifocality (**Fig. 5**).[87]

PROGNOSIS

Several factors are known to affect morbidity, mortality, and prognosis in patients diagnosed with PPGL. Among them, catecholamine hypersecretion, histologic parameters, *SDHB* mutation, methylation patterns, infiltrative growth, incomplete resection, and metastatic disease all contribute to increased morbidity and mortality.[34,37,44,88,89] The presence of metastases worsens the prognosis by decreasing the overall 5-year survival rate to less than 60%. Metastatic disease involving the liver or lungs decreases the survival time to less than 5 years.[90] Early detection, complete tumor resection, and appropriate clinical follow-up are key management strategies for patients with PPGL.

SUMMARY

Most PPGLs are biologically low-risk neuroendocrine neoplasms with characteristic histologic and immunohistochemical features rendering them, for the most part, especially in the context of preoperative predictive study (imaging/metabolic) modalities, readily identifiable. The complexities regarding their genetic profiling, risk stratification, syndromic association, and, importantly, their potential for biological aggression, require pathologists to extend their knowledge beyond the basic recognition of their histologic parameters. Multidisciplinary care, including pretreatment testing, treatment, diagnosis, and follow-up, and genetic testing/counseling are essential for patients with PPGL. Because pathologists may play the initial role in the diagnosis of PPGL, it is essential for them to know the diagnostic parameters, spectrum of biological behaviors, and next steps for determining underlying genetic alterations in this tumor type. In doing so, pathologists will be key allies in developing appropriate, patient-specific care plans that may expand to additional family members.

REFERENCES

1. Andersen GS. The incidence rate of phaeochromocytoma and Conn's syndrome in Denmark, 1977-1981. J Hum Hypertens 1988;2(3):187–9.
2. Fernandez-Calvet L, Garcia-Mayor RVG. Incidence of pheochromocytoma in South Galicia, Spain. J Intern Med 1994;236(6):675–7.
3. Holland J, Chandurkar V. A retrospective study of surgically excised phaeochromocytomas in Newfoundland, Canada. Indian J Endocrinol Metab 2014;18(4):542–5.
4. Young WF. The incidentally discovered adrenal mass. N Engl J Med 2007;356:601–10.
5. Hart MN, Cyrus A. Hyaline globules of the adrenal medulla. Am J Clin Pathol 1968;49(3):387–91.
6. Dekker A, Oehrle JS. Hyaline globules of the adrenal medulla of man. A product of lipid peroxidation? Arch Pathol 1971;91(4):353–64.

7. Montuenga LM, Guembe L, Burrell MA, et al. The diffuse endocrine system: from embryogenesis to carcinogenesis. Prog Histochem Cytochem 2005; 38(2):155–272.
8. Tischler AS, De Krijger RR, Gill A, et al. Phaeochromocytoma. In: Lloyd RV, Osamura RY, Kloppel G, et al, editors. WHO classification of the tumours of endocrine organs. 4th edition. Lyon (France): International Agency for Research on Cancer); 2017. p. 181–9.
9. Favier J, Amar L, Gimenez-Roqueplo AP. Paraganglioma and phaeochromocytoma: from genetics to personalized medicine. Nat Rev Endocrinol 2015; 11(2):101–11.
10. Pacak K, Wimalawansa S. Pheochromocytoma and paraganglioma. Endocr Pract 2015;21(3):406–12.
11. Eisenhofer G, Lenders J, Pacak K. Biochemical diagnosis of pheochromocytoma. Front Horm Res 2004;31(1):76–106.
12. Lenders J, Eisenhofer G, Mannelli M, et al. Phaechromocytoma. Lancet 2005;366(9486):665–75.
13. Calhoun DA, Jones D, Textor S, et al. Resistant hypertension: diagnosis, evaluation, and treatment a scientific statement from the american heart association professional education committee of the council for high blood pressure research. Circulation 2008;117(25):e510–26.
14. Guérin M, Guillemot J, Thouënnon E, et al. Granins and their derived peptides in normal and tumoral chromaffin tissue: implications for the diagnosis and prognosis of pheochromocytoma. Regul Pept 2010;165(1):21–9.
15. Baguet J-P, Hammer L, Mazzuco TL, et al. Circumstances of discovery of phaeochromocytoma: a retrospective study of 41 consecutive patients. Eur J Endocrinol 2004;150(5):681–6.
16. Young WF, Maddox DE. Spells: in search of a cause. Mayo Clin Proc 1995;70(8):757–65.
17. Nijhoff MF, Dekkers OM, Vleming LJ, et al. ACTH-producing pheochromocytoma: clinical considerations and concise review of the literature. Eur J Intern Med 2009;20(7):682–5.
18. Bayraktar F, Kebapcilar L, Kocdor MA, et al. Cushing's syndrome due to ectopic CRH secretion by adrenal pheochromocytoma accompanied by renal infarction. Exp Clin Endocrinol Diabetes 2006; 114(8):444–7.
19. Loehry CA, Kingham JGC, Whorwell PJ. Watery diarrhoea and hypokalaemia associated with a phaeochromocytoma. Postgrad Med J 1975;51(596): 416–9.
20. Pacak K, Jochmanova I, Prodanov T, et al. New syndrome of paraganglioma and somatostatinoma associated with polycythemia. J Clin Oncol 2013; 31(13):1690–8.
21. Yang C, Zhuang Z, Fliedner SMJ, et al. Germ-line PHD1 and PHD2 mutations detected in patients with pheochromocytoma/paraganglioma-polycythemia. J Mol Med 2015;93(1):93–104.
22. Erickson D, Kudva YC, Ebersold MJ, et al. Benign paragangliomas: Clinical presentation and treatment outcomes in 236 patients. J Clin Endocrinol Metab 2001;86(11):5210–6.
23. Piccini V, Rapizzi E, Bacca A, et al. Head and neck paragangliomas: genetic spectrum and clinical variability in 79 consecutive patients. Endocr Relat Cancer 2012;19(2):149–55.
24. Lenders JWM, Duh QY, Eisenhofer G, et al. Pheochromocytoma and paraganglioma: An endocrine society clinical practice guideline. J Clin Endocrinol Metab 2014;99(6):1915–42.
25. Tischler AS, De Krijger RR. Pathology of pheochromocytoma and paraganglioma. Endocr Relat Cancer 2015;22:T123–33.
26. Shin W-Y, Groman GS, Berkman JI. Pheochromocytoma with angiomatous features. A case report and ultrastructural study. Cancer 1977;40(1):275–83.
27. Lam KY, Lo CY. Composite pheochromocytoma-ganglioneuroma of the adrenal gland: An uncommon entity with distinctive clinicopathologic features. Endocr Pathol 1999;10(4):343–52.
28. Ilona Linnoila R, Keiser HR, Steinberg SM, et al. Histopathology of benign versus malignant sympathoadrenal paragangliomas: Clinicopathologic study of 120 cases including unusual histologic features. Hum Pathol 1990;21(11):1168–80.
29. Baisakh MR, Mohapatra N, Adhikary SD, et al. Malignant peripheral nerve sheath tumor of adrenal gland with heterologus osseous differentiation in a case of von Recklinghausen's disease. Indian J Pathol Microbiol 2014;57(1):130–2.
30. Namekawa T, Utsumi T, Imamoto T, et al. Composite pheochromocytoma with a malignant peripheral nerve sheath tumor: case report and review of the literature. Asian J Surg 2016;39(3):187–90.
31. Khan A, Solomon S, Childress R. Composite pheochromocytoma-ganglioneuroma: a rare experiment of nature. Endocr Pract 2009;5(2):115–8.
32. Chetty R, Pillay P, Jaichand V. Cytokeratin expression in adrenal phaeochromocytomas and extra-adrenal paragangliomas. J Clin Pathol 1998;51(6):477–8.
33. Salmenkivi K, Haglund C, Arola J, et al. Increased expression of tenascin in pheochromocytomas correlates with malignancy. Am J Surg Pathol 2001; 25(11):1419–23.
34. Kimura N, Takayanagi R, Takizawa N, et al. Pathological grading for predicting metastasis in phaeochromocytoma and paraganglioma. Endocr Relat Cancer 2014;21(3):405–14.
35. Kimura N, Watanabe T, Noshiro T, et al. Histological grading of adrenal and extra-adrenal pheochromocytomas and relationship to prognosis: a clinicopathological analysis of 116 adrenal pheochromocytomas and 30 extra-adrenal sympathetic paragangliomas

including 38 malignant tumors. Endocr Pathol 2005; 16(1):23–32.
36. Thompson LDR. Pheochromocytoma of the adrenal gland scaled score (PASS) to separate benign from malignant neoplasms: a clinicopathologic and immunophenotypic study of 100 cases. Am J Surg Pathol 2002;26(5):551–66.
37. Kimura N, Takekoshi K, Naruse M. Risk stratification on pheochromocytoma and paraganglioma from laboratory and clinical medicine. J Clin Med 2018; 7(9):E242.
38. Strong VE, Kennedy T, Al-Ahmadie H, et al. Prognostic indicators of malignancy in adrenal pheochromocytomas: clinical, histopathologic, and cell cycle/apoptosis gene expression analysis. Surgery 2008; 143(6):759–68.
39. Agarwal A, Mehrotra PK, Jain M, et al. Size of the tumor and pheochromocytoma of the adrenal gland scaled score (PASS): Can they predict malignancy? World J Surg 2010;34(12):3022–8.
40. Gao B, Meng F, Bian W, et al. Development and validation of pheochromocytoma of the adrenal gland scaled score for predicting malignant pheochromocytomas. Urology 2006;68(2):282–6.
41. Koh JM, Ahn SH, Kim H, et al. Validation of pathological grading systems for predicting metastatic potential in pheochromocytoma and paraganglioma. PLoS One 2017;12(11):e0187398.
42. Stenman A, Zedenius J, Juhlin CC. The value of histological algorithms to predict the malignancy potential of pheochromocytomas and abdominal paragangliomas—A meta-analysis and systematic review of the literature. Cancers (Basel) 2019;11(2):E225.
43. Neumann HPH, Bausch B, McWhinney SR, et al. Germ-line mutations in nonsyndromic pheochromocytoma. N Engl J Med 2002;346(19):1459–66.
44. Amar L, Bertherat J, Baudin E, et al. Genetic testing in pheochromocytoma or functional paraganglioma. J Clin Oncol 2005;23(34):8812–8.
45. Brito JP, Asi N, Bancos I, et al. Testing for germline mutations in sporadic pheochromocytoma/paraganglioma: a systematic review. Clin Endocrinol (Oxf) 2015;82(3):338–45.
46. Martucci VL, Pacak K. Pheochromocytoma and paraganglioma: diagnosis, genetics, management, and treatment. Curr Probl Cancer 2014;38(1):7–41.
47. Crona J, Taïeb D, Pacak K. New perspectives on pheochromocytoma and paraganglioma: toward a molecular classification. Endocr Rev 2017;38(6):489–515.
48. Fishbein L, Leshchiner I, Walter V, et al. Comprehensive molecular characterization of pheochromocytoma and paraganglioma. Cancer Cell 2017;31(2):181–93.
49. Jochmanova I, Pacak K. Genomic landscape of pheochromocytoma and paraganglioma. Trends Cancer 2018;4(1):6–9.
50. Koch CA, Huang SC, Moley JF, et al. Allelic imbalance of the mutant and wild-type RET allele in MEN 2A-associated medullary thyroid carcinoma. Oncogene 2001;20(53):7809–11.
51. Gimenez-Roqueplo AP, Dahia PL, Robledo M. An update on the genetics of paraganglioma, pheochromocytoma, and associated hereditary syndromes. Horm Metab Res 2012;44(5):328–33.
52. Haissaguerre M, Courel M, Caron P, et al. Normotensive incidentally discovered pheochromocytomas display specific biochemical, cellular, and molecular characteristics. J Clin Endocrinol Metab 2013; 98(11):4346–54.
53. Crona J, Verdugo AD, Granberg D, et al. Next-generation sequencing in the clinical genetic screening of patients with pheochromocytoma and paraganglioma. Endocr Connect 2016;2(2):104–11.
54. Banks KC, Moline JJ, Marvin ML, et al. 10 rare tumors that warrant a genetics referral. Fam Cancer 2013;12(1):1–18.
55. Astuti D, Latif F, Dallol A, et al. Gene mutations in the succinate dehydrogenase subunit SDHB cause susceptibility to familial pheochromocytoma and to familial paraganglioma. Am J Hum Genet 2002; 69(1):49–54.
56. Mannelli M, Simi L, Gaglianò MS, et al. Genetics and biology of pheochromocytoma. Exp Clin Endocrinol Diabetes 2007;115(3):160–5.
57. Niemann S, Muller U. Mutations in SDHC cause autosomal dominant paraganglioma, type 3. Nat Genet 2000;26(3):268–70.
58. Baysal BE, Ferrell RE, Willett-Brozick JE, et al. Mutations in SDHD, a mitochondrial complex II gene, in hereditary paraganglioma. Science 2000; 287(5454):848–51.
59. Sanchez Cifuentes A, Candel Arenas MF, Albarracín Marín-Blazquez A. Hereditary paraganglioma-pheochromocytoma syndrome. Med Clin (Barc) 2018;151(10):e57–8.
60. Walther MM, Keiser HR, Linehan WM. Pheochromocytoma: evaluation, diagnosis, and treatment. World J Urol 2002;17(1):35–9.
61. Moline J, Eng C. Multiple endocrine neoplasia type 2: an overview. Genet Med 2011;13(9):755–64.
62. Guilmette J, Nosé V. Hereditary and familial thyroid tumours. Histopathology 2018;72(1):70–81.
63. Modigliani E, Vasen HM, Raue K, et al. Pheochromocytoma in multiple endocrine neoplasia type 2: European study. J Intern Med 1995;238(4):363–7.
64. Moraitis A, Martucci V, Pacak K. Genetics, diagnosis, and management of medullary thyroid carcinoma and pheochromocytoma/paraganglioma. Endocr Pract 2014;20(2):176–87.
65. King KS, Pacak K. Familial pheochromocytomas and paragangliomas. Mol Cell Endocrinol 2013; 386(1–2):92–100.
66. Richard S, Gardie B, Couvé S, et al. Von Hippel-Lindau: how a rare disease illuminates cancer biology. Semin Cancer Biol 2013;23(1):26–37.

67. Lonser RR, Glenn GM, Walther M, et al. von Hippel-Lindau disease. Lancet 2003;361(9374):2059–67.
68. Walther MM, Reiter R, Keiser HR, et al. Clinical and genetic characterization of pheochromocytoma in von Hippel- Lindau families: Comparison with sporadic pheochromocytoma gives insight into natural history of pheochromocytoma. J Urol 1999;162(3Pt 1):659–64.
69. Maher ER, Neumann HP, Richard S. von Hippel-Lindau disease: a clinical and scientific review. Eur J Hum Genet 2011;19(6):617–23.
70. Tsang SH, Sharma T. Von Hippel-Lindau disease. Adv Exp Med Biol 2018;1085(1):123–35.
71. Chou A, Toon C, Pickett J, et al. Von Hippel-Lindau syndrome. Front Horm Res 2013;41(1):30–49.
72. Eisenhofer G, Walther MM, Huynh TT, et al. Pheochromocytomas in von Hippel-Lindau syndrome and multiple endocrine neoplasia type 2 display distinct biochemical and clinical phenotypes. J Clin Endocrinol Metab 2001;86(5):1999–2008.
73. Neumann H, Berger DP, Sigmund G, et al. Pheochromocytomas, multiple endocrine neoplasia type 2, and von Hippel-Lindau Disease. N Engl J Med 2002;329(21):1531–8.
74. Brauch H, Hoeppner W, Jähnig H, et al. Sporadic pheochromocytomas are rarely associated with germline mutations in the vhl tumor suppressor gene or the ret protooncogene. J Clin Endocrinol Metab 1997;82(12):4101–4.
75. Van der Harst E, De Krijger RR, Dinjens WNM, et al. Germline mutations in the vhl gene in patients presenting with phaeochromocytomas. Int J Cancer 1998;77(3):337–40.
76. Friedrich CA. Von Hippel-Lindau syndrome. A pleomorphic condition. Cancer 1999;86(suppl 11): 2478–82.
77. Varshney N, Kebede AA, Owusu-Dapaah H, et al. A review of Von Hippel-Lindau syndrome. J Kidney Cancer VHL 2017;4(3):20–9.
78. Welander J, Söderkvist P, Gimm O. Genetics and clinical characteristics of hereditary pheochromocytomas and paragangliomas. Endocr Relat Cancer 2011;18(6):R253–76.
79. Wu J, Williams JP, Rizvi TA, et al. Plexiform and dermal neurofibromas and pigmentation are caused by NF1 loss in desert hedgehog-expressing cells. Cancer Cell 2008;13(2):105–16.
80. Bausch B, Koschker AC, Fassnacht M, et al. Comprehensive mutation scanning of NF1 in apparently sporadic cases of pheochromocytoma. J Clin Endocrinol Metab 2006;91(9):3478–81.
81. Machens A, Brauckhoff M, Gimm O, et al. Risk-oriented approach to hereditary adrenal pheochromocytoma. Front Horm Res 2006;1073(1):417–28.
82. Huson SM, Compston DAS, Harper PS. A genetic study of von Recklinghausen neurofibromatosis in south east Wales. II Guidelines for genetic counselling. J Med Genet 1989;26(11):712–21.
83. Peczkowska M, Kowalska A, Sygut J, et al. Testing new susceptibility genes in the cohort of apparently sporadic phaeochromocytoma/paraganglioma patients with clinical characteristics of hereditary syndromes. Clin Endocrinol (Oxf) 2013;79(6):817–23.
84. Kimura N, Watanabe T, Fukase M, et al. Neurofibromin and NF1 gene analysis in composite pheochromocytoma and tumors associated with von Recklinghausen's disease. Mod Pathol 2002;15(3): 183–8.
85. Pasini B, Stratakis CA. SDH mutations in tumorigenesis and inherited endocrine tumours: lesson from the phaeochromocytoma-paraganglioma syndromes. J Intern Med 2009;266(1):19–42.
86. Benn DE, Robinson BG, Clifton-Bligh RJ. Clinical manifestations of paraganglioma syndromes types 1-5. Endocr Relat Cancer 2015;22(4):T91–103.
87. Fliedner SMJ, Lehnert H, Pacak K. Metastatic paraganglioma. Semin Oncol 2010;37(6):627–37.
88. Kimura N, Takekoshi K, Horii A, et al. Clinicopathological study of SDHB mutation-related pheochromocytoma and sympathetic paraganglioma. Endocr Relat Cancer 2014;21(3):L13–6.
89. Blank A, Schmitt AM, Korpershoek E, et al. SDHB loss predicts malignancy in pheochromocytomas/ sympathethic paragangliomas, but not through hypoxia signalling. Endocr Relat Cancer 2010;17(4): 919–28.
90. Pacak K, Eisenhofer G, Ahlman H, et al. Pheochromocytoma: recommendations for clinical practice from the first international symposium. Nat Clin Pract Endocrinol Metab 2007;3(2):92–102.

A Diagnostic Approach to Adrenocortical Tumors

Anjelica Hodgson, MD[a], Sara Pakbaz, MD[b], Ozgur Mete, MD[c,d,*]

KEYWORDS

- Adrenal gland • Cushing syndrome • Primary aldosteronism • Virilism and feminization
- Adrenal cortical adenoma • Adrenal cortical carcinoma • Nodular cortical disease • IGF-2

Key points

- Confirmation of adrenocortical origin, distinction of benign from malignant lesions, providing prognostic information in adrenocortical carcinoma, and correlation of laboratory results with clinicopathologic findings are among the critical responsibilities of pathologists who evaluate adrenocortical lesions.
- Several scoring schemes and algorithms have traditionally been used to distinguish adrenocortical adenomas from carcinomas.
- Immunohistochemical biomarkers and molecular diagnostics can distinguish adrenocortical carcinomas from adrenocortical adenomas and can also provide important prognostic information.
- Advances in molecular biology have resulted in better understanding of the pathogenesis and molecular characteristics of adrenocortical tumors.

ABSTRACT

Adrenocortical tumors range from primary bilateral micronodular or macronodular forms of adrenocortical disease to conventional adrenocortical adenomas and carcinomas. Accurate classification of these neoplasms is critical given the varied pathogenesis, clinical behavior, and outcome of these different lesions. Confirmation of adrenocortical origin, diagnosing malignancy, providing relevant prognostic information in adrenocortical carcinoma, and correlation of laboratory results with clinicopathologic findings are among the important responsibilities of pathologists who evaluate these lesions. This article focuses on a practical approach to the evaluation of adrenocortical tumors with an emphasis on clinical and imaging findings, morphologic characteristics, and multifactorial diagnostic schemes and algorithms.

OVERVIEW

Adrenocortical tumors (ACTs), as the name implies, originate within the adrenal cortex. The cortex makes up the outer portion of the adrenal gland and is composed of 3 histologic zones: zona glomerulosa (ZG), zona fasciculata (ZF), and zona reticularis (ZR). Each zone possesses specific histomorphologic and ultrastructural features as well as distinct functional capabilities related to hormone production.[1]

Disclosure: The authors have nothing to disclose.
[a] Department of Laboratory Medicine and Pathobiology, The University of Toronto, 1 King's College Circle, Medical Sciences Building, Toronto, Ontario M5S1A8, Canada; [b] Department of Pathology, University Health Network, The University of Toronto, 200 Elizabeth Street, 11th Floor, Toronto, Ontario M5G2C4, Canada; [c] Department of Pathology, University Health Network, 200 Elizabeth Street, 11th Floor, Toronto, Ontario M5G2C4, Canada; [d] Department of Laboratory Medicine and Pathobiology, The University of Toronto, Toronto, Ontario, Canada
* Corresponding author.
E-mail address: ozgur.mete2@uhn.ca

Surgical Pathology 12 (2019) 967–995
https://doi.org/10.1016/j.path.2019.08.005

Because of the increasing use of diagnostic imaging, lesions arising in the adrenal cortex, both symptomatic and asymptomatic, are being identified with growing frequency. Once an adrenocortical nodule is identified, the diagnostic considerations that must be considered range from indolent and benign, such as adrenal cortical adenoma (ACA), to often aggressive and malignant, such as adrenal cortical carcinoma (ACC). In addition to these well-recognized conventional entities, advances in molecular biology and identification of clonality in the setting of bilateral nodular forms of adrenocortical hyperplasia have brought entities such as primary bilateral macronodular adrenocortical disease (also known as primary bilateral macronodular adrenocortical hyperplasia [PBMAH]) and primary pigmented micronodular adrenocortical disease (PPNAD) into the spectrum of clonal lesions to be considered under the adrenocortical neoplasia umbrella. Accurate classification of ACTs is critical given the varied pathogenesis, clinical behavior, and outcome of these lesions.

In this article, an approach to the evaluation of ACTs is discussed, with an emphasis on important clinical information along with macroscopic and microscopic features, diagnostic scoring schemes, molecular biology, and ancillary tests.

CLINICAL, BIOCHEMICAL, AND RADIOLOGICAL FEATURES OF ADRENOCORTICAL TUMORS

Adrenal nodules are common, with an estimated 10% of the population thought to harbor some sort of adrenal cortical lesion.[2] These lesions span a proliferative spectrum on which adrenocortical hyperplasia (a reversible and genetically stable process), clonal nodules of PBMAH and PPNAD (irreversible processes with distinct genetic signatures), ACA, and ACC must be considered. A distinct functional adrenocortical lesion lacking features of malignancy is designated an ACA, whereas incidentally discovered nonfunctional adrenocortical nodules less than 1.0 cm are often designated as cortical nodular disease (**Fig. 1**). There is evidence to suggest that an adrenocortical nodule as small as 3 to 5 mm may indeed be clonal[3,4]; therefore, the concept of cortical nodular disease also encompasses small adenomas.

ACAs are more common than ACCs; about 5% of the general population is estimated to harbor an ACA, whereas ACCs are seen in less than 2 per million people.[2,5,6] With the exception of familial cases, ACCs typically present in the fourth and fifth decades of life and more commonly in

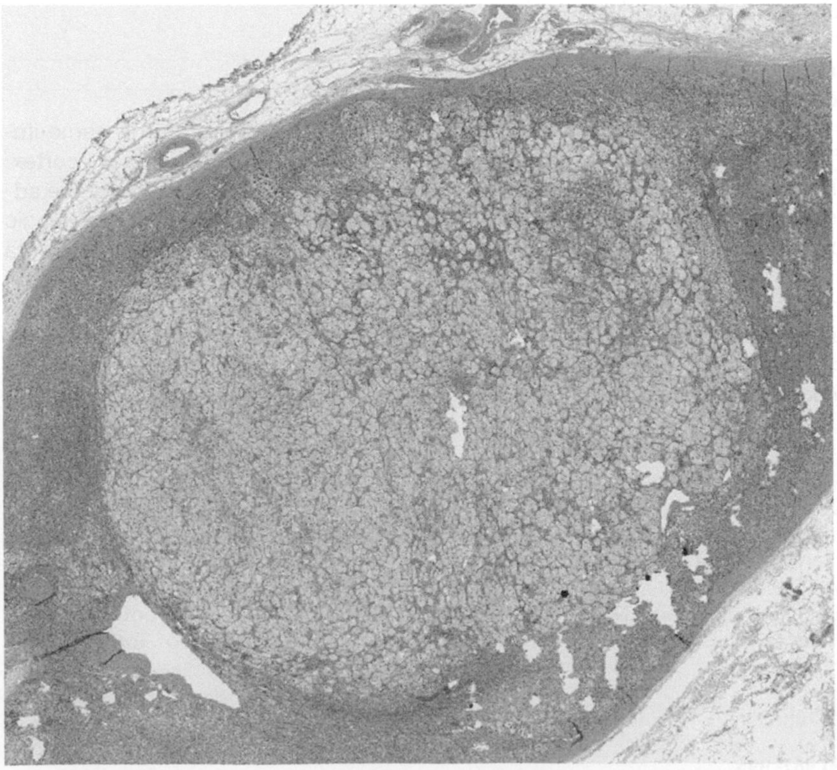

Fig. 1. Cortical nodular disease. A 0.5-cm clear cell–rich cortical nodular proliferation, consistent with cortical nodular disease. These proliferations refer to incidentally discovered nonfunctional benign adrenocortical nodules less than 1.0 cm.

women, whereas ACAs occur in all age groups and affect men and women equally. Given that primary adrenocortical lesions arise from hormone-producing cells, it is no surprise that these lesions may be hormonally active and cause clinical signs and symptoms related to hormone excess. Based on the presence or absence of hormonal activity, ACTs are classified as functional or nonfunctional, respectively. Several hormones can be produced by functional ACTs, including mineralocorticoids (aldosterone), glucocorticoids (cortisol), and sex steroids (androgens). **Table 1** summarizes the key clinical, biochemical, and clinicopathologic features of functioning ACTs.[6–12] Importantly, primary aldosteronism is extremely rare in ACCs, whereas virilization and sex hormone excess are

Table 1
Brief overview of clinical, biochemical, and pathologic features of functional adrenocortical proliferations

	Associated Endocrinopathies		
	Mineralocorticoid Excess (Primary Aldosteronism)	**Glucocorticoid Excess (Adrenal Cushing Syndrome)**	**Sex Steroid Excess (Feminization and Virilization Syndrome)**
Clinical Features	Third-sixth decade; equal male/female ratio Hypertension with hypokalemia or normokalemia; nonspecific symptoms including muscle weakness, easy fatigability, headache, palpitations, nocturia, polyuria, and polydipsia	Any age; women affected more commonly than men Central obesity, facial rounding, hirsutism, easy bruising, skin striae, poor wound healing, muscle weakness, hypertension, hyperglycemia, osteoporosis in adulthood; weight gain and growth failure in childhood; subclinical Cushing syndrome	Variable clinical findings based on the patient's age, gender, and level of hormone excess; virilization in women (increased muscle mass and facial hair, deep voice and amenorrhea); in prepuberty age (pubic hair growth); feminization in men (gynecomastia and impotence)
Biochemical Aspects	Increased plasma aldosterone and high plasma aldosterone/renin ratio following an aldosterone suppression test Preoperative bilateral adrenal venous sampling for aldosterone/cortisol ratio or lateralization index with or without cosyntropin stimulation	Increased cortisol level in at least 2 endocrine assays (ie, baseline morning and evening measurements of 24-h urinary free cortisol, serum free cortisol, or late-night salivary free cortisol), autonomy confirmed by a dexamethasone suppression test. Plasma ACTH is also measured	Increased level of DHEA, DHEA-S, androstenedione, dihydrotestosterone, testosterone, estrogen, hydroxyprogesterone, or estradiol Neonatal screening and biochemical tests for glucocorticoid deficiency and salt wasting crisis are required when CAH is suspected
Clinicopathologic Aspects	Bilateral ZG hyperplasia (most common, around 60%) Unilateral ZG hyperplasia (2%) ACA (30%–40%) ACC (1%)	ACTH-dependent ACH (80%) ACTH-independent ACH (2%) (eg, PBMAH[a] and PPNAD[b]) ACA (10%) ACC (8%)	Classic and nonclassic CAH ACT (adults often manifest with ACC in the absence of congenital adrenal hyperplasia)

Abbreviations: ACH, adrenocortical hyperplasia; ACTH, adrenocorticotrophic hormone; CAH, congenital adrenocortical hyperplasia; DHEA, dehydroepiandrosterone; DHEA-S, dehydroepiandrosterone sulfate.
[a] Primary bilateral macronodular adrenocortical hyperplasia.
[b] Primary pigmented micronodular adrenocortical disease.

almost always related to malignancy in adults, in the absence of congenital adrenal hyperplasia.[9–11] Expression of 2 or more hormones by an ACT is seen more frequently in ACCs, with the most common synchronous combination being sex steroid and cortisol secretion.

Adrenal lesions are often discovered by imaging studies intended to evaluate for some other disease process. When discovered incidentally, these lesions are commonly referred to as incidentalomas.[13] Once discovered, abdominal computed tomography (CT) is the general imaging modality of choice to evaluate adrenal cortical lesions.[14] The features that should be assessed include tumor size, appearance (ie, integrity and invasiveness), heterogeneity, lipid content, and the rate of washout after intravenous administration of contrast. In neonates with congenital adrenal hyperplasia, adrenal ultrasonography is useful.[15] Some studies have suggested that chemical-shift MRI may be the preferred imaging modality in young patients or in cases in which a patient with an iodinated contrast allergy is found to have an indeterminate adrenal mass on unenhanced CT.[14,15]

Radiological findings of bilateral nodular adrenocortical disease are variable. In PBMAH, massive bilateral enlargement is a characteristic finding.[16] Unlike PBMAH, CT and MRI findings can sometimes underestimate the extent of, and possibly miss, primary bilateral micronodular adrenocortical disease.[17] In these scenarios, the use of functional imaging studies (eg, noriodocholesterol scintigraphy or PET-CT scans) can be helpful in identifying the bilateral nature of the disease; functional imaging studies may be of particular value especially in the setting of normal CT scans with abnormal biochemical findings.[17] From a biochemical perspective, patients with PPNAD often show a characteristic paradoxic response to a dexamethasone suppression (Liddle test) with an increase in 17-hydroxycorticosteroid and urinary free cortisol.[18]

In the case of biochemically active ACTs, imaging studies may be used to locate the hypersecreting tumor, although, in some scenarios, locating the lesion is sometimes difficult, especially in some cases of primary aldosteronism. In these cases, adrenal vein sampling (AVS) to assess aldosterone/cortisol ratios in both adrenal veins is considered the gold standard in order to lateralize the side of a hyperfunctioning tumor[6,9]; however, this invasive technique often yields borderline results. In addition, in cases in which the ACT cosecretes cortisol and aldosterone, the characteristic hormone gradient may be lost. Recent evidence has shown that the use of molecular adrenal imaging studies (eg, metomidate PET-CT) along with AVS can be helpful in identifying the source of primary aldosteronism.[19,20] In patients with hypercortisolism, the diagnosis of adrenal Cushing syndrome is considered only after exclusion of adrenocorticotrophic hormone (ACTH) –dependent disease (eg, pituitary or ectopic source of ACTH). Because of this, brain MRI to look for a pituitary tumor, bilateral inferior petrosal sinus sampling in nonvisible pituitary lesions, and a chest and abdominal/pelvic CT scan may be required.[14]

The common radiological features of ACTs are summarized in **Table 2**. Note that indeterminate

Table 2
Imaging characteristics of benign and malignant adrenocortical tumors

Radiological Characteristics	Benign	Malignant
Tumor size	Often <4–6 cm	Often $\geq$4–6 cm
Tumor appearance	Well delineated; round with regular border	Ill-defined, irregular border; areas of necrosis
Tumor heterogeneity	Homogeneous enhancement	Heterogeneous enhancement
Lipid content and density appearance on unenhanced CT	Lipid rich Low density on unenhanced CT ($\leq$10 Hounsfield units)	Lipid poor High density on unenhanced CT (>10 Hounsfield units)
Contrast enhancement and washout pattern 15 min after intravenous administration of contrast[a]	Enhanced with rapid washout ($\geq$40%) after 15 min	Enhanced with less washout (15%–25%) after 15 min
Chemical-shift MRI	Loss of signal intensity on the out-of-phase image	No loss of signal intensity on the out-of-phase image

[a] Hypervascular metastatic tumors such as renal cell carcinoma and hepatocellular carcinoma can have rapid washout mimicking an adrenocortical adenoma.

radiological adrenocortical lesions are commonly reported,[14,21,22] although detailed descriptions of those findings are beyond the scope of this article.

MORPHOLOGIC DIAGNOSIS OF ADRENOCORTICAL TUMORS

GROSS EXAMINATION

Complete morphologic assessment of ACTs begins with a review of the available clinical, biochemical, and radiological information, followed by a thorough gross examination of the adrenalectomy resection specimen. It is important to note what type of surgery has been done, because some specimens may be more fragmented than others.[23] An increasing number of surgical centers are performing morcellation procedures at the time of laparoscopic adrenalectomy when removing small tumors considered to be ACAs based on preoperative imaging. From a pathologic perspective, this is obviously not ideal. However, care should be taken to evaluate the same parameters as in an intact resection specimen whenever possible.[24]

When evaluating an adrenalectomy specimen, the usual principles of macroscopic examination apply, including specimen painting, margin identification, specimen measurement, and specimen weighing. When looking at the cut surface of the specimen, the tumor as well as the nontumor adrenal parenchyma must be carefully evaluated. In adults, the normal adrenal cortex has an average thickness of at least 2 mm.[10] In patients with a cortisol-secreting lesion, the cortex becomes thin (also known as atrophy of the cortex) because of negative feedback inhibition by the autonomous cortisol secretion on the hypothalamic-pituitary-adrenal axis.[10,25] Failure to recognize this finding may have critical consequences because this information can be lifesaving if hormone replacement therapy was not provided to the patient postoperatively.[25] Among patients with subclinical Cushing syndrome, some may be undetected preoperatively. Any additional nodularity, their measurements, and the presence or absence of associated pigmentation within the cortex besides the main lesion should also be commented on and sampled adequately for microscopic examination. The appearance and distribution of the medulla should also be described. If feasible, photographs of both the intact and serial sections of the specimen should be taken; rarely, having gross images to review can be critical in the assessment of a resection specimen.

The tumor should be accurately measured and its relationship to the capsule should be scrutinized with any gross disruption or invasion into periadrenal tissue noted. Ideally, periadrenal adipose tissue should be dissected away for accurate weighing of the tumor although sometimes, this is not always possible. Both benign and malignant ACTs frequently present as solitary masses, although multifocal ACTs can also occur. ACAs are more commonly 5 cm or less, whereas ACCs are often significantly larger and often weigh more than 100 g,[26] although exceptions have been reported. ACCs may show a vague multinodular appearance reflective of the heterogeneity often seen microscopically, which represents a potential pitfall in the examination of these lesions, because undersampling may miss areas of the tumor that are dictating biological behavior.

Most commonly, ACAs are well delineated and homogeneous, but they infrequently show hemorrhage and cystic degeneration (**Fig. 2**). Most are yellow-gold (frequently in aldosterone-producing ACAs), reflecting their lipid-rich nature (see **Fig. 2**A), whereas oncocytic ACTs or ACTs with oncocytic change (see **Fig. 2**B) have a distinct red-brown appearance. So-called black adenomas have also been described (see **Fig. 2**C); these lesions get their distinctive color from lipofuscin accumulation. The micronodules (<1 cm) of PPNAD and some forms of primary micronodular adrenocortical disease may also show a variable degree of pigmentation.

In contrast, ACCs are more often heterogeneous and may show fibrous bands. In addition, hemorrhage, necrosis, and calcification are commonly identified. They may be well circumscribed or show an irregular border and infiltration into adjacent structures. When locally invasive, ACCs tend to invade regional venous structures (**Fig. 3**), adipose tissue surrounding the adrenal gland, and adjacent organs such as the kidney.[27]

In addition to sampling the tumor proper for microscopic examination, it is critical to sample the tumor interface with adjacent tissue, because the authors have found this to be the area where invasive growth and angioinvasion are most evident. As for every resection specimen, lymph nodes should be entirely submitted when present.

MICROSCOPIC EXAMINATION

Traditionally, ACTs are thought to arise from the different zones of the adrenal cortex and, as such, they most often recapitulate the cellular morphology characteristic of different adrenocortical cells. For example, it is common for ACAs to be composed of corded/nested lipid-rich cells with abundant vacuolated clear cytoplasm and low nuclear/cytoplasmic ratio reminiscent of the

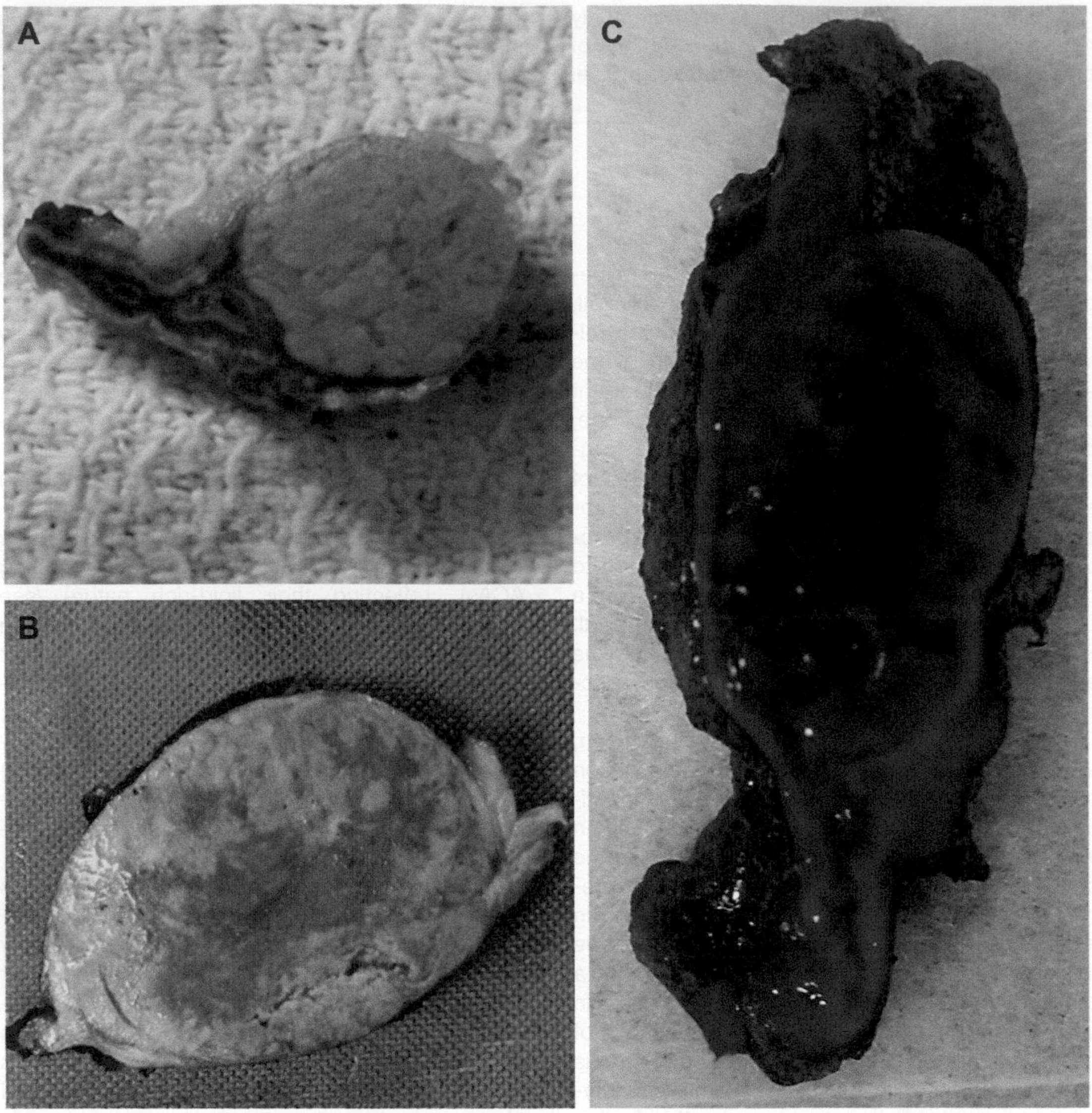

Fig. 2. Gross findings in adrenocortical adenomas. Conventional adenomas are often well-delineated and homogeneous cortical lesions (*A–C*). Most are yellow, as seen in most aldosterone-producing adenomas (*A*). Some tumors show variable degree of oncocytic change, which imparts a red-brown appearance grossly. Note the nontumorous cortical atrophy; this finding distinguishes cortisol-producing tumors from aldosterone-producing adenomas (*B*). Black adenomas have distinctive dark-brown color (*C*).

ZF, in addition to more compact or eosinophilic cells reminiscent of the ZR layer.

Depending on the hormonal functionality of the ACT being evaluated, genotypic-phenotypic features of the tumor and specific changes within the nontumor cortex may be apparent. For example, ACAs producing aldosterone are likely to be the most heterogeneous group among ACAs. Depending on their underlying molecular biology, they can show combinations of different cell types, including lipid-rich (ZF-like) cells, lipid-poor compact (ZR-like) cells, smaller cells resembling ZG-like cells, and compact cells with overlapping features of ZG-like and ZR-like cells (**Figs. 4** and **5**). The native ZG is commonly hyperplastic, so-called paradoxical ZG layer hyperplasia (**Fig. 6**), and may show micronodular proliferations that are now recognized as aldosterone-producing cell clusters (APCCs) (**Fig. 7**), a new concept in primary aldosteronism.[28] When treated with spironolactone, an antagonist of aldosterone, aldosterone-producing ACAs, in addition to the background parenchyma, show characteristic eosinophilic concentric lamellated intracellular

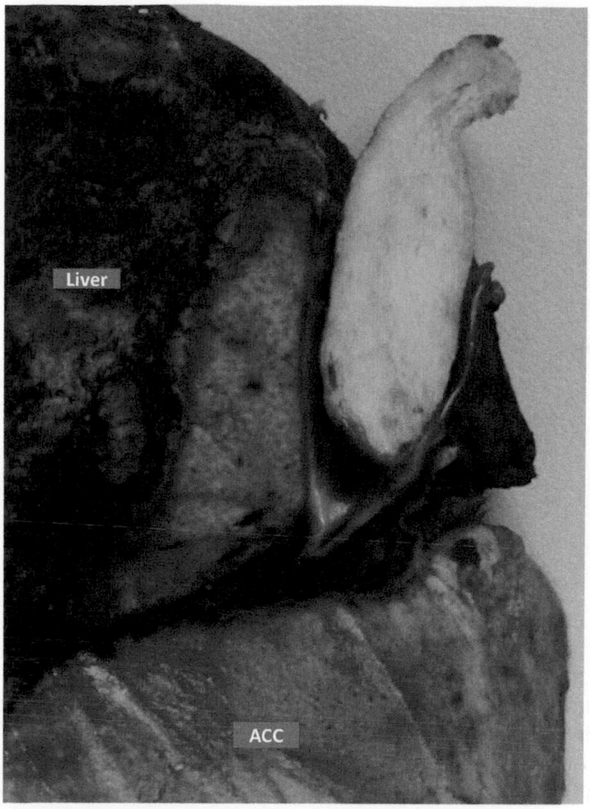

Fig. 3. Gross findings in adrenocortical carcinomas (ACC). These tumors are often heterogeneous with areas of hemorrhage. They may be well circumscribed or show an irregular border and infiltration into adjacent structures, including large venous structures as shown here.

inclusions called spironolactone bodies (see **Figs. 5** and **7**; **Fig. 8**). It has been reported that spironolactone bodies are not seen when eplerenone is administered (aldosterone receptor antagonist).[29]

In adrenal Cushing syndrome, there is a spectrum of cortisol-producing proliferations from bilateral micronodules (<1 cm) and macronodules (>1 cm) with their distinct molecular alterations

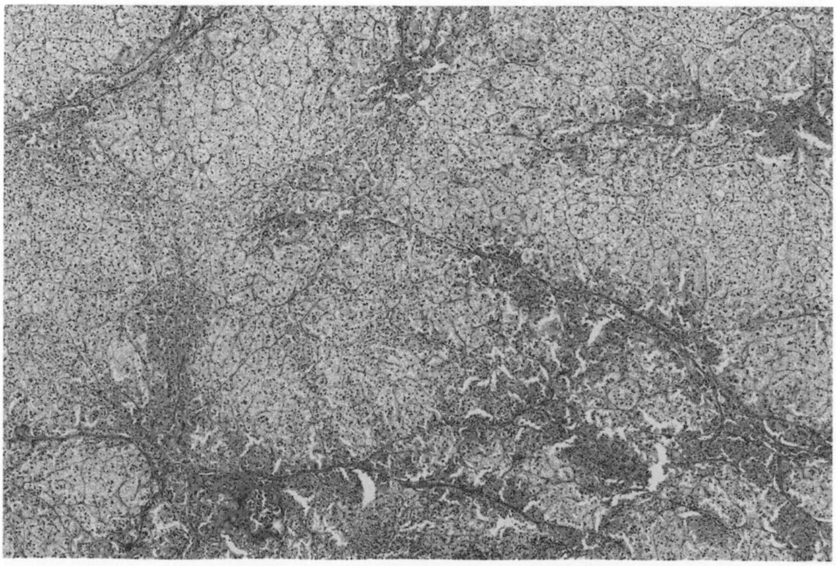

Fig. 4. Clear cell–rich adrenocortical adenoma in primary aldosteronism. Aldosterone-producing adenomas can show combinations of different cell types, including lipid-rich (zona fasciculata–like) cells, lipid-poor compact (zona reticularis–like) cells, smaller cells resembling zona glomerulosa–like cells, and compact cells with overlapping features of ZG-like and zona reticularis–like cells. Shown is a clear cell–rich adenoma that is more commonly seen in tumors with *KCNJ5* mutations.

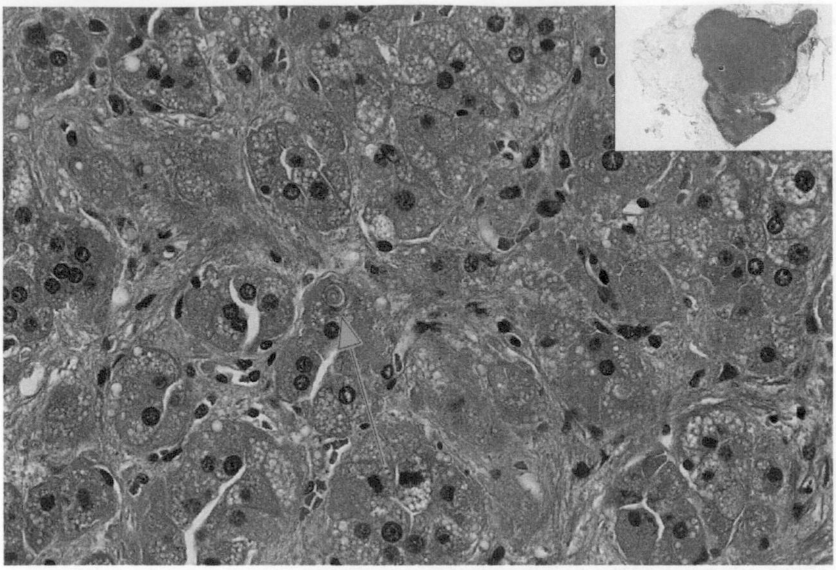

Fig. 5. Spironolactone bodies in aldosterone-producing adenoma. Some aldosterone-producing adenomas are enriched in cells lacking ZF-like clear cell pre dominance. These tumors tend to be more frequent in *KCNJ5* wild-type adenomas. Shown is an aldosterone-producing adenoma treated with spironolactone. The tumor cells also show intracytoplasmic eosinophilic concentric lamellated inclusions called spironolactone bodies (*arrow*).

representing PPNAD and PBMAH, respectively.[4,28,30,31] Conceptually, the bilateral micronodular or macronodular disease can be regarded as multifocal ACAs, given their clonal nature. ACCs have been described in the context of PPNAD.[32,33] Morphologically, PPNAD is composed of bilateral cortical micronodules composed of pigmented compact cell–rich proliferations with variable degrees of cortical atrophy in the intervening cortex. Sometimes, isolated nonpigmented or weakly/variably pigmented micronodular proliferations can also occur in the setting of Cushing syndrome. Tumor nodules identified in PBMAH are composed of cortical proliferations composed mainly of lipid-rich cells and variable amounts of compact cells that represent multiple nodules mostly exceeding 1 cm and irregular enlargement of both adrenal glands.[28] Conventional cortisol-secreting ACAs show various morphologic features ranging from pure clear cell tumors to mixed clear and compact cell ACTs. The autonomous neoplastic cortisol secretion from the adrenal gland shuts down the hypothalamic corticotropin-releasing hormone, resulting in resting corticotrophs via Crooke hyaline change in addition to a lack of ACTH-mediated trophic changes in both adrenal glands. Consistently, the background adrenal

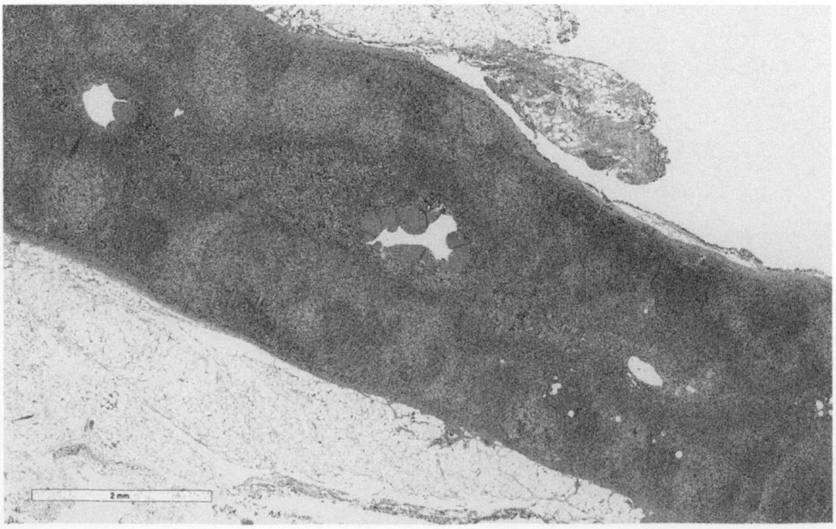

Fig. 6. ZG layer hyperplasia is characterized by the presence of continuous and/or multilayered ZG layer. In some cases, aldosterone-producing cell clusters can be seen in association with ZG layer hyperplasia.

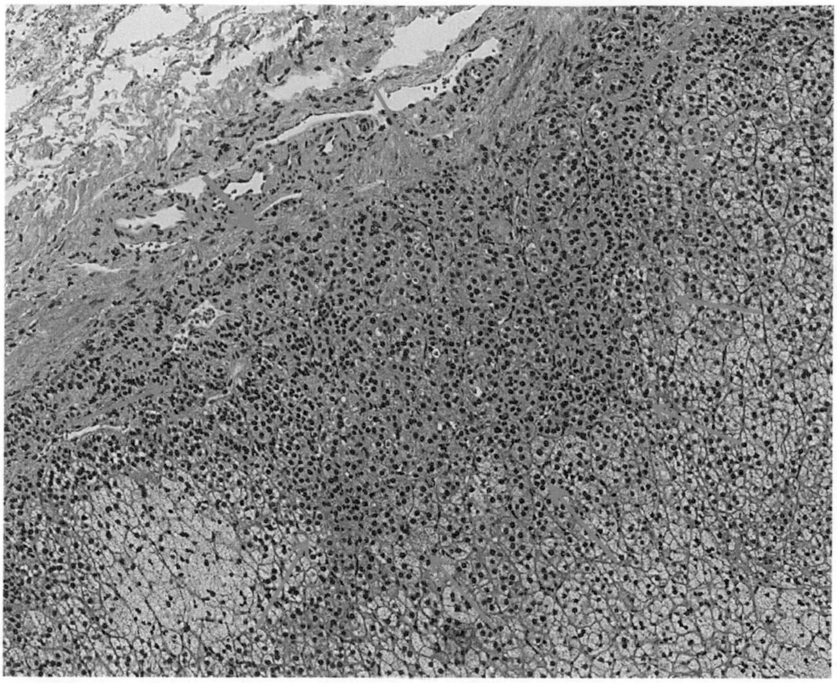

Fig. 7. APCCs are microscopic aldosterone-producing cortical proliferations originating from the ZG layer and extending into the ZF layer. The identification of somatic alterations implicated in the calcium/calmodulin kinase pathway supports their clonal (neoplastic) nature. Shown is an APCC that contains spironolactone bodies. Arrows outline the APCC.

cortex and/or internodular adrenal cortex become atrophic because of the absence of the ZR layer along with a thinned ZF layer (**Fig. 9**). Sex hormone–secreting ACTs, in contrast with ACTs secreting other hormones, usually tend to be enriched in compact eosinophilic cells normally seen in the ZF. Nonfunctional ACAs can also show morphologic heterogeneity.

Several morphologic changes can be observed in both ACAs and ACCs, including oncocytic and myxoid changes as well as myelolipomatous change. Tumors are designated as mixed oncocytic ACTs when the cortical neoplasm shows 50% to 90% oncocytic change, whereas the term pure oncocytic ACT is applied to those tumors that show greater than 90% oncocytic

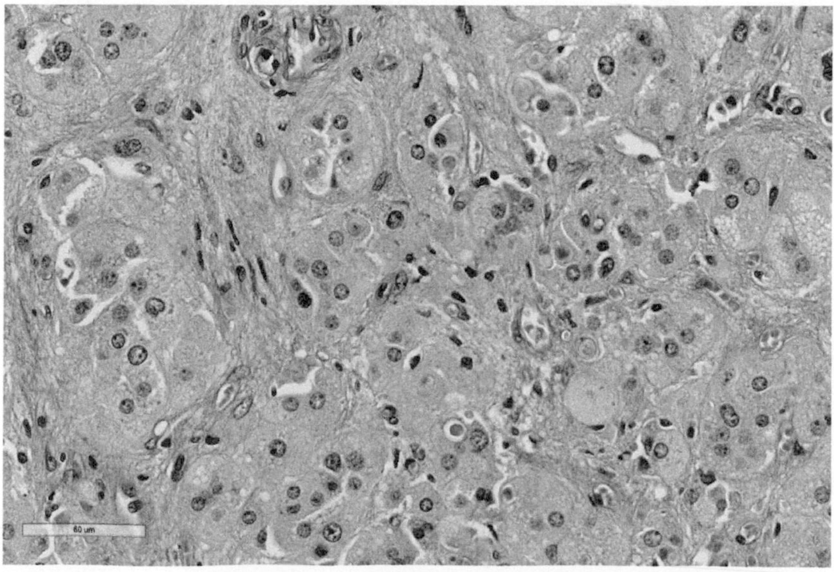

Fig. 8. Luxol fast blue (LFB) histochemistry. Because of their high phospholipid content, spironolactone bodies can be distinguished from potential mimics using LFB.

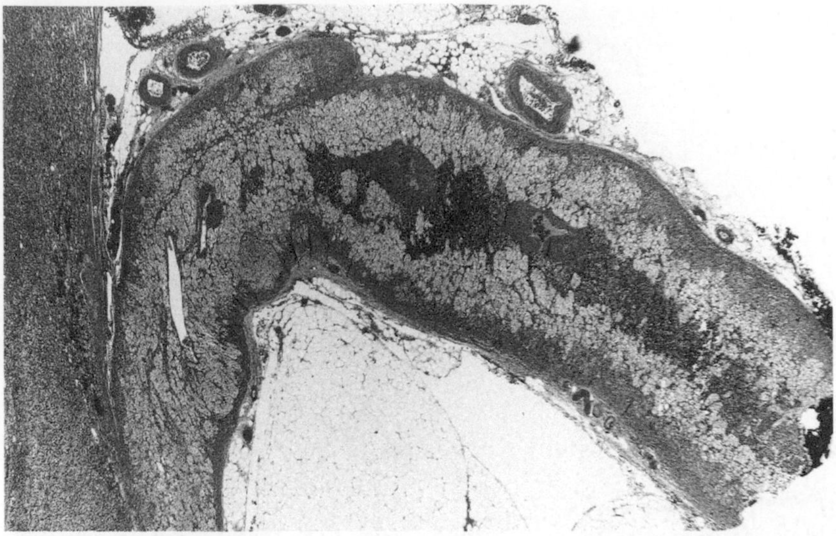

Fig. 9. Nontumorous cortical atrophy. In the absence of exogenous cortisol administration, nontumorous cortical atrophy distinguishes cortisol-producing adrenocortical tumors from those that produce aldosterone.

change.[34,35] Some rare changes, especially myxoid changes, are more common in ACCs. Sarcomatoid areas can be seen in ACCs and, when identified, can cause confusion with other malignant tumors in the differential diagnosis, particularly primary or secondary (metastatic) sarcomas. Given the range of morphologic heterogeneity, 4 histologic variants of ACC are currently recognized: conventional (**Fig. 10**), oncocytic (**Fig. 11**), myxoid (**Fig. 12**), and sarcomatoid.[27] ACCs can also show a combination of these variants (**Fig. 13**).

To aid in establishing a diagnosis of ACC, several multifactorial scoring schemes/algorithms have been described that evaluate several features that have been associated with poor outcome (**Fig. 14**). In 1984, Weiss[36,37] proposed the first diagnostic scheme, colloquially known as the Weiss criteria. The original Weiss criteria focused on the assessment of 9 features: high nuclear grade (Fuhrman grading system), mitotic rate more than 5 mitoses per 50 high-power fields (**Fig. 15**), atypical mitotic figures, less than 25% clear cells, diffuse architecture (defined as patternless sheets exceeding 30% of the tumor; nested/alveolar, columnar, trabecular, or cordlike areas are defined as nondiffuse growth), tumor necrosis (**Fig. 16**), venous invasion (**Fig. 17**), sinusoidal invasion, and capsular invasion. Of the 43 cases in the original Weiss series, none of the 24 tumors

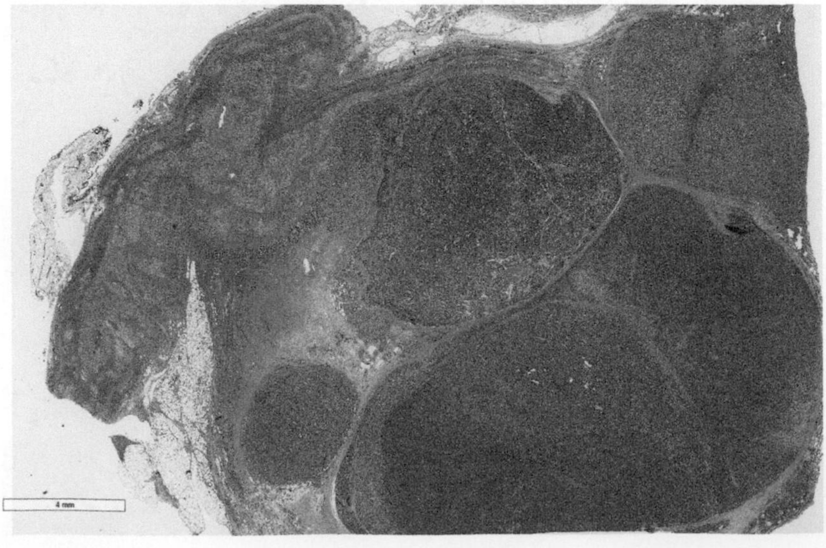

Fig. 10. Conventional adrenocortical carcinoma.

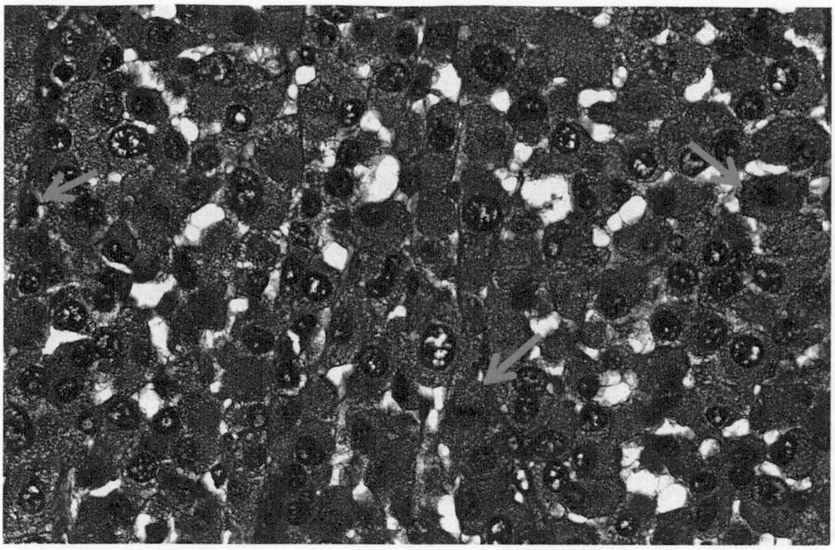

Fig. 11. Oncocytic adrenocortical carcinoma (*arrows* indicate mitotic figures).

meeting 2 or fewer criteria metastasized or recurred, whereas all but 1 of the remaining 19 cases meeting 4 or more criteria either metastasized or recurred.[36] The original Weiss criteria have since been modified because of the lack of reproducibility and interpretive difficulties. The modified Weiss criteria (by Aubert and colleagues[26]) were thought to be more reproducible and easier to apply because they called for the assessment of 5 instead of 9 criteria.

Because the Weiss criteria include some features of malignancy that are morphologically inherent to pure oncocytic ACTs (eg, diffuse growth pattern, scarcity of clear cells, and prominent nucleoli leading to high-grade nuclear scoring), the Lin-Weiss-Bisceglia criteria[38] were described with an increased focus on invasiveness and mitotic count and less focus on some other morphologic features defined in the Weiss criteria. The Lin-Weiss-Bisceglia criteria[38] use a major and minor criteria framework to classify oncocytic ACTs for which the presence of 1 major criteria (mitotic rate >5 mitoses per 50 high-power fields, atypical mitotic figures, venous invasion) indicates malignancy (**Fig. 18**) and the presence of 1 to 4 minor criteria (tumor size >10 cm and/or weight >200 g, necrosis, sinusoidal invasion, capsular invasion) indicates a tumor of uncertain malignant potential. Oncocytic ACAs should not show any of the major or minor criteria.

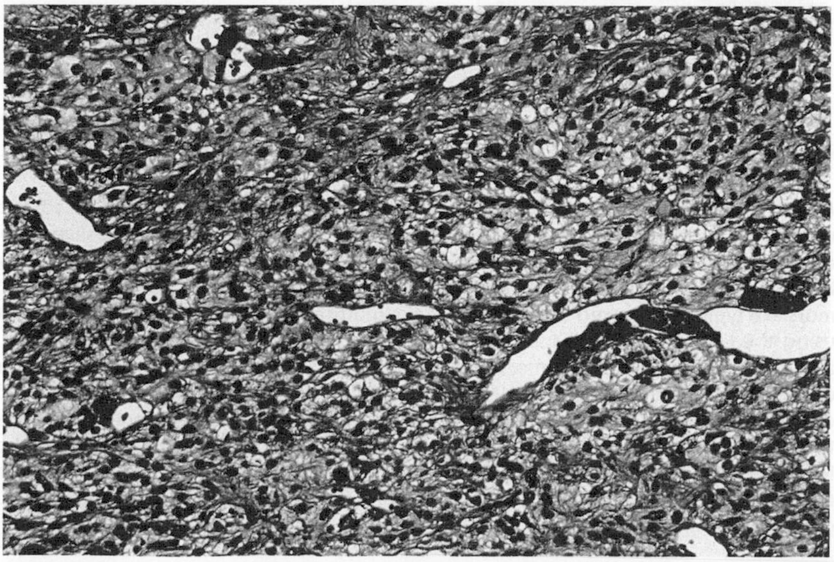

Fig. 12. Myxoid adrenocortical carcinoma.

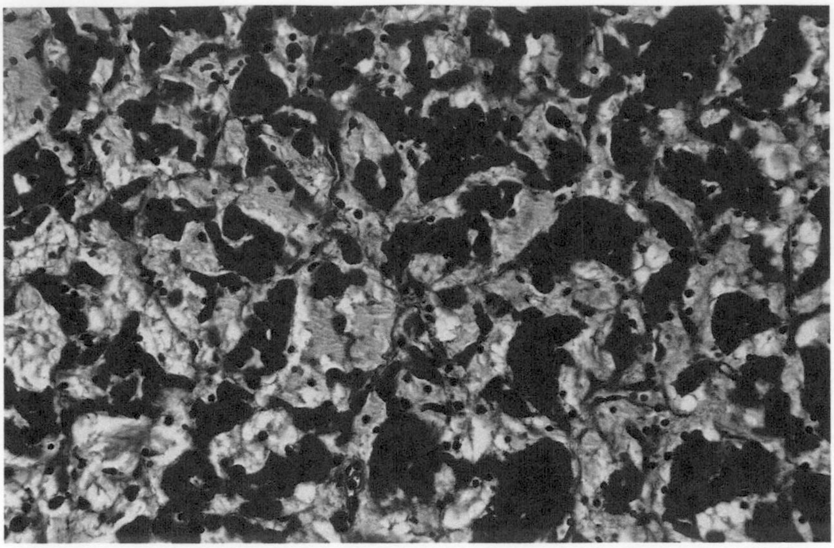

Fig. **13.** Adrenocortical carcinoma with myxoid and oncocytic change.

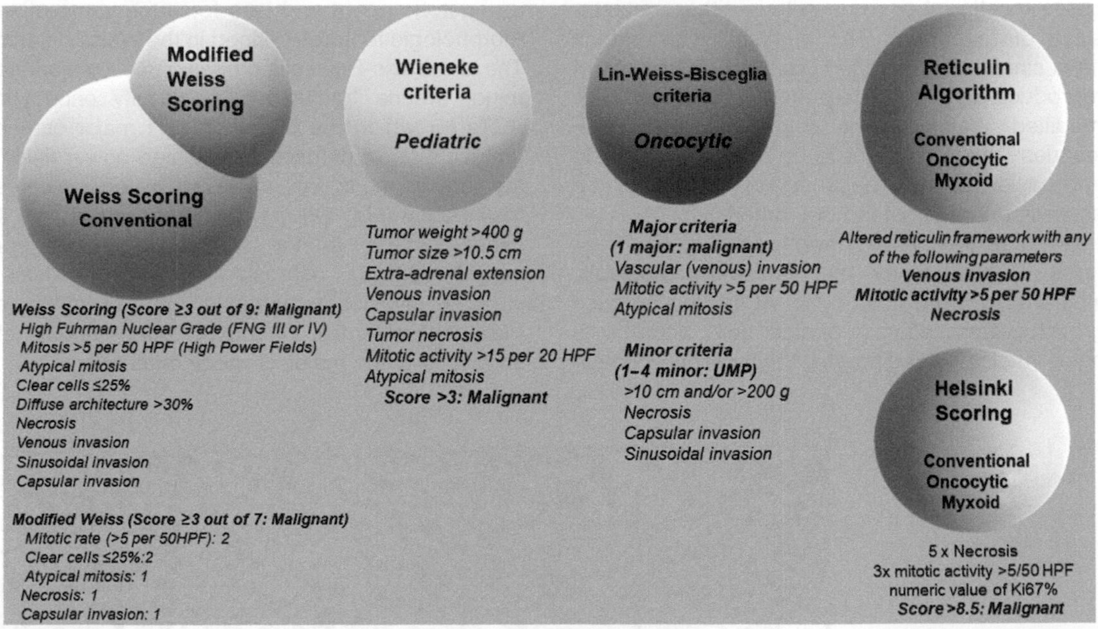

Modified Weiss Scoring
Weiss Scoring
Conventional
Wieneke criteria
Pediatric
Lin-Weiss-Bisceglia criteria
Oncocytic
Reticulin Algorithm
Conventional
Oncocytic
Myxoid
Weiss Scoring (Score ≥3 out of 9: Malignant)
High Fuhrman Nuclear Grade (FNG III or IV)
Mitosis >5 per 50 HPF (High Power Fields)
Atypical mitosis
Clear cells ≤25%
Diffuse architecture >30%
Necrosis
Venous invasion
Sinusoidal invasion
Capsular invasion
Modified Weiss (Score ≥3 out of 7: Malignant)
Mitotic rate (>5 per 50HPF): 2
Clear cells ≤25%:2
Atypical mitosis: 1
Necrosis: 1
Capsular invasion: 1
Tumor weight >400 g
Tumor size >10.5 cm
Extra-adrenal extension
Venous invasion
Capsular invasion
Tumor necrosis
Mitotic activity >15 per 20 HPF
Atypical mitosis
Score >3: Malignant
Major criteria
(1 major: malignant)
Vascular (venous) invasion
Mitotic activity >5 per 50 HPF
Atypical mitosis
Minor criteria
(1–4 minor: UMP)
>10 cm and/or >200 g
Necrosis
Capsular invasion
Sinusoidal invasion
Altered reticulin framework with any of the following parameters
Venous invasion
Mitotic activity >5 per 50 HPF
Necrosis
Helsinki Scoring
Conventional
Oncocytic
Myxoid
5 x Necrosis
3x mitotic activity >5/50 HPF
numeric value of Ki67%
Score >8.5: Malignant

Fig. 14. Multifactorial diagnostic schemes to aid in making the diagnosis of adrenocortical carcinoma. Several multifactorial scoring schemes/algorithms have been described to evaluate several features that have been associated with poor outcome in adrenocortical carcinomas. The Weiss and modified Weiss scoring schemes have been used to distinguish conventional adrenocortical carcinomas identified in adults. Pediatric adrenocortical tumors are typically assessed using the Wieneke multifactorial system. Oncocytic adrenocortical tumors are assessed using the Lin-Weiss-Bisceglia scoring scheme. The reticulin algorithm can be applied to conventional, oncocytic, and myxoid adrenocortical tumors identified in adults. The Helsinki scoring scheme can distinguish malignancy in conventional adrenocortical tumors in adults. This approach also provides prognostic information. Although the data on myxoid adrenocortical tumors are limited, recent evidence suggests that the diagnostic performance of the Helsinki scoring system in oncocytic adrenocortical tumors was not as good as the Lin-Weiss-Bisceglia system. However, the Helsinki score was able to predict poor prognostic subgroups of oncocytic adrenocortical carcinomas. Generated from Dr. Ozgur Mete's USCAP 2019 Endocrine Pathology Society Companion Meeting Lecture on Challenges in Adrenal Cortical Pathology. HPF, high-power field; UMP, uncertain malignant potential.

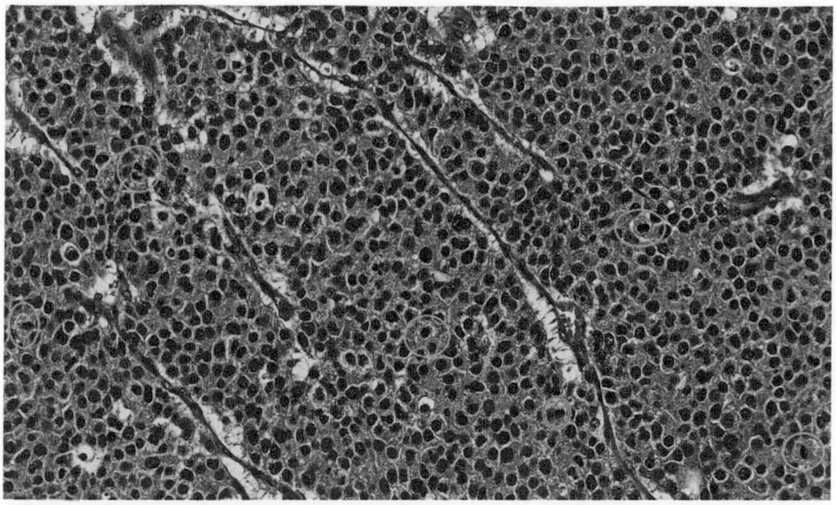

Fig. 15. Increased mitotic activity. An accurate assessment of mitotic activity is important when evaluating cortical neoplasms. Increased mitotic activity is defined as a mitotic count exceeding 5 per 50 HPF. Adrenocortical carcinomas are categorized as high grade or low grade based on mitotic counts from hot spots, depending on whether up to 20 (low grade) or more than 20 mitoses (high grade) are seen per 50 HPF. Shown is an adrenocortical carcinoma with increased mitotic activity. Mitotic figures are circled.

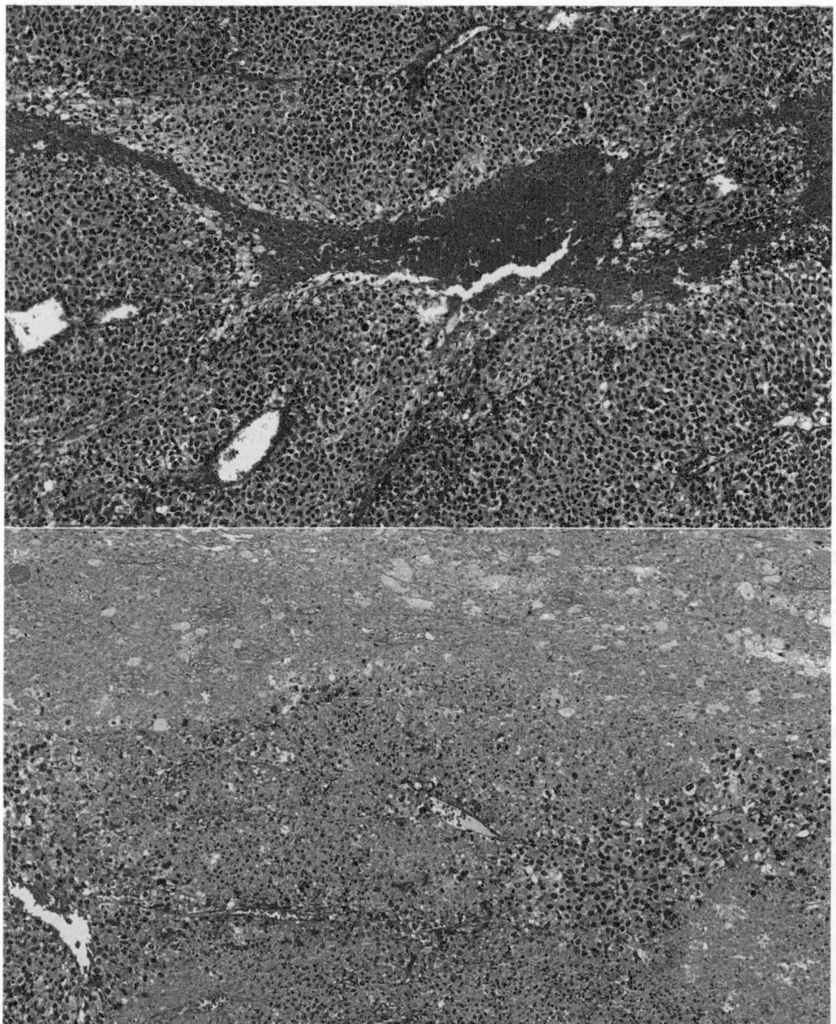

Fig. 16. Tumor necrosis. The upper and lower parts of this composite photomicrograph show focal coagulative and geographic necrosis in adrenocortical carcinomas, respectively.

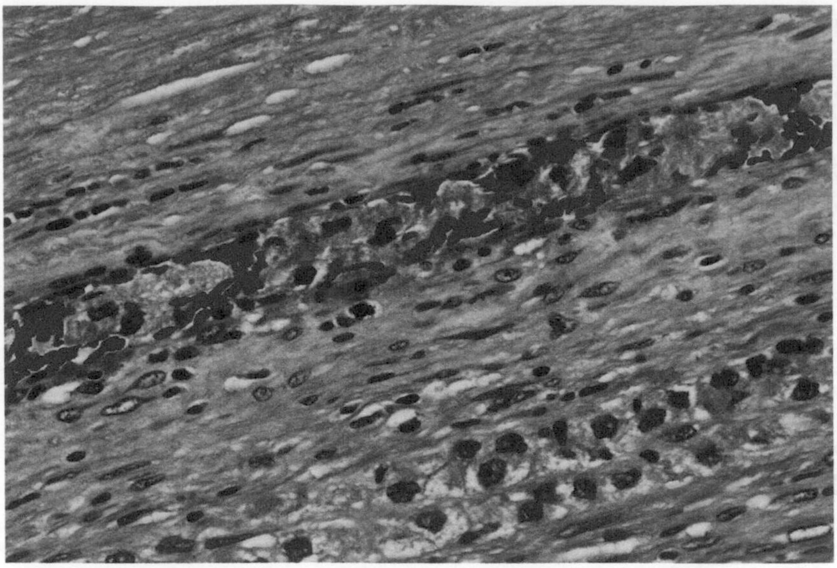

Fig. 17. Vascular invasion (angioinvasion). Tumor cells invading through a vessel wall and/or intravascular tumor cells admixed with fibrinoid material qualify for vascular invasion.

The first algorithm to consider the use of a histochemical stain as a requirement in the morphologic evaluation of ACTs is the reticulin algorithm. This algorithm is gaining significant popularity among diagnosticians because of the objective nature of evaluating the tumor reticulin network combined with the limited number of features needed to define malignancy.[39–41] ACAs typically show preserved reticulin framework (**Fig. 19**). When an altered reticulin network in an ACT is identified (**Fig. 20**) in combination with 1 or more parameters (vascular invasion, tumor necrosis, or mitotic activity >5 per 50 high-power fields), the diagnosis of ACC can be made.[39–41] In addition to conventional forms of ACCs, recent series have also underscored the usefulness of the reticulin algorithm in oncocytic[34,35,40–42] and myxoid ACTs.[40] Because the distinction of myxoid ACCs can be challenging using the Weiss parameters,[43] the reticulin algorithm may add value to the diagnostic work-up. Of note, a multicentric validation series of 245 ACTs also included 2 cases of pediatric ACT.[40] Although the interpretation of the reticulin histochemistry is often an easy task for diagnosticians, they should be aware of the common pitfalls related to its interpretation (discussed later).

Ki67 labeling index has been shown to be prognostically significant in ACCs (discussed later).[44] The Helsinki scoring system, proposed in 2015[45]

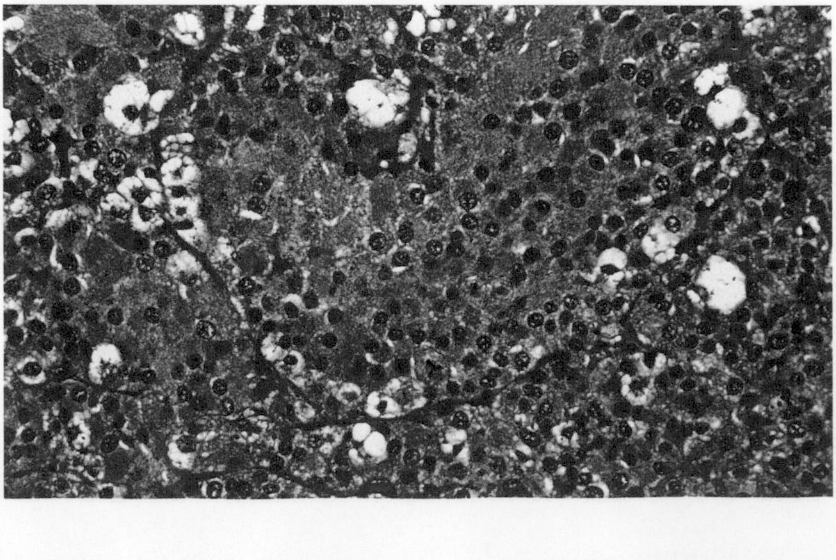

Fig. 18. Atypical mitotic figure. Shown is a tripolar mitotic figure in an adrenocortical carcinoma.

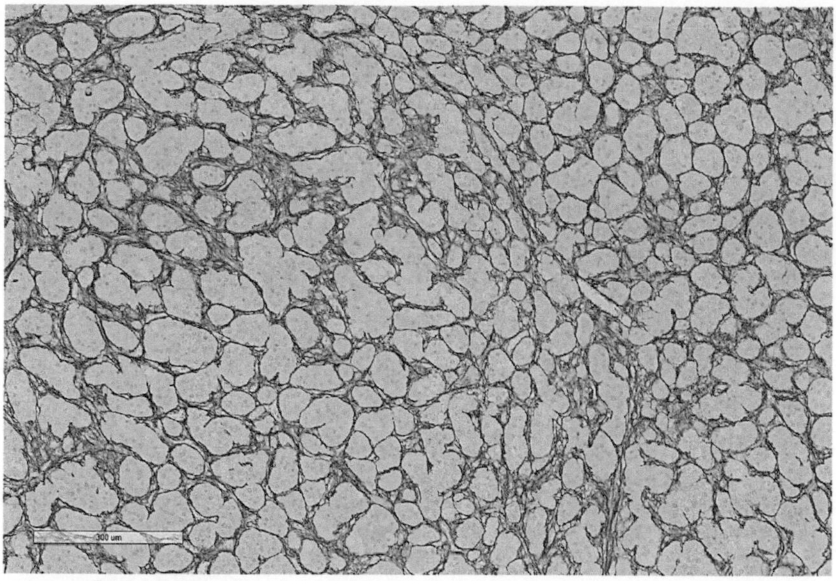

Fig. 19. Reticulin histochemistry in adrenocortical adenomas. A preserved reticulin framework is a feature of adrenocortical adenomas.

and subsequently validated in a later series,[46] has incorporated the role of the Ki67 labeling index into its criteria for malignancy along with mitotic rate (>5 per 50 high-power fields) and presence/absence of necrosis. The Helsinki system uses a weighted-point system: 5 points are awarded if necrosis is present and 3 points are awarded if more than 5 mitoses are seen in 50 high-power fields. The value of the Ki67 index (percentage positive tumor nuclei from hot spots) is used as the third scoring component. A score greater than 8.5 indicates a malignant lesion. Of note, the Ki67 index should be evaluated in the area of highest proliferative activity; no visual assessment is allowed, and, ideally, the evaluation should be done by an automated image analysis software nuclear algorithm. The Italian validation series included oncocytic (mixed and pure tumors) and myxoid ACCs in addition to conventional ACCs.[46] In this validation cohort, oncocytic ACCs (diagnosed based on the Lin-Weiss-Bisceglia criteria) had a Helsinki score ranging from 3 to 79.[46] Although there were only a few myxoid tumors from which to draw a reliable conclusion, the Helsinki score of 19 or greater captured a significant proportion of aggressive forms of oncocytic ACCs.[46] In a recent multicenter French cohort, the diagnostic performance of the Helsinki scoring scheme in oncocytic ACTs was not as good as other schemes, but the Helsinki score was more useful in the prediction of poor prognostic subgroups of oncocytic ACCs.[35] These findings have pointed out the diagnostic limitations of this scoring system; however, further studies are still needed to expand the diagnostic limitations of this scheme.

Although rare,[47] pediatric ACTs often represent a diagnostic conundrum because it has been shown that some histologic features typically associated with malignancy in adult adrenocortical neoplasms do not necessarily correlate with poor outcome in pediatric patients. Although this may partially be related to differences in application of some cardinal features of malignancy among diagnosticians, the Wieneke system[48] was devised to better delineate benign from malignant ACTs in the pediatric setting. The Wieneke system incorporates some traditional prognostic variables (atypical mitoses, vascular invasion, capsular invasion, tumor necrosis, mitotic rate >15 per 20 high-power fields) into its scoring algorithm, in addition to gland size and weight as well as tumor involvement of local structures, including vena cava and other extra-adrenal structures. When 4 parameters are met, a diagnosis of pediatric ACC can be made. An assignment of uncertain malignant potential can be made with a score of 3, whereas a score of 1 or 2 is thought to suggest a benign course. This approach to pediatric ACTs has also been evaluated in subsequent series.[49–51]

It has been the observation of our team members that areas suggestive of adenoma-to-carcinoma tumor progression exist in some ACTs (O.M., author observation). Moreover, ACA-like low-proliferative regions can be seen admixed with nodular areas with high-grade proliferation. These lesions can be particularly challenging for diagnosticians, especially when limited representative sampling was performed from the tumor. Even so, there are very rare ACTs that are in a diagnostic gray zone and, in those cases, some diagnosticians use the term atypical or borderline

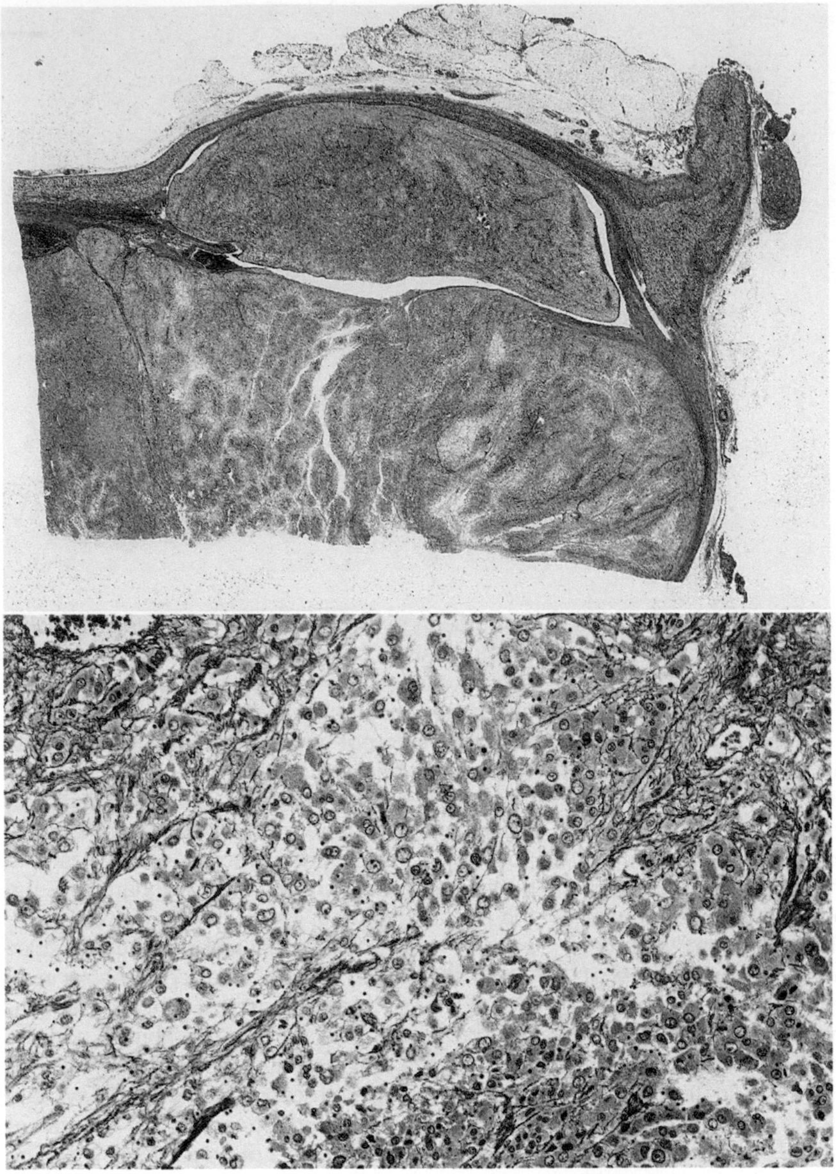

Fig. 20. Reticulin histochemistry in adrenocortical carcinomas. Loss of the reticulin framework is often seen in adrenocortical carcinomas. The upper photomicrograph represents an adrenal cortical carcinoma with altered reticulin framework (low magnification). The lower photomicrograph represents the high magnification of this tumor showing loss of reticulin framework.

adrenocortical neoplasm, whereas others apply the term ACT of uncertain malignant potential (UMP) for similar presentations. When the rare diagnosis of an ACT-UMP is being considered, additional sections should be submitted of the entire periphery of the tumor along with the central portion, and a diligent search including serial/deeper sections should be conducted to evaluate for features of malignancy. The diagnostic work-up of an ACT is no longer restricted to conventional histomorphology. There are several immunohistochemical biomarkers that can be useful in establishing a diagnosis of malignancy.[41,52] Similarly, the diagnosis and prognostication of ACC is now possible when applying various molecular biology techniques in the evaluation of an ACT[53] (discussed later).

Once a diagnosis of malignancy has been established, ACCs are further categorized as high grade or low grade based on mitotic counts from hot spots, depending on whether up to 20 (low grade) or more than 20 mitoses (high grade) are seen per 50 high-power fields. This approach stems from the original article by Weiss and colleagues,[37] but this has been adopted in the past decade in several practices given its prognostic significance.[52,54–56] Volante and colleagues[39] also showed that ACCs can be further prognosticated combining tumor stage and mitotic activity (≤9 per 50 high-power fields vs >9 per 50 high-power fields). Mete and colleagues also showed that the cutoff of 10 mitoses per 50 high-power fields had a better performance in the correlation of disease-free survival in ACCs.[41]

In practice, most ACCs are easily separated from ACAs, especially when they are widely invasive and highly proliferative. Overall, it has been reported that vascular invasion (see **Fig. 17**), defined as tumor cells invading through a vessel wall and/or intravascular tumor cells admixed with thrombus, is the strongest diagnostic parameter and predictive of poor outcome,[41] and thus it is reasonable to suggest that every case should be thoroughly scrutinized to rule this finding in or out, even in cases that are obviously malignant.

HISTOCHEMISTRY IN THE DIAGNOSIS OF ADRENOCORTICAL TUMORS

The use of histochemistry in benign ACTs is limited. In the setting of primary aldosteronism, Luxol fast blue (see **Fig. 8**) can be used to identify spironolactone bodies.[9] Histochemistry has gained popularity with the introduction of the reticulin algorithm because the algorithm is now regarded as a simple and reproducible method that can be used to separate ACAs from ACCs (see **Figs. 19** and **20**); however, clinicians should recognize pitfalls and pearls in the interpretation of reticulin findings. Although validation of the reticulin algorithm in large series of pediatric ACCs is currently lacking, this algorithmic approach has been shown to aid in making the diagnosis of conventional as well as oncocytic[34,40,41] and myxoid variants.[40] The backbone of the reticulin algorithm is the reticulin histochemical stain (most commonly Gordon-Sweet-Silver). Assessment of this staining in ACTs evaluates both quantitative (loss of continuity in reticulin fibers) and qualitative (abnormal reticulin network with irregular thickness of fibers, frayed appearance, or pericellular pattern leading to a meshlike appearance) changes.[40,41] Qualitative alterations in some ACTs may be the source of underestimation of malignancy because clinicians may encounter ACCs rich in areas of meshlike pericellular reticulin staining that can be mistaken for an unaltered reticulin framework. By being aware of this potential pitfall, additional careful examination of the reticulin histochemistry can solve this quandary because ACCs tend to show variable degrees of reticulin disruption even in the presence of qualitative changes.[41] Although the quantitative alterations are most helpful,[41] ACAs with areas of degeneration (eg, hemorrhage, extensive post-biopsy changes) can also show variable disruption of the reticulin framework. Furthermore, examples of very focal loss of reticulin staining and foci of incomplete or complete pericellular pattern have also been described in some ACAs.[41] Therefore, altered reticulin framework should be taken into consideration along with other histologic findings as well as biomarker profiling when evaluating an ACT.

IMMUNOHISTOCHEMISTRY IN THE DIAGNOSIS OF ADRENOCORTICAL TUMORS

Immunohistochemistry has become an integral component of the diagnostic work-up of ACTs. Biomarkers are routinely used to address various clinical needs, including confirmation of the adrenocortical origin, distinction of functional tumors, supporting the diagnosis of malignancy, providing prognostic and theranostic information in ACCs, and facilitating the screening process for germline pathogenesis.[52] Relevant immunohistochemical biomarkers are summarized in **Box 1**.

Several locoregional (eg, renal cell carcinoma, pheochromocytoma, epithelioid perivascular epithelioid cell neoplasms, sarcoma) and metastatic neoplasms (eg, melanoma, hepatocellular carcinoma) can simulate ACTs. Therefore, the confirmation of cortical origin should be considered in all ACTs, especially in the absence of adrenocortical hormone excess. Failure to confirm adrenocortical origin resulting in misdiagnoses has clearly been shown as being one of the major lessons from consultations practices.[57] To confirm adrenocortical origin, steroidogenic factor-1 (SF-1) (**Fig. 21**), a transcription factor characteristic of steroidogenic tissues, is the most specific diagnostic biomarker.[52] Negativity for SF-1 in sarcomatoid components of ACCs[58] as well as in ACTs with suboptimal tissue fixation are important pitfalls in the interpretation of SF-1 staining.

Once adrenocortical origin has been established, several biomarkers can be used to aid in distinguishing ACA from ACC, especially with challenging surgical specimens and particularly in the evaluation of core biopsy material. Mete and colleagues[41] reported that juxtanuclear insulinlike growth factor 2 (IGF-2) (**Fig. 22**) staining optimized at 1:3000 to 1:6000 dilutions was the most useful diagnostic biomarker of adult ACCs because this pattern of staining was absent in ACAs. The juxtanuclear Golgi pattern is thought to reflect impairment in translation and processing of the IGF-2 molecule in the Golgi apparatus, which results in IGF-2 overexpression.[41,59]

Box 1
Summary of practical immunohistochemistry in the assessment of adrenocortical tumors

Adrenal cortical confirmatory biomarkers

Steroidogenic factor-1 (most specific), Melan-A, calretinin, alpha-inhibin, synaptophysin

Functionality-related biomarkers

Cytochrome P (CYP) 11B2, CYP11B1, HSD3B1 and HSD3B2 (3β-hydroxysteroid dehydrogenase type 1 and type 2)

Pathogenic biomarkers

Insulinlike growth factor 2 (juxtanuclear staining), p53 (overexpression or global loss), beta-catenin (diffuse nuclear pattern)

Proliferation-related biomarkers

Ki67 (MIB1 antibody), phosphohistone-H3

Prognostic biomarkers

Ki67, p53, beta-catenin (diffuse nuclear pattern), DAXX, ATRX

Germline susceptibility screening biomarkers

Menin (multiple endocrine neoplasia type 1 [MEN1] syndrome), p27 (MEN4 syndrome), p53 (Li-Fraumeni syndrome), MMR (mismatch repair) proteins (Lynch syndrome), beta-catenin and APC (familial adenomatous polyposis [FAP] syndrome), succinate dehydrogenase subunit B (SDHB; familial paraganglioma syndrome caused by *SDHx*)

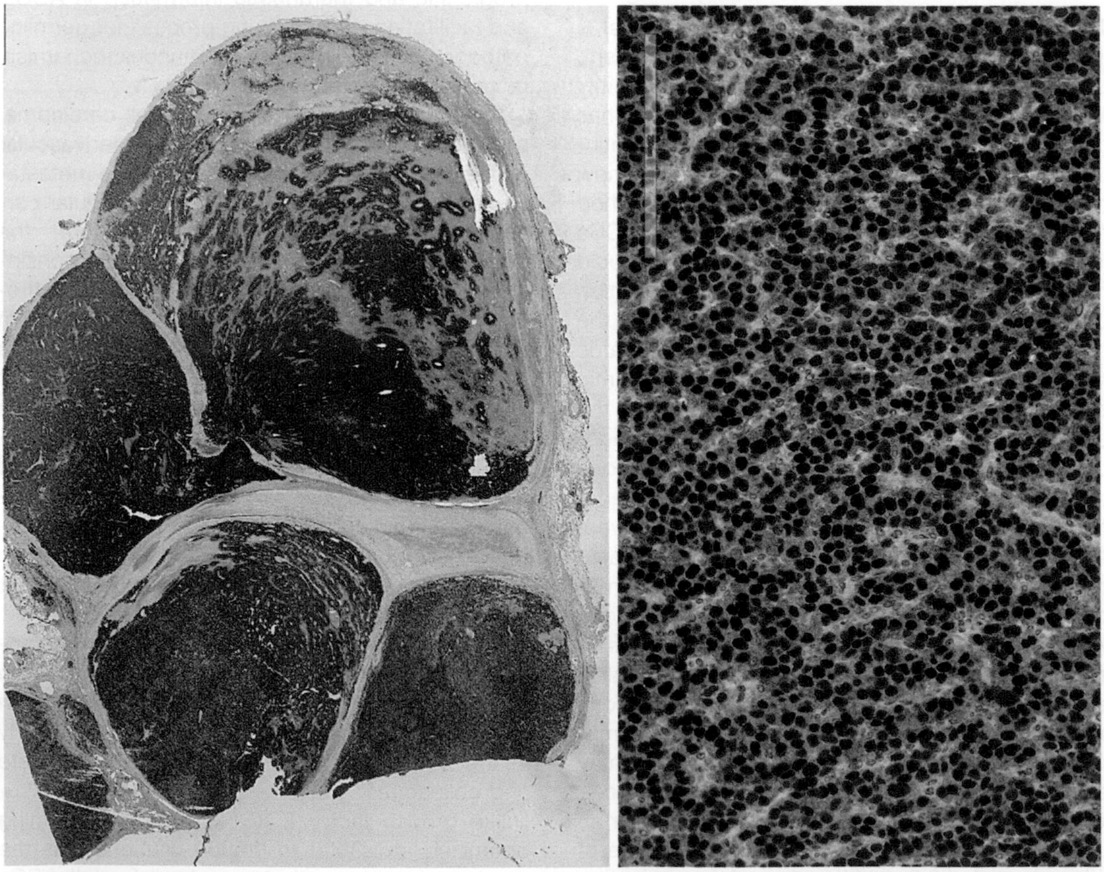

Fig. 21. Confirmation of adrenocortical origin. Several biomarkers have been proposed to confirm adrenal cortical origin, including synaptophysin, alpha-inhibin, Melan-A, and calretinin. However, among these, SF-1 stands out as the best biomarker to confirm cortical origin. Shown is diffuse nuclear SF-1 staining in an adrenocortical carcinoma. The left side of the composite photomicrograph illustrates SF-1 positivity in an adrenocortical carcinoma (low magnification). The right side of this composite photomicrograph represents high magnification of SF-1 expression in the same tumor.

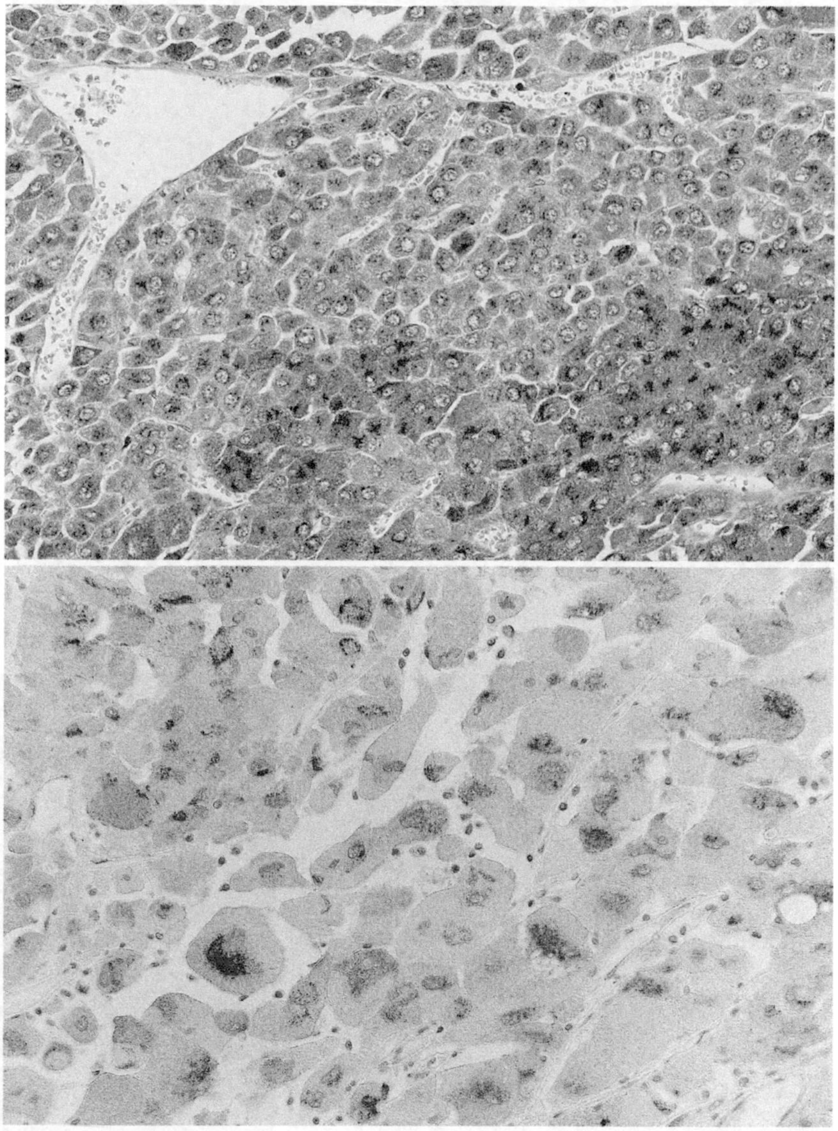

Fig. 22. IGF-2 immunohistochemistry. Juxtanuclear IGF-2 immunostaining is a feature of adrenocortical carcinoma. Shown are conventional (*upper*) and oncocytic (*lower*) adrenocortical carcinoma with juxtanuclear IGF-2 staining.

Abnormal p53 immunoexpression is a well-known marker of malignancy in several organs. Although pediatric ACCs tend to show more frequent *TP53* alterations,[60–63] overexpression (more frequent) (**Fig. 23**) or global loss as a result of *TP53* gene mutation has been seen in about 20% to 25% of adult ACCs.[60,62] Aberrant expression has been associated with high-grade proliferative features and tumor aggressiveness.[62,63]

Diffuse nuclear and cytoplasmic beta-catenin expression (**Fig. 24**) reflecting the activation of the Wnt pathway can be a feature of ACCs.[41] This finding alone should not warrant a diagnosis of malignancy because ACAs can also harbor *CTNNB1* mutations and show activation of the Wnt pathway.[28] In addition, patients with familial adenomatous polyposis (FAP) can also manifest with ACTs, including ACAs. In contrast, there is a general consensus that ACCs with diffuse cytoplasmic and nuclear beta-catenin reactivity are more frequently associated with a poor prognosis.[63–65]

As proliferation-driven neoplasms, an accurate assessment of cell proliferation biomarkers in ACTs is a crucial clinical task for pathologists assessing these tumors. Several biomarkers have been used to do this, such as Ki67, phosphohistone-H3 (PHH3), p53, BUB1B, HURP, and NEK2.[41,52] PHH3 (**Fig. 25**) can be considered to distinguish mitotic figures from apoptotic or cells with crush artifact; thus, it can assist mitotic count[66] to enable accurate mitotic tumor grading.

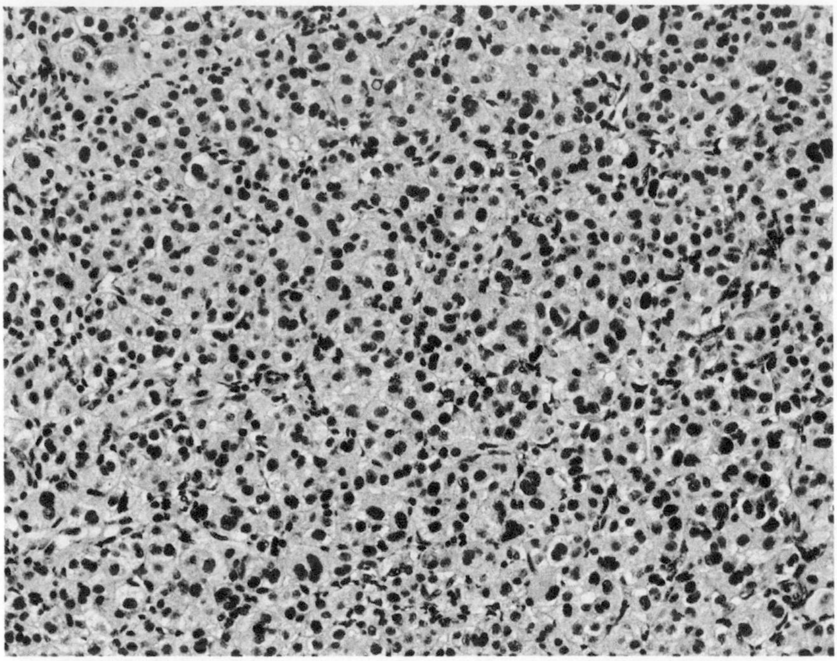

Fig. 23. p53 immunohistochemistry. Shown is p53 overexpression in an adrenocortical carcinoma.

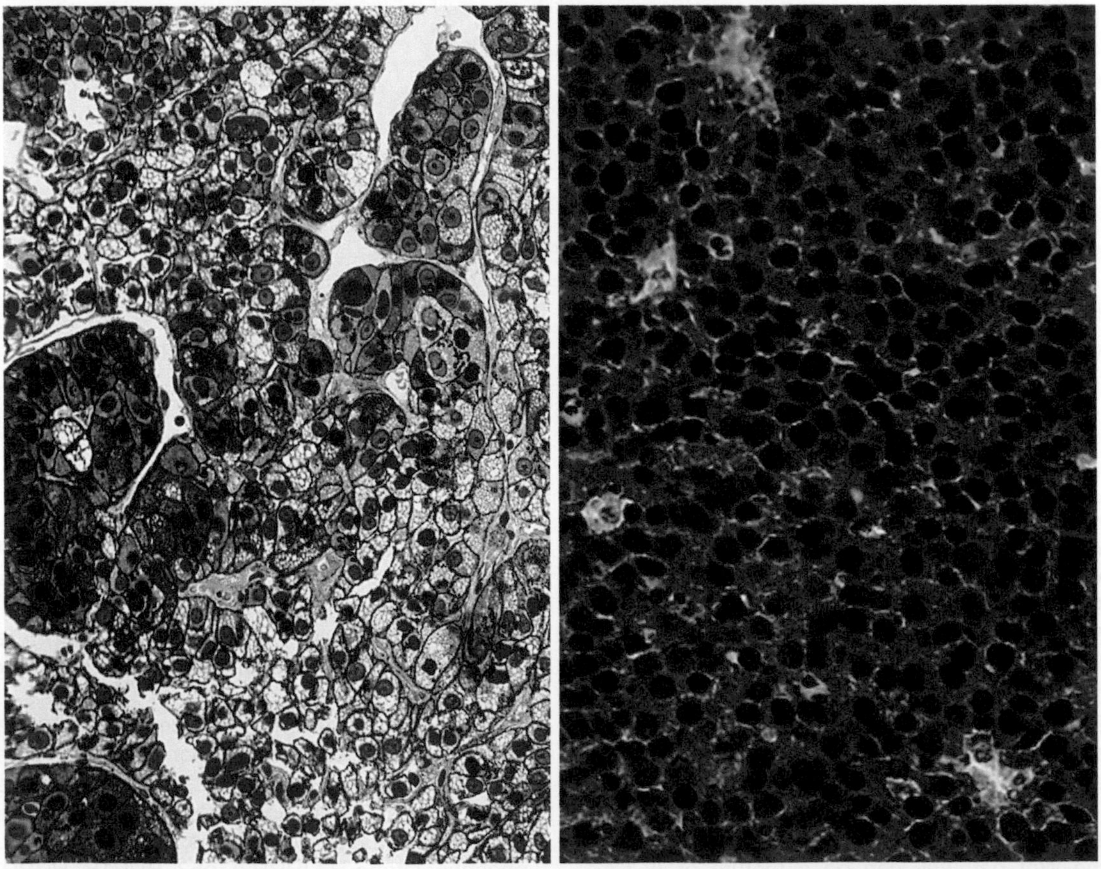

Fig. 24. Beta-catenin immunohistochemistry. Beta-catenin reactivity can be variable in adrenocortical neoplasms. Not all adrenocortical carcinomas manifest with nuclear and cytoplasmic beta-catenin expression; some adrenocortical carcinomas display variable nuclear staining (*left*). Diffuse nuclear and cytoplasmic beta-catenin expression in adrenocortical carcinoma (*right*). Diffuse nuclear and cytoplasmic beta-catenin reactivity alone does not warrant a diagnosis of malignancy; however, adrenocortical carcinomas with diffuse cytoplasmic and nuclear beta-catenin reactivity are more frequently associated with a poor prognosis.

Ki67 is one of the most important biomarkers and is readily available in almost all pathology laboratories. Most ACCs show a Ki67 proliferation exceeding 5%[41] (**Fig. 26**). The MIB1 antibody (anti–human Ki67 monoclonal antibody) is considered the gold standard for this assessment.[63] The management of patients with ACCs requires the knowledge of an accurate Ki67 labeling index along with other tumor characteristics.[67] Several pitfalls and pearls exist in the assessment of the Ki67 proliferation index. Because ACCs are well known to display intratumoral proliferative heterogeneity (see **Fig. 26**), the first step in obtaining an accurate and meaningful Ki67 labeling index is the selection of the right tumor block based on high mitotic density seen in hematoxylin-eosin–stained sections. Tumor blocks with poor tissue fixation can result in impaired detection of nuclear antigen. If there is any concern regarding tissue fixation, multiple blocks should be assessed. Although the antibody and staining methods used can vary from one laboratory to another, visual assessment is no longer an acceptable option for the analysis of the Ki67 in ACCs.[68,69] Manual counting or automated image analysis nuclear algorithms from hot spots of nuclear labeling (preferably 1000–2000 tumor cells) should be assessed in ACCs (**Fig. 27**). Some studies have classified ACCs into 3 groups: low-risk (grade 1), intermediate-risk (grade 2), and high-risk (grade 3) categories based on the Ki-67 index with different cutoffs (<10%, 10%–19%, ≥20%; or <20%, 20%–50%, >50%).[66,70] Overall, Ki67 labeling index is considered an important factor in prognosticating ACCs[66,70,71] as well as in determining the need for adjuvant therapies.[52,67] A recent French series of pediatric ACCs also highlighted the impact of Ki67 because pediatric ACCs with poor prognosis had 2 of the following parameters: Ki67 greater than 15%, mitotic activity greater than 15 per 20 high-power fields, vascular invasion, tumor necrosis, and adrenal capsule invasion.[49]

Regarding other prognostic biomarkers of ACCs, ATRX and DAXX (proteins that regulate telomere elongation) have been previously studied.[41,72] Global loss of DAXX and ATRX are commonly seen in ACCs and loss of DAXX is more frequent in disease-free patients.[41] Some biomarkers associated with DNA damage repair (eg, PBK) as well as the phosphatidylinositol 3 kinase (PI3K) signaling pathway (eg, PTEN and phospho-mTOR [mammalian target of rapamycin]) have also been investigated for diagnostic and prognostic purposes in ACCs; other biomarkers have been reported to predict response to mitotane or other chemotherapy regimens; however, further studies are needed to expand the use of these biomarkers in routine practice.[73]

Antibodies against key enzymes involved in the steroidogenic pathway can be used to assess the functionality of ACTs[28,74] (**Fig. 28**). Among these, monoclonal antibodies against HSD3B1/2 (3β-hydroxysteroid dehydrogenase type 1 and type 2) and CYP11B1/2 (cytochrome P450 family 11 subfamily B member 1 and member 2) have shown promise. CYP11B1 is typically expressed in the ZF layer, whereas CYP11B2

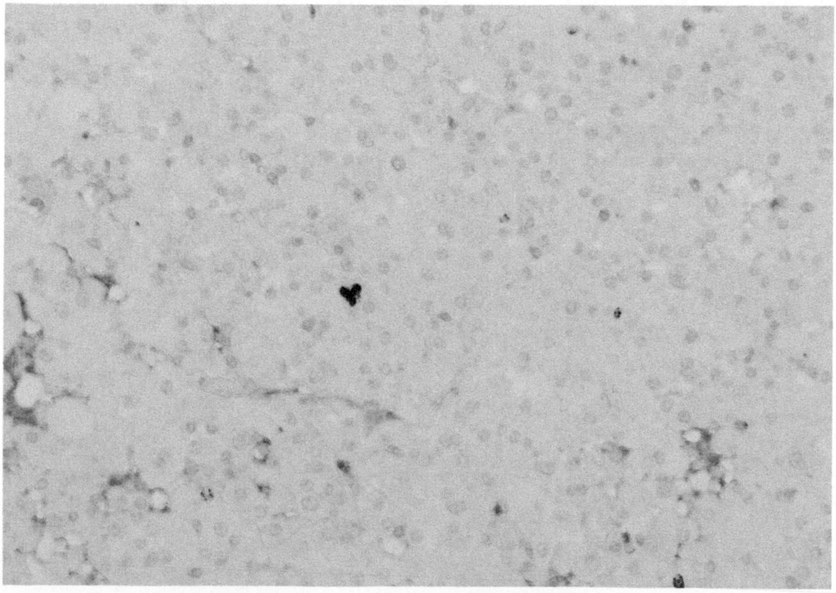

Fig. 25. PHH3 immunohistochemistry. PHH3 can be used to facilitate counting mitotic figures, because it also allows distinction of mitotic figures from apoptotic bodies and cells with crush artifact. Shown is an atypical mitotic figure using PHH3.

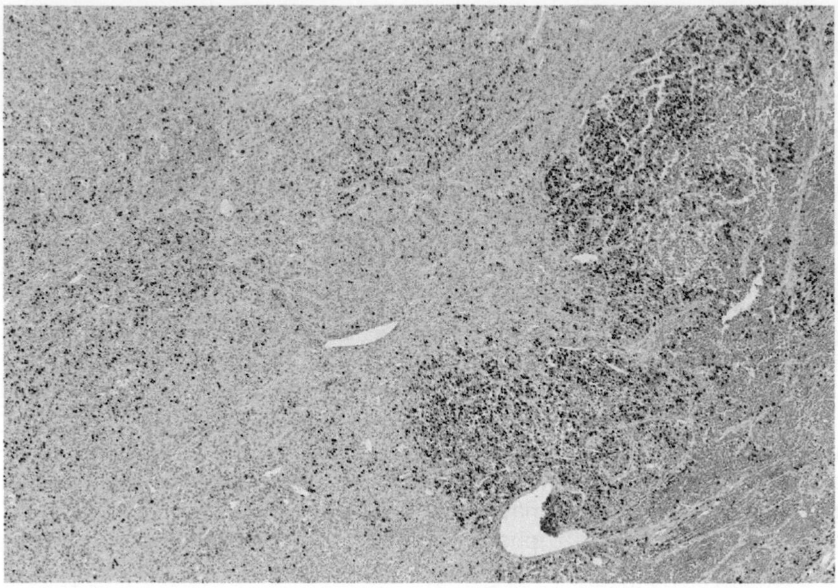

Fig. 26. Ki67 immunohistochemistry in adrenocortical neoplasms. Adrenocortical carcinomas are proliferation-driven neoplasms; most adrenocortical carcinomas have a Ki67 labeling index that exceeds 5%; however, these tumors often show intratumoral proliferative heterogeneity. Shown is Ki67 staining pattern in an adrenocortical carcinoma.

(aldosterone synthase) expression is exclusive to the ZG layer. In primary aldosteronism, the distinction of functional sites can be challenging and the use of CYP11B2 can assist in the functional assessment.[6,28,52,74] ZG hyperplasia and sites of APCCs can be located using CYP11B2, especially in the absence of an adrenal mass.[75]

In general, family history, early onset, bilaterality, and multifocality are features that suggest germline susceptibility, and exclusion of an underlying disorder is required. Most ACTs occurring in adults are sporadic, whereas pediatric tumors are more frequently associated with germline disease.[6,52] Menin, p27, p53, beta-catenin, MMR (mismatch repair) proteins, and succinate dehydrogenase subunit B (SDHB) immunohistochemistry can assist screening of adrenal manifestations of multiple endocrine neoplasia type 1 (MEN1),[6,52,76] MEN4,[6,52] Li-Fraumeni,[61,77] FAP,[78] Lynch,[79] and familial paraganglioma syndromes.[80] Other syndromes, including Beckwith-Wiedemann syndrome (*IGF-2*, *H19* at the 11p15 locus), Carney complex (*PRKAR1A*),

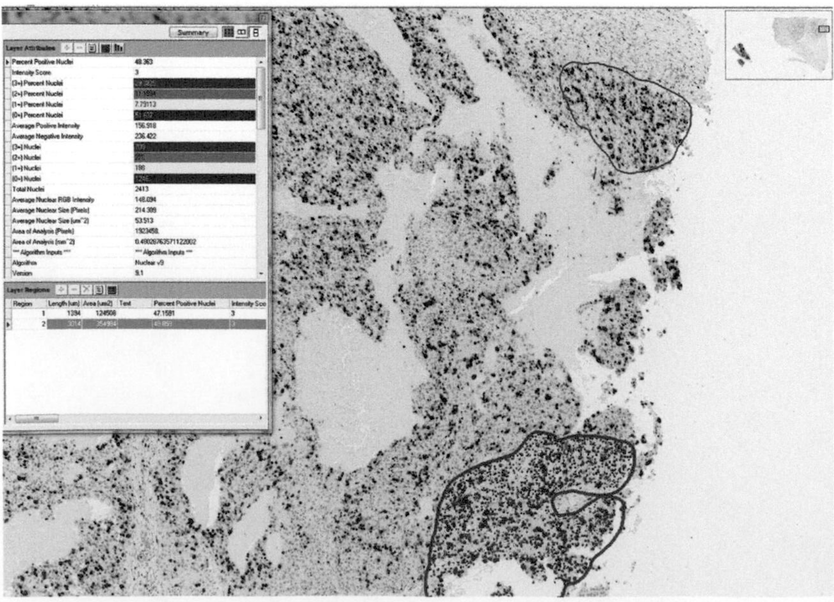

Fig. 27. Assessment of Ki67 immunohistochemistry. Accurate assessment of the Ki67 labeling index is of clinical significance because this information has prognostic and therapeutic implications. Visual assessment is no longer an acceptable option for the analysis of the Ki67 in adrenocortical carcinomas. Manual counting or automated image analysis nuclear algorithms from hot spots of nuclear labeling should be considered. Shown is the assessment of Ki67 using an automated image analysis nuclear algorithm.

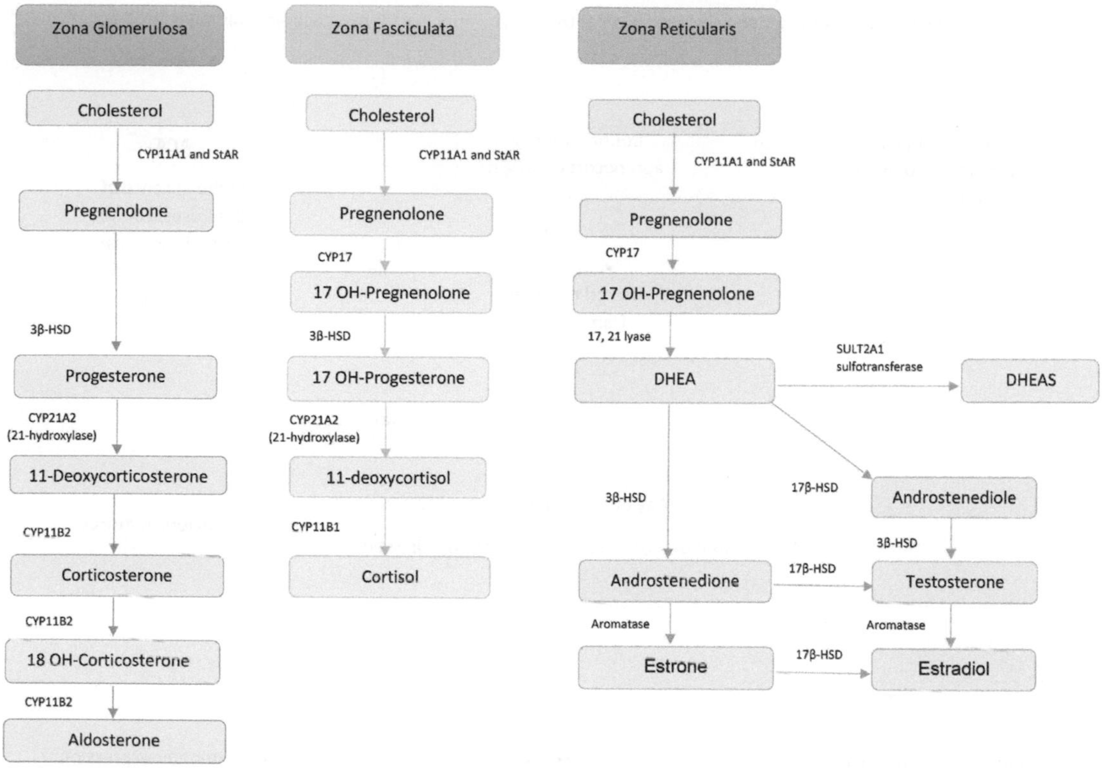

Fig. 28. The steroidogenic pathway. Immunohistochemical antibodies against key enzymes involved in the steroidogenic pathway can be used to assess the functionality of an adrenocortical neoplasm. Among these, monoclonal antibodies against HSD3B1/2 (3β-hydroxysteroid dehydrogenase type 1 and type 2) and CYP11B1/2 (cytochrome P450 family 11 subfamily B member 1 and member 2) have shown promise.

and neurofibromatosis type 1 (*NF1*), may be associated with ACCs.[32,81,82]

ULTRASTRUCTURAL EXAMINATION IN THE DIAGNOSIS OF ADRENOCORTICAL TUMORS

Ultrastructural examination has limited value in the modern surgical pathology of the adrenal cortex. Despite its limited utility, ultrastructural examination may be useful in identifying aldosterone-producing proliferations that show platelike or lamellar mitochondrial cristae, in contrast with nonfunctional and cortisol-producing cells that show tubulovesicular cristae.[6]

MOLECULAR BIOLOGY IN ADRENOCORTICAL NEOPLASMS

The past decade has seen significant progress in the understanding of adrenocortical tumorigenesis as well as the cellular mechanisms implicated in primary aldosteronism and adrenal Cushing syndrome. Most aldosterone-producing ACAs and APCCs are associated with increased transcription of CYP11B2 because of molecular alterations leading to aberrant activation of the calcium/calmodulin kinase pathway.[28,83,84] Among these, *KCNJ5* mutations are the most common alterations, followed by *ATP1A1*, *ATP2B3*, and *CACNA1D* mutations.[28,85–89] Unlike primary aldosteronism, most cortisol-producing ACAs harbor molecular alterations (most common *PRKACA* mutations, followed by *PRKAR1A*, *GNAS*, *PDE8B*, *PDE11A*, *PRKACB*, and *MC2R* mutations) implicated in the cyclic AMP (cAMP)/protein kinase A (PKA) pathway.[10,28,90,91] As seen in the example of Carney complex–related PPNAD, multiple microscopic ACAs identified in bilateral primary micronodular adrenocortical disease arise in the background of germline mutations (most commonly inactivating *PRKAR1A* mutations) that result in aberrant signaling of the cAMP/PKA pathway.[10,28,92,93] In contrast, around 55% of PBMAH manifests with germline *ARMC5* mutations.[94] Alterations in *MEN1*, *APC*, *FH*, *PDE8B*, and *PDE11A* have also been reported in PBMAH.[93,95–99] In contrast, *CTNNB1* mutations are more frequently implicated in nonfunctioning ACAs; these also occur in primary aldosteronism

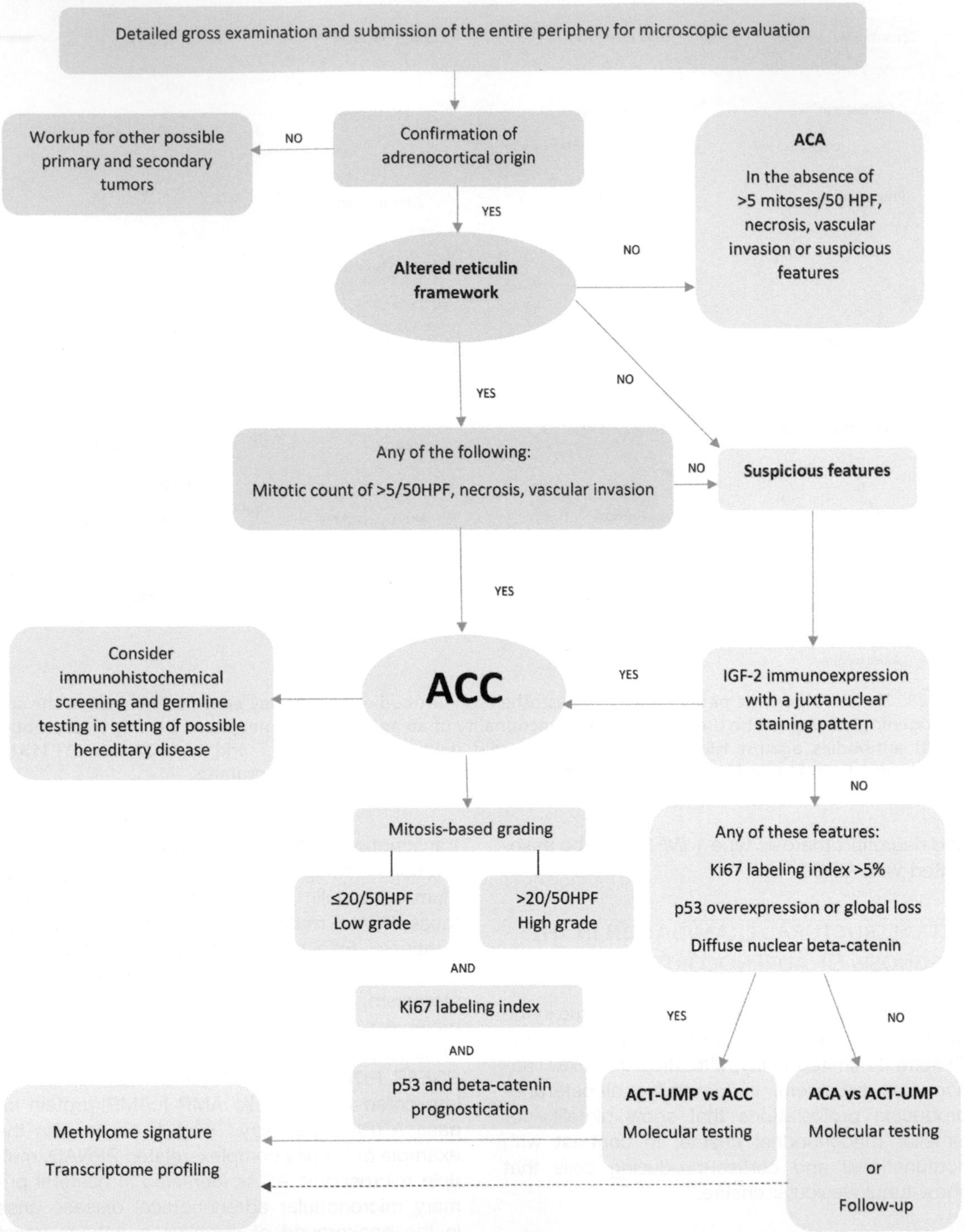

Fig. 29. Integrated practical approach to adult adrenocortical tumors with no extra-adrenal spread. Following careful macroscopic examination and an initial microscopic assessment that includes confirmation of adrenocortical origin of the lesion in question, evaluation of the reticulin framework is a critical step in the diagnostic approach to adrenocortical tumors. Suspicious features in the setting of a preserved reticulin framework include mitotically active tumors with fewer than 5 mitoses per 50 HPFs, presence of necrosis, adrenocortical tumors with suspicious but not unequivocal vascular invasion, and/or other invasive growth features. In these situations, IGF-2 immunohistochemistry is often useful. The additional immunohistochemical application of Ki67, p53, and beta-catenin as well as molecular testing can also be helpful in further classifying the challenging neoplasms. In addition to serving a diagnostic purpose, the use of Ki67, p53, and beta-catenin also has a prognostic role in the evaluation of adrenocortical carcinomas.

or adrenal Cushing syndrome.[28] Advances have generated several genotype-phenotype correlations in functioning ACAs.[28]

Gene expression profiles based on transcriptome (gene expression) profiling, exome or whole-genome sequencing and single nucleotide polymorphism arrays, miRnome (microRNA expression) analysis, chromosomal alterations, and methylome (DNA-methylation) signatures have expanded the molecular landscape of ACTs by highlighting distinct diagnostic and prognostic signatures of ACCs. Transcriptome studies have shown that ACCs can be distinguished from ACAs based on differential gene expression profiles.[64,65] Among these, upregulation of *IGF-2* stands out as one of the most important diagnostic characteristics of ACCs,[64,65] irrespective of tumor cytomorphology, proliferative grade, and prognosis. The absence of *IGF-2* alterations in adult ACAs makes IGF-2 a reliable candidate to be used in the distinction of ACCs. This finding is translated in paranuclear IGF-2 immunoreactivity in adult ACCs, as discussed earlier. Loss of heterozygosity (11p15) involving the *IGF-2* locus has also been noted in 91% of pediatric ACTs, underscoring its role in tumorigenesis.[100]

Transcriptome profiling has also shed light on the prognostic heterogeneity of ACCs by defining the bad and the good prognostic gene expression clusters.[64,65] *CTNNB1* and *TP53* alterations, along with overexpression of cell cycle–related genes, have been specifically seen in the bad prognostic transcriptome clusters.

Subsequent studies have identified common drivers, chromosomal alterations, and miRnome profiles implicated in the pathogenesis of ACCs.[53,101,102] The Wnt/beta-catenin signaling pathway (eg, *ZNRF3*, *CTNNB1*) has been found to be the most frequently altered pathway in ACCs.[53,101,102] Other common driver genes have been implicated in the PKA pathway (eg, *PRKAR1A*), cell cycle regulation (eg, *TP53*, *RB1*, *CDKN2A*, *CDK4*, *MDM2*) as well as the chromatin remodeling (eg, *MEN1*, *DAXX*, *ATRX*) and chromosome maintenance (eg, *TERT*, *TERF2*).[53,101,102] *CTNNB1* mutations are almost mutually exclusive from *TP53* mutations. When comparing primary tumor tissue with metastatic clones, a 2.8-fold higher mutation rate was identified in addition to increased mutational heterogeneity among metastatic sites.[103]

The Cancer Genome Atlas (TCGA) study identified whole-genome doubling as a sign of tumor progression in ACC.[53] The integrated genomics from ENSAT (the European Network for the Study of Adrenal Tumors)[101] and TCGA[53] series have further refined the spectrum of prognostic molecular clusters of transcriptome data series. Transcriptome clusters have been correlated with ENSAT molecular prognostic subgroups based on methylome and miRnome signatures.[101] The TCGA series defined 3 distinct molecular prognostic clusters that could be predicted using a 68-CpG probe DNA-methylation signature.[53] ACCs with high-CpG island methylator phenotype (CIMP) status were enriched in the worst prognostic subgroups in both ENSAT and TCGA series.[53,101] Similarly, tumors within the high proliferative category and steroid phenotype were enriched in the worst prognostic TCGA cluster.[53] A recent series identified the *G0S2* (G0/G1 Switch 2) methylation as a hallmark of biologically aggressive and rapidly recurrent ACCs with high-CIMP status, irrespective of the tumor grade.[104] The same series underscored the role of *BUB1B-PINK1* score (based on expression of *BUB1B* and *PINK1*), which also showed prognostic impact in earlier studies[64,105] in the prognostication and treatment rationalization of ACCs with unmethylated *G0S2* status.[104]

Heterogeneity and diagnostic challenges in pediatric ACCs have currently limited the characterization of these lesions, although it has been shown that synchronous *TP53* and *ATRX* mutations and associated genomics changes predict poor prognosis.[100]

MAKING THE RIGHT DIAGNOSIS: USING AN ALGORITHMIC APPROACH

Practicing pathologists who are not exposed frequently to ACTs may be uncomfortable during the handling of such specimens. A systematic approach is often helpful in rendering the correct diagnosis. Although the use of ancillary tools can be helpful, detailed examination of morphologic findings is still the basis of any evaluation. This article proposes a practical integrated algorithmic approach to ACTs to tackle some of these common diagnostic challenges (**Fig. 29**).

REFERENCES

1. Val P, Martinez A. Editorial: adrenal cortex: from physiology to disease. Front Endocrinol 2016;7:1–2.
2. Young WF. Clinical practice. The incidentally discovered adrenal mass. N Engl J Med 2007;356:601–10.
3. van Nederveen FH, de Krijger RR. Precursor lesions of the adrenal gland. Pathobiology 2007;74:285–90.
4. Mete O, Asa SL. Precursor lesions of endocrine system neoplasms. Pathology 2013;45:316–30.

5. Erickson LA, Rivera M, Zhang J. Adrenocortical carcinoma: review and update. Adv Anat Pathol 2014;21:151–9.
6. Duan K, Giordano TJ, Mete O. Adrenal cortical proliferations. In: Mete O, Asa SL, editors. Endocrine pathology. United Kingdom: Cambridge University Press; 2016. p. 602–27.
7. Funder JW, Carey RM, Fardella C, et al. Case detection, diagnosis, and treatment of patients with primary aldosteronism: an endocrine society clinical practice guideline. J Clin Endocrinol Metab 2008;93:3266–81.
8. Stowasser M. Update in primary aldosteronism. J Clin Endocrinol Metab 2015;100:1–10.
9. Duan K, Mete O. Clinicopathologic correlates of primary aldosteronism. Arch Pathol Lab Med 2015; 139:948–54.
10. Duan K, Gomez Hernandez K, Mete O. Clinicopathological correlates of adrenal Cushing's syndrome. J Clin Pathol 2015;68:175–86.
11. El-Maouche D, Arlt W, Merke DP. Congenital adrenal hyperplasia. Lancet 2017;390:2194–210.
12. Sasano H. The adrenal cortex. In: Stefaneanu L, Sasano H, Kovacs K, editors. Molecular and Cellular Endocrine Pathology. London: Arnold; 2000. p. 221–52.
13. Grumbach MM, Biller BMK, Braunstein GD, et al. Management of the clinically inapparent adrenal mass ('incidentaloma'). Ann Intern Med 2003;138: 424–9.
14. Francis IR. Distinguishing benign from malignant adrenal masses. Cancer Imaging 2003;3:102–10.
15. Daneman D, Daneman A. Diagnostic imaging of the thyroid and adrenal glands in childhood. Endocrinol Metab Clin North Am 2005;34:745–68.
16. Doppman JL, Nieman LK, Travis WD, et al. CT and MR imaging of massive macronodular adrenocortical disease: a rare cause of autonomous primary adrenal hypercortisolism. J Comput Assist Tomogr 1991;15:773–9.
17. Vezzosi D, Tenenbaum F, Cazabat L, et al. Hormonal, radiological, NP-59 scintigraphy, and pathological correlations in patients with cushing's syndrome due to primary pigmented nodular adrenocortical disease (PPNAD). J Clin Endocrinol Metab 2015;100:4332–8.
18. Louiset E, Stratakis CA, Perraudin V, et al. The paradoxical increase in cortisol secretion induced by dexamethasone in primary pigmented nodular adrenocortical disease involves a glucocorticoid receptor-mediated effect of dexamethasone on protein kinase A catalytic subunits. J Clin Endocrinol Metab 2009;94:2406–13.
19. Mendichovszky IA, Powlson AS, Manavaki R, et al. Targeted molecular imaging in adrenal disease-an emerging role for metomidate PET-CT. Diagnostics (Basel) 2016;6, [pii:E42].
20. O'Shea PM, O'Donoghue D, Bashari W, et al. 11 C-Metomidate PET/CT is a useful adjunct for lateralisation of primary aldosteronism in routine clinical practice. Clin Endocrinol (Oxf) 2019. https://doi.org/10.1111/cen.13942.
21. Dunnick NR, Korobkin M. Imaging of adrenal incidentalomas: current status. AJR Am J Roentgenol 2002;179:559–68.
22. Francis IR, Mayo-Smith WW. Adrenal imaging. In: Hodler J, Kubik-Huch RA, von Schulthess GK, editors. Diseases of the abdomen and pelvis 2018-2021. Cham (Switzerland): Springer International Publishing; 2018. p. 85–90.
23. Zografos GN, Vasiliadis G, Farfaras AN, et al. Laparoscopic surgery for malignant adrenal tumors. JSLS 2009;13:196–202.
24. McNicol AM. A diagnostic approach to adrenal cortical lesions. Endocr Pathol 2008;19:241–51.
25. Mete O, Asa SL. Morphological distinction of cortisol-producing and aldosterone-producing adrenal cortical adenomas: not only possible but a critical clinical responsibility. Histopathology 2012; 60:1015–6, [author reply: 1016–7].
26. Aubert S, Wacrenier A, Leroy X, et al. Weiss system revisited: a clinicopathologic and immunohistochemical study of 49 adrenocortical tumors. Am J Surg Pathol 2002;26:1612–9.
27. Lloyd RV, Osamura RY, Kloppel G, et al. WHO classification of tumours of endocrine organs. 4th edition. Lyon (France): WHO Press; 2017.
28. Mete O, Duan K. The many faces of primary aldosteronism and cushing syndrome: a reflection of adrenocortical tumor heterogeneity. Front Med 2018;5:54.
29. Patel KA, Calomeni EP, Nadasdy T, et al. Adrenal gland inclusions in patients treated with aldosterone antagonists (Spironolactone/Eplerenone): incidence, morphology, and ultrastructural findings. Diagn Pathol 2014;9:147.
30. Lowe KM, Young WF, Lyssikatos C, et al. Cushing syndrome in carney complex: clinical, pathologic, and molecular genetic findings in the 17 affected mayo clinic patients. Am J Surg Pathol 2017;41: 171–81.
31. Stratakis CA, Boikos SA. Genetics of adrenal tumors associated with Cushing's syndrome: a new classification for bilateral adrenocortical hyperplasias. Nat Clin Pract Endocrinol Metab 2007;3: 748–57.
32. Morin E, Mete O, Wasserman JD, et al. Carney complex with adrenal cortical carcinoma. J Clin Endocrinol Metab 2012;97:E202–6.
33. Anselmo J, Medeiros S, Carneiro V, et al. A large family with Carney complex caused by the S147G PRKAR1A mutation shows a unique spectrum of disease including adrenocortical cancer. J Clin Endocrinol Metab 2012;97:351–9.

34. Duregon E, Volante M, Cappia S, et al. Oncocytic adrenocortical tumors: diagnostic algorithm and mitochondrial DNA profile in 27 cases. Am J Surg Pathol 2011;35:1882–93.
35. Renaudin K, Smati S, Wargny M, et al. Clinicopathological description of 43 oncocytic adrenocortical tumors: importance of Ki-67 in histoprognostic evaluation. Mod Pathol 2018;31:1708–16.
36. Weiss LM. Comparative histologic study of 43 metastasizing and nonmetastasizing adrenocortical tumors. Am J Surg Pathol 1984;8:163–9.
37. Weiss LM, Medeiros LJ, Vickery AL. Pathologic features of prognostic significance in adrenocortical carcinoma. Am J Surg Pathol 1989;13:202–6.
38. Bisceglia M, Ludovico O, Di Mattia A, et al. Adrenocortical oncocytic tumors: report of 10 cases and review of the literature. Int J Surg Pathol 2004;12:231–43.
39. Volante M, Bollito E, Sperone P, et al. Clinicopathological study of a series of 92 adrenocortical carcinomas: from a proposal of simplified diagnostic algorithm to prognostic stratification. Histopathology 2009;55:535–43.
40. Duregon E, Fassina A, Volante M, et al. The reticulin algorithm for adrenocortical tumor diagnosis: a multicentric validation study on 245 unpublished cases. Am J Surg Pathol 2013;37:1433–40.
41. Mete O, Gucer H, Kefeli M, et al. Diagnostic and prognostic biomarkers of adrenal cortical carcinoma. Am J Surg Pathol 2018;42:201–13.
42. Fonseca D, Murthy SS, Tagore KR, et al. Diagnosis of adrenocortical tumors by reticulin algorithm. Indian J Endocrinol Metab 2017;21:734–7.
43. Papotti M, Volante M, Duregon E, et al. Adrenocortical tumors with myxoid features: a distinct morphologic and phenotypical variant exhibiting malignant behavior. Am J Surg Pathol 2010;34:973–83.
44. Morimoto R, Satoh F, Murakami O, et al. Immunohistochemistry of a proliferation marker Ki67/MIB1 in adrenocortical carcinomas: Ki67/MIB1 labeling index is a predictor for recurrence of adrenocortical carcinomas. Endocr J 2008;55:49–55.
45. Pennanen M, Heiskanen I, Sane T, et al. Helsinki score-a novel model for prediction of metastases in adrenocortical carcinomas. Hum Pathol 2015;46:404–10.
46. Duregon E, Cappellesso R, Maffeis V, et al. Validation of the prognostic role of the 'Helsinki Score' in 225 cases of adrenocortical carcinoma. Hum Pathol 2017;62:1–7.
47. Lalli E, Figueiredo BC. Pediatric adrenocortical tumors: what they can tell us on adrenal development and comparison with adult adrenal tumors. Front Endocrinol 2015;6:1–9.
48. Wieneke JA, Thompson LDR, Heffess CS. Adrenal cortical neoplasms in the pediatric population: a clinicopathologic and immunophenotypic analysis of 83 patients. Am J Surg Pathol 2003;27:867–81.
49. Picard C, Orbach D, Carton M, et al. Revisiting the role of the pathological grading in pediatric adrenal cortical tumors: results from a national cohort study with pathological review. Mod Pathol 2018. https://doi.org/10.1038/s41379-018-0174-8.
50. Das S, Sengupta M, Islam N, et al. Weineke criteria, Ki-67 index and p53 status to study pediatric adrenocortical tumors: Is there a correlation? J Pediatr Surg 2016;51:1795–800.
51. Chatterjee G, DasGupta S, Mukherjee G, et al. Usefulness of Wieneke criteria in assessing morphologic characteristics of adrenocortical tumors in children. Pediatr Surg Int 2015;31:563–71.
52. Mete O, Asa SL, Giordano TJ, et al. Immunohistochemical biomarkers of adrenal cortical neoplasms. Endocr Pathol 2018;29:137–49.
53. Zheng S, Cherniack AD, Dewal N, et al. Comprehensive pan-genomic characterization of adrenocortical carcinoma. Cancer Cell 2016;29:723–36.
54. Miller BS, Gauger PG, Hammer GD, et al. Proposal for modification of the ENSAT staging system for adrenocortical carcinoma using tumor grade. Langenbecks Arch Surg 2010;395:955–61.
55. Assié G, Antoni G, Tissier F, et al. Prognostic parameters of metastatic adrenocortical carcinoma. J Clin Endocrinol Metab 2007;92:148–54.
56. Giordano TJ. The argument for mitotic rate-based grading for the prognostication of adrenocortical carcinoma. Am J Surg Pathol 2011;35:471–3.
57. Duregon E, Volante M, Bollito E, et al. Pitfalls in the diagnosis of adrenocortical tumors: a lesson from 300 consultation cases. Hum Pathol 2015;46:1799–807.
58. Papathomas TG, Duregon E, Korpershoek E, et al. Sarcomatoid adrenocortical carcinoma: a comprehensive pathological, immunohistochemical, and targeted next-generation sequencing analysis. Hum Pathol 2016;58:113–22.
59. Schmitt A, Saremaslani P, Schmid S, et al. IGFII and MIB1 immunohistochemistry is helpful for the differentiation of benign from malignant adrenocortical tumours. Histopathology 2006;49:298–307.
60. Reincke M, Karl M, Travis WH, et al. p53 mutations in human adrenocortical neoplasms: immunohistochemical and molecular studies. J Clin Endocrinol Metab 1994;78:790–4.
61. Wasserman JD, Novokmet A, Eichler-Jonsson C, et al. Prevalence and functional consequence of TP53 mutations in pediatric adrenocortical carcinoma: a children's oncology group study. J Clin Oncol 2015;33:602–9.
62. Waldmann J, Patsalis N, Fendrich V, et al. Clinical impact of TP53 alterations in adrenocortical carcinomas. Langenbecks Arch Surg 2012;397:209–16.

63. Jouinot A, Bertherat J. Management of endocrine disease: adrenocortical carcinoma: differentiating the good from the poor prognosis tumors. Eur J Endocrinol 2018;178:R215–30.
64. de Reyniès A, Assié G, Rickman DS, et al. Gene expression profiling reveals a new classification of adrenocortical tumors and identifies molecular predictors of malignancy and survival. J Clin Oncol 2009;27:1108–15.
65. Giordano TJ, Kuick R, Else T, et al. Molecular classification and prognostication of adrenocortical tumors by transcriptome profiling. Clin Cancer Res 2009;15:668–76.
66. Duregon E, Molinaro L, Volante M, et al. Comparative diagnostic and prognostic performances of the hematoxylin-eosin and phospho-histone H3 mitotic count and Ki-67 index in adrenocortical carcinoma. Mod Pathol 2014;27:1246–54.
67. Fassnacht M, Dekkers O, Else T, et al. European Society of Endocrinology Clinical Practice Guidelines on the management of adrenocortical carcinoma in adults, in collaboration with the European Network for the Study of Adrenal Tumors. Eur J Endocrinol 2018;179:G1–46.
68. Papathomas TG, Pucci E, Giordano TJ, et al. An international Ki67 reproducibility study in adrenal cortical carcinoma. Am J Surg Pathol 2016;40: 569–76.
69. Lu H, Papathomas TG, van Zessen D, et al. Automated Selection of Hotspots (ASH): enhanced automated segmentation and adaptive step finding for Ki67 hotspot detection in adrenal cortical cancer. Diagn Pathol 2014;9:216.
70. Beuschlein F, Weigel J, Saeger W, et al. Major prognostic role of Ki67 in localized adrenocortical carcinoma after complete resection. J Clin Endocrinol Metab 2015;100:841–9.
71. Yamazaki Y, Nakamura Y, Shibahara Y, et al. Comparison of the methods for measuring the Ki-67 labeling index in adrenocortical carcinoma: manual versus digital image analysis. Hum Pathol 2016; 53:41–50.
72. Heaphy CM, de Wilde RF, Jiao Y, et al. Altered telomeres in tumors with ATRX and DAXX mutations. Science 2011;333:425.
73. Ross JS, Wang K, Rand JV, et al. Next-generation sequencing of adrenocortical carcinoma reveals new routes to targeted therapies. J Clin Pathol 2014;67:968–73.
74. Gomez-Sanchez CE, Gomez-Sanchez EP. Immunohistochemistry of the adrenal in primary aldosteronism. Curr Opin Endocrinol Diabetes Obes 2016; 23:242–8.
75. Yamazaki Y, Nakamura Y, Omata K, et al. Histopathological classification of cross-sectional image-negative hyperaldosteronism. J Clin Endocrinol Metab 2017;102:1182–92.
76. Skogseid B, Rastad J, Gobl A, et al. Adrenal lesion in multiple endocrine neoplasia type 1. Surgery 1995;118:1077–82.
77. Wagner J, Portwine C, Rabin K, et al. High frequency of germline p53 mutations in childhood adrenocortical cancer. J Natl Cancer Inst 1994; 86:1707–10.
78. Smith TG, Clark SK, Katz DE, et al. Adrenal masses are associated with familial adenomatous polyposis. Dis Colon Rectum 2000;43:1739–42.
79. Raymond VM, Everett JN, Furtado LV, et al. Adrenocortical carcinoma is a lynch syndrome-associated cancer. J Clin Oncol 2013;31:3012–8.
80. Else T, Lerario AM, Everett J, et al. Adrenocortical carcinoma and succinate dehydrogenase gene mutations: an observational case series. Eur J Endocrinol 2017;177:439–44.
81. Menon RK, Ferrau F, Kurzawinski TR, et al. Adrenal cancer in neurofibromatosis type 1: case report and DNA analysis. Endocrinol Diabetes Metab Case Rep 2014;2014:140074.
82. Henry I, Jeanpierre M, Couillin P, et al. Molecular definition of the 11p15.5 region involved in Beckwith-Wiedemann syndrome and probably in predisposition to adrenocortical carcinoma. Hum Genet 1989;81:273–7.
83. Omata K, Anand SK, Hovelson DH, et al. Aldosterone-producing cell clusters frequently harbor somatic mutations and accumulate with age in normal adrenals. J Endocr Soc 2017;1: 787–99.
84. Omata K, Satoh F, Morimoto R, et al. Cellular and genetic causes of idiopathic hyperaldosteronism. Hypertension 2018;72:874–80.
85. Monticone S, Else T, Mulatero P, et al. Understanding primary aldosteronism: impact of next generation sequencing and expression profiling. Mol Cell Endocrinol 2015;399:311–20.
86. Seidel E, Scholl UI. Intracellular molecular differences in aldosterone- compared to cortisol-secreting adrenal cortical adenomas. Front Endocrinol 2016;7:75.
87. Åkerström T, Crona J, Delgado Verdugo A, et al. Comprehensive re-sequencing of adrenal aldosterone producing lesions reveal three somatic mutations near the KCNJ5 potassium channel selectivity filter. PLoS One 2012;7:e41926.
88. Tan GC, Negro G, Pinggera A, et al. Aldosterone-producing adenomas: histopathology-genotype correlation and identification of a novel CACNA1D mutation. Hypertension 2017;70:129–36.
89. Nanba K, Chen AX, Omata K, et al. Molecular heterogeneity in aldosterone-producing adenomas. J Clin Endocrinol Metab 2016;101:999–1007.
90. Lodish M, Stratakis CA. A genetic and molecular update on adrenocortical causes of Cushing syndrome. Nat Rev Endocrinol 2016;12:255–62.

91. Espiard S, Knape MJ, Bathon K, et al. Activating PRKACB somatic mutation in cortisol-producing adenomas. JCI Insight 2018;3.
92. Kamilaris CDC, Faucz FR, Voutetakis A, et al. Carney complex. Exp Clin Endocrinol Diabetes 2019;127:156–64.
93. Hannah-Shmouni F, Faucz FR, Stratakis CA. Alterations of Phosphodiesterases in Adrenocortical Tumors. Front Endocrinol 2016;7:111.
94. Assié G, Libé R, Espiard S, et al. ARMC5 mutations in macronodular adrenal hyperplasia with Cushing's syndrome. N Engl J Med 2013;369:2105–14.
95. Yoshida M, Hiroi M, Imai T, et al. A case of ACTH-independent macronodular adrenal hyperplasia associated with multiple endocrine neoplasia type 1. Endocr J 2011;58:269–77.
96. Libé R, Fratticci A, Coste J, et al. Phosphodiesterase 11A (PDE11A) and genetic predisposition to adrenocortical tumors. Clin Cancer Res 2008;14:4016–24.
97. Matyakhina L, Freedman RJ, Bourdeau I, et al. Hereditary leiomyomatosis associated with bilateral, massive, macronodular adrenocortical disease and atypical cushing syndrome: a clinical and molecular genetic investigation. J Clin Endocrinol Metab 2005;90:3773–9.
98. Hsiao H-P, Kirschner LS, Bourdeau I, et al. Clinical and genetic heterogeneity, overlap with other tumor syndromes, and atypical glucocorticoid hormone secretion in adrenocorticotropin-independent macronodular adrenal hyperplasia compared with other adrenocortical tumors. J Clin Endocrinol Metab 2009;94:2930–7.
99. Gaujoux S, Pinson S, Gimenez-Roqueplo A-P, et al. Inactivation of the APC gene is constant in adrenocortical tumors from patients with familial adenomatous polyposis but not frequent in sporadic adrenocortical cancers. Clin Cancer Res 2010;16: 5133–41.
100. Pinto EM, Chen X, Easton J, et al. Genomic landscape of paediatric adrenocortical tumours. Nat Commun 2015;6:6302.
101. Assié G, Letouzé E, Fassnacht M, et al. Integrated genomic characterization of adrenocortical carcinoma. Nat Genet 2014;46:607–12.
102. Juhlin CC, Goh G, Healy JM, et al. Whole-exome sequencing characterizes the landscape of somatic mutations and copy number alterations in adrenocortical carcinoma. J Clin Endocrinol Metab 2015;100:E493–502.
103. Gara SK, Lack J, Zhang L, et al. Metastatic adrenocortical carcinoma displays higher mutation rate and tumor heterogeneity than primary tumors. Nat Commun 2018;9:4172.
104. Mohan DR, Lerario AM, Else T, et al. Targeted assessment of G0S2 methylation identifies a rapidly recurrent, routinely fatal molecular subtype of adrenocortical carcinoma. Clin Cancer Res 2019;25(11):3276–88.
105. Fragoso MCBV, Almeida MQ, Mazzuco TL, et al. Combined expression of BUB1B, DLGAP5, and PINK1 as predictors of poor outcome in adrenocortical tumors: validation in a Brazilian cohort of adult and pediatric patients. Eur J Endocrinol 2012;166: 61–7.

Treatment of Adrenocortical Carcinoma

Anand Vaidya, MD, MMSc[a,*], Matthew Nehs, MD[b,c], Kerry Kilbridge, MD[b,c,d]

KEYWORDS

• Adrenocortical carcinoma • Adrenal • Mitotane • Adrenal cortex • Cancer

Key points

- Adrenocortical carcinoma (ACC) is a rare cancer that is usually associated with a poor prognosis.
- ACC can often grow rapidly and produce excess adrenal hormones that contribute to morbidity
- Surgery is the cornerstone of therapy and currently the only avenue for a potential cure
- Adjuvant systemic medical therapies, such as mitotane, chemotherapy, and radiation, also are reviewed.

ABSTRACT

Adrenocortical carcinoma (ACC) is a rare malignancy with a poor prognosis. ACC is capable of secreting excess adrenocortical hormones, which can compound morbidity and compromise clinical outcomes. By the time most ACCs are diagnosed, there is usually locoregional or metastatic disease. Surgery is the most important treatment to offer possibility of cure or prolong survival. Several adjuvant therapies are used depending on grade and stage of the tumor and other patient-related factors. This review provides an overview of treatment approaches for ACC, highlighting evidence to support each treatment and acknowledging where more data and research are needed to improve care.

OVERVIEW

Adrenocortical carcinoma (ACC) is a rare malignancy, with an estimated incidence of 1 million to 2 million cases per year.[1–3] ACC most commonly diagnosed in the fifth to seventh decades of life, but it can arise at any age. Although most ACCs are considered sporadic and without a known cause, a minority of cases are attributable to known hereditary predispositions, including Li-Fraumeni syndrome, Lynch syndrome, multiple endocrine neoplasia type 1, and familial adenomatous polyposis.[1,4–6] The prognosis of ACC is usually poor; by the time ACC is diagnosed, a majority of patients have locally or systemically advanced disease, often with hormonal hypersecretion that increases morbidity. The combination of its rarity and generally short survival time has resulted in few prospective or randomized trials, and, therefore, most best practices for ACC therapy are driven by lower grades of evidence and consensus opinion. Surgery is the most important treatment modality and the only avenue to achieve cure. Adjuvant systemic therapies usually are used, depending on the stage and grade of the tumor, to influence progression-free survival and overall survival.

Disclosures: M. Nehs and K. Kilbridge have nothing to disclose. A. Vaidya has been a consultant and/or scientific advisory board member for Corcept Therapeutics, Ionis Pharmaceuticals, Selenity Therapeutics, HRA Pharma, and Orphagen Pharmaceuticals.

[a] Division of Endocrinology Diabetes, and Hypertension, Department of Medicine, Center for Adrenal Disorders, Brigham and Women's Hospital, Harvard Medical School, 25 Shattuck Street, Boston, MA 02115, USA; [b] Brigham and Women's Hospital, Harvard Medical School, 25 Shattuck Street, Boston, MA 02115, USA; [c] Department of Surgery, Dana-Farber Cancer Institute, 450 Brookline Avenue, Boston, MA 02215, USA; [d] Lank Center for Genitourinary Oncology, Dana-Farber Cancer Institute, 450 Brookline Avenue, Boston, MA 02215, USA

* Corresponding author. Brigham and Women's Hospital, Harvard Medical School, 25 Shattuck Street, Boston, MA 02115.

E-mail address: anandvaidya@bwh.harvard.edu

Surgical Pathology 12 (2019) 997–1006
https://doi.org/10.1016/j.path.2019.08.010

This article provides a brief overview of the approach to treating ACC. This review is designed specifically to provide an overview for pathologists who wish to better understand how ACC is treated and how pathologic parameters influence treatment decisions. More comprehensive guidelines on ACC treatment are available elsewhere.[1]

CLINICAL PRESENTATION AND EVALUATION

ACC is a unique malignancy in that it can autonomously secrete one, or multiple, adrenal cortical hormones that can substantially compound morbidity. ACC is consequently commonly diagnosed either during the evaluation of hypercortisolism or Cushing syndrome, hyperandrogenism, or primary aldosteronism or during the evaluation of a concerning adrenal mass that was incidentally discovered on imaging.[7,8] Imaging characteristics of ACC typically include a heterogeneous and often large adrenal mass that also may exhibit calcifications, hemorrhage/necrosis, and poor contrast washout characteristics on delayed computed tomography.[7,8] Less commonly, ACC is diagnosed during the evaluation of nonspecific symptoms that raise concern for a malignancy, such as weight loss, fevers, night sweats, back or flank pain, or abdominal fullness. More than half of ACCs have clinically relevant adrenal hormone excess, although it is likely that most ACCs secrete subclinical levels of adrenal cortical hormones or their intermediate metabolites.[9] The most effective approach to mitigating the adverse effects of hypercortisolism, hyperandrogenism, and hyperaldosteronism is a complete surgical resection. When this cannot be accomplished, medical therapies directed at inhibiting or blocking cortisol, the use of mineralocorticoid antagonists, and supportive care may be necessary.

The clinical evaluation of ACC involves measurements to assess adrenocortical hormone excess and cross-sectional imaging. A biopsy is often tempting to make a tissue diagnosis but is strongly discouraged because the heterogeneity of ACC can result in nonmalignant or uninterpretable results that can be falsely reassuring. Additionally, there is a theoretic risk for seeding the needle track.[7,8,10] When the imaging appearance of an adrenal mass is concerning for ACC, a surgical resection should be strongly considered for diagnosis, prognostication, and treatment.[7,8]

HISTOPATHOLOGIC EVALUATION AND STAGING

Although a clinical evaluation often strongly suggests ACC (ie, a large heterogeneous adrenal mass with Cushing syndrome and hyperandrogenism), definitive diagnosis is made by histopathologic examination. The most commonly used histopathologic tool to make the distinction between an adrenocortical adenoma and ACC uses Weiss criteria on hematoxylin-eosin–stained slides.[11,12] Three or more of the following Weiss criteria are strongly indicative of ACC: high nuclear grade, more than 5 mitoses per 50 high-power fields, atypical mitotic figures, less than 25% clear cells, diffuse architecture, necrosis, venous invasion, sinusoidal invasion, and capsular invasion. To complement the Weiss criteria, several other classification systems exist and can be useful for borderline tumors.[13–17] For more details regarding the histopathologic evaluation of adrenocortical tumors, please see the article by Anjelica Hodgson and colleagues', "A Diagnostic Approach to Adrenocortical Tumors," in this issue.

The prognosis for ACC is poor, with an overall survival of less than 5 years from the time of diagnosis. The prognosis varies greatly, however, by the stage and grade of disease and the treatment center that is coordinating care.[1,2] Widely accepted staging criteria include the American Joint Committee on Cancer and the European Network for the Study of Adrenal Tumors (ENSAT); both criteria are similar. Stage I ACC is defined as T1, N0, M0, where the primary tumor is $\leq$ 5cm in size. Stage II ACC is defined as T2, N0, M0 where the primary tumor is > 5 cm in size. Stage III ACC is defined as T1-T2, N1, M0 or T3-T4, N0-N1, M0 where a primary tumor of any size has infiltrated surrounding periadrenal tissue or invaded adjacent organs or there is tumor thrombus in the inferior vena cava or renal vein or there is involvement of lymph nodes. Stage IV ACC is defined as T1-T4, N0-N1, M1 where there is evidence of distant metastases regardless of other factors.[1] The only cure for ACC is complete surgical resection, whereas nonsurgical therapies (discussed later) are not curative and can have poor efficacy and/or be toxic.

Stage I and stage II ACC have 5-year survival rates of 60% to 80% respectively because they are most amenable to complete surgical resection; however, detection of ACC at these stages is not common.[1,2] ACC is most commonly detected with locoregional disease (stage III) or advanced disease (stage IV), where despite adjuvant therapies the overall survival rates at 5 years are 30% to 50% and less than 25%, respectively.[1,2,18] For these reasons and the fact that expertise in ACC care is not widespread, it is strongly recommended that patients with ACC be treated by multidisciplinary teams at highly experienced centers.[1,7] A complete surgical resection by an experienced surgical team is critical for optimal outcomes and a multidisciplinary approach to adjuvant systemic and localized therapies by an experienced medical team can amplify these gains.

Key Points
ON CLINICAL PRESENTATION AND HISTOPATHOLOGIC EVALUATION AND STAGING

- ACC can autonomously secrete one or multiple adrenal cortical hormones that can substantially compound morbidity.
- The prognosis for ACC is poor, with an overall survival of less than 5 years from the time of diagnosis.
- Tumor stage, grade, and Ki-67 proliferative index are the parameters most predictive of the prognosis and survival.

SURGERY

A complete surgical resection (R0 resection) is currently the only known pathway to cure in ACC. Incomplete surgical resections are associated with better long-term outcomes and survival than no resection at all[2]; therefore, it is strongly recommended that highly experienced surgical teams evaluate and assess each case of ACC.

PERIOPERATIVE SURGICAL PLANNING

A contrast-enhanced abdominal CT scan is an essential part of the preoperative work-up to assess for tumor size, necrosis, invasion into surrounding organs, lymphadenopathy, and a patient's body habitus (**Fig. 1**). Obesity and excess retroperitoneal fat (as are often seen in patients with ACC-related Cushing syndrome) can compound the difficulty of exposure and necessitate a larger surgical exposure, such as a thoracoabdominal incision. These large incisions have increased morbidity and pain in the postoperative recovery period, but they may provide the only exposure that allows for a safe and oncologically sound resection. All patients with Cushing syndrome or cortisol hypersecretion should be suspected of having suppression of the contralateral adrenal gland and, therefore, may have adrenal insufficiency postoperatively. This can be effectively addressed with intraoperative and postoperative hydrocortisone supplementation, ideally in conjunction with experienced anesthesiology and endocrinology teams.

SURGICAL APPROACH

Radical adrenalectomy should be performed by surgeons with considerable experience with adrenal or oncologic surgery.[1] ACCs often are large invasive masses that are stuck to surrounding tissues and organs; therefore, the surgical team should assess the tumor's characteristics when planning the surgical approach.

There are no large randomized trials comparing open to laparoscopic adrenalectomy for ACC. Early reports of laparoscopic resection of ACC had increased rates of tumor capsule disruption and spillage, and a meta-analysis from 2016 showed a significantly higher rate of peritoneal carcinomatosis with a laparoscopic approach.[19] Several retrospective case series, however, have reported no difference in mortality when comparing a laparoscopic approach for tumors less than 10 cm.[19,20] If invasion is seen during laparoscopic adrenalectomy, conversion to an open/radical approach is generally undertaken, in line with standard oncologic principles. In the absence of randomized controlled trial data, consensus guidelines recommend open surgery for known or suspected ACC as the gold standard approach.[1] This may be particularly important for stage I and stage II tumors, where an R0 resection and cure is still possible.[21] Open surgery allows for wide exposure and en bloc resection of the adrenal mass, perinephric fat, and surrounding organs that may be involved (eg, spleen, pancreas, and kidney). Furthermore, open surgery increases the ability to sample surrounding lymph nodes, which is important for accurate staging.

The surgical approach to the adrenal mass depends greatly on the side and size of the tumor. Left-sided ACCs generally are adherent or invasive to the spleen, pancreas, left kidney, splenic flexure of the colon, and/or stomach. The surgical exposure and approach should consider that these organs may need to be resected at the time of the operation. Often, the tail of the pancreas and spleen need to be excised in order to gain exposure to the left adrenal mass (**Fig. 2**). It is less common for the parenchyma of the left kidney to be invaded by tumor; however, the blood supply to the left kidney (left renal artery and/or vein) often is involved, which necessitates left nephrectomy

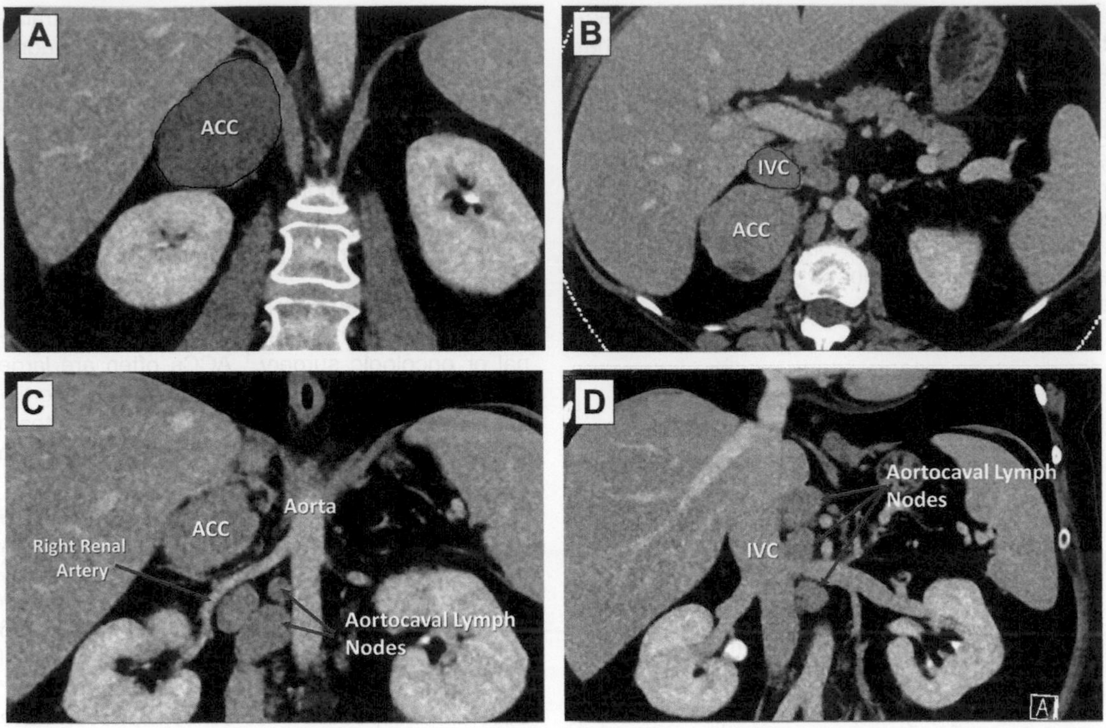

Fig. 1. CT scan images from a 47-year-old woman with metastatic right-sided ACC. (*A*) Coronal view showing an 8-cm right-sided ACC. (*B*) Relationship of the ACC to the IVC. (*C*) Relationship of the tumor to the renal artery and aortocaval lymph nodes. (*D*) Aortocaval lymphadenopathy near the insertion of the left renal vein.

as part of the resection (**Fig. 3**). Lymph nodes that are commonly involved include the para-aortic, left renal, and splenic nodes; however, ACC can spread to contralateral nodal basins as well.

Right-sided ACCs can invade the right kidney, liver, and inferior vena cava (IVC). Aortocaval lymph node metastases are a common location of lymphadenopathy for right-sided ACC (see **Fig. 1**C, D). If the ACC invades the IVC (often along the right adrenal vein), a portion of the IVC along with tumor thrombus needs to be excised. This can require complete isolation of the retrohepatic IVC and/or cardiopulmonary bypass. Invasion of the liver may require an en bloc resection of the adrenal tumor with the right lobe of the liver.

COMPLICATIONS

The risks and complications of adrenalectomy greatly depend on which adrenal gland is involved. The risks of left-sided multivisceral resections include renal failure/insufficiency, pancreatic fistula, postsplenectomy sepsis, and/or delayed gastric emptying. The main risk of resection of a right-sided ACC is massive life-threatening bleeding from injury to the IVC. Para-aortic lymph node dissection also can include the risk of chyle leak from damage to the cisterna chyli and retroperitoneal lymphatics. Complications that are common to both left and right open adrenal resections include wound infection, hernia, bleeding, and adrenal insufficiency in addition to perioperative cardiovascular morbidity, such as myocardial infarction and deep venous thrombosis or venous thromboembolism.

Key Points
FOR SURGERY

- Complete surgical resection is the only known avenue for a potential cure of ACC.
- Open radical adrenalectomy performed by surgeons with considerable experience with adrenal or oncologic surgery is the preferred approach.
- ACC can be adherent and invasive to local surroundings, thereby increasing the complication rates.

ADJUVANT MITOTANE THERAPY

Mitotane is a derivative of the insecticide dichlorodiphenyltrichloroethane (DDT).[22] For decades it

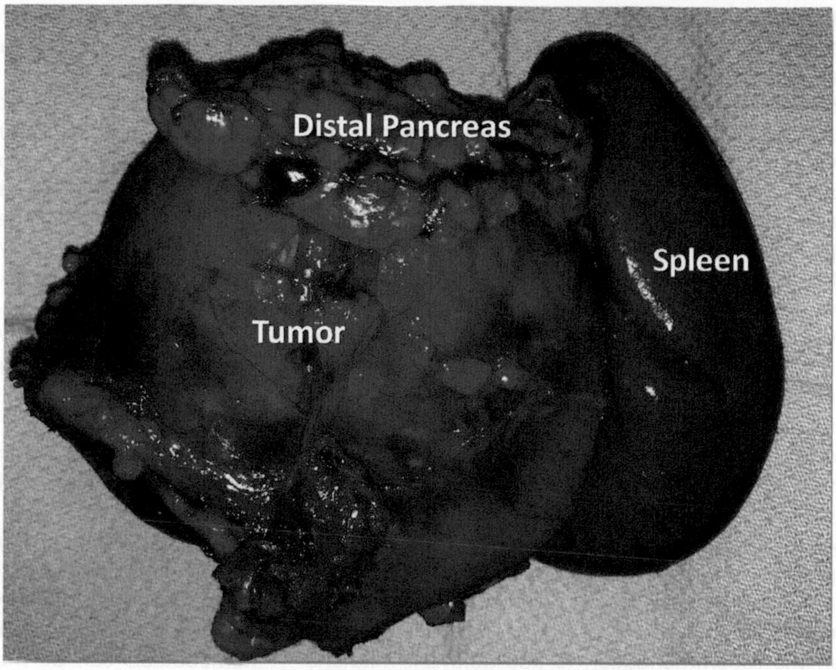

Fig. 2. Gross specimen from a 34-year-old woman with a 9-cm left-sided ACC. En bloc resection of the distal pancreas and spleen were required in order to obtain adequate surgical exposure.

had been considered to have adrenolytic properties; however, newer data and clinical observations suggest that it may be adrenostatic, at least in some instances.[23] Adjuvant mitotane therapy is recommended for patients after complete surgical resection who have either stage III or stage IV disease and/or high-grade disease of any stage (Ki67 index >10%). Although pathologists generally grade ACC according to the mitotic count, treatment algorithms often rely on Ki-67 proliferative index, with a Ki-67 proliferative index less than or equal to 10% considered low grade and a Ki-67 proliferative index greater than 10% considered high grade. Therefore, it is important for pathologists to include a Ki-67 proliferative index in the pathology report. Newer evidence suggests that mitotane monotherapy, or in combination with chemotherapy, may continue to provide benefit for patients with recurrent metastatic disease.[18,24,25] For patients with stage I or stage

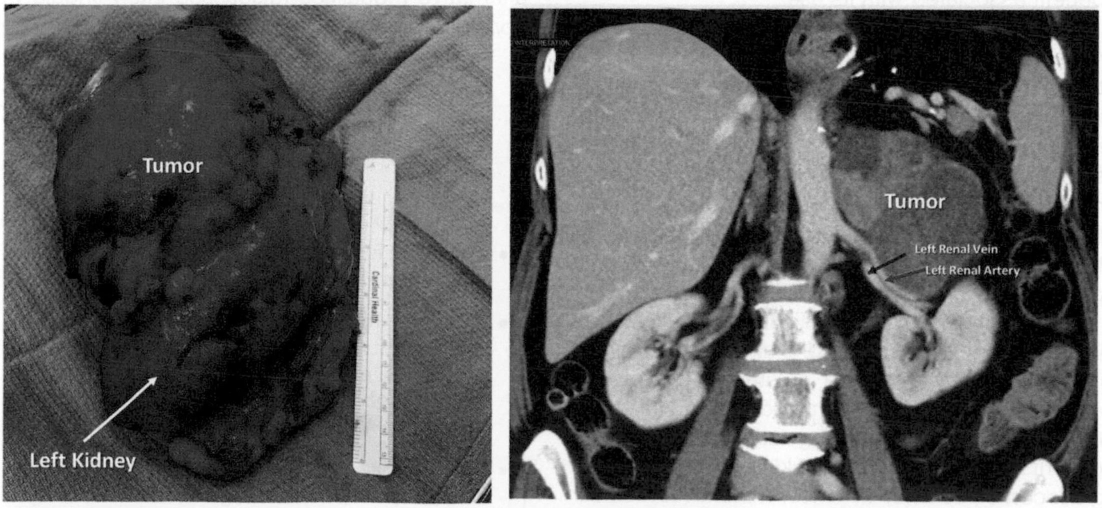

Fig. 3. Gross specimen and CT scan from a 68-year-old woman with an 8-cm left-sided ACC. The tumor did not invade the parenchyma of the left kidney but it was densely adherent to the renal artery (*red arrow*) and renal vein (*blue arrow*), necessitating the removal of the kidney in order to obtain an R0 resection.

II disease that is low grade (Ki67 ≤10%), after an R0 resection, there is no evidence-based recommendation on whether adjuvant mitotane may be beneficial. In these instances, case-by-case decisions to initiate adjuvant mitotane are made after weighing a multitude of patient-specific factors and balancing them with potential adverse effects (discussed later). There currently is an ongoing prospective randomized trial that is evaluating the efficacy of adjuvant mitotane compared with no mitotane in low-risk ACC (stages I–III and Ki67 <10% after R0 resection; ADIUVO trial).

It is important to recognize that there are currently no prospective studies or randomized trials evaluating the efficacy of mitotane. The landmark evidence to support its use comes from retrospective cohort studies that showed that adjuvant mitotane therapy was associated with significantly prolonged recurrence-free survival, and possibly greater overall survival compared with no adjuvant therapy among patients with locoregional/stage III ACC.[26,27] These data have resulted in the recommendation to use adjuvant mitotane monotherapy for high-grade disease and stage III or greater disease and combination mitotane plus chemotherapy in advanced and recurrent ACC (discussed later).[18,26] Adjuvant mitotane therapy generally is continued for approximately 2 years unless limited by severe or intolerable adverse events and/or substantial recurrences in disease despite optimal mitotane dosing; however, anecdotal reports suggest that long-term continuation of mitotane therapy may reduce or maintain the burden of disease in select subgroups.[24,25] Patients with metastatic ACC may continue mitotane indefinitely if it is tolerated and there seems to be clinical benefit associated with its use.

Among the most common adverse effects are nausea, vomiting, diarrhea, and generalized fatigue.[1] Neurologic complications can arise, particularly when mitotane doses and levels are high, including ataxia, memory loss, lethargy, and depression. Liver toxicity can occur at any level or dose of mitotane and can range from a mild transaminitis to overt hepatic dysfunction and liver failure. Mitotane can cause substantial hypercholesterolemia, pancytopenia, and drug-induced skin rash.

Several endocrinopathies are known to be induced by mitotane. Adrenal insufficiency is induced due to inhibition of steroidogenesis by mitotane and possibly also an adrenolytic effect on the remaining contralateral gland. For this reason, patients on mitotane should be treated with glucocorticoids and, at times, mineralocorticoids. Hypothyroidism may occur, although the pattern of laboratories can indicate either primary or secondary hypothyroidism. For this reason, many patients on mitotane need supplemental thyroid hormone. Mitotane can induce a primary or secondary hypogonadism in men with or without gynecomastia, and it has been observed to cause endometrial hypertrophy. Both of these reproductive abnormalities require careful monitoring and have unclear ramifications. Insufficient treatment of these endocrinopathies can cause fatigue, hypotension, depression, and other symptoms that may limit the intensity of therapy or be misattributed to other factors. To further compound these endocrine alterations, mitotane increases hepatic globulin synthesis and secretion, including that of cortisol-binding globulin, thyroid hormone-binding globulin, and sex-hormone binding globulin. Further, mitotane increases cytochrome P450 3A4 (CYP3A4) activity, which is responsible for the metabolism of supplemental hormone therapy and many other routine medications. For all these reasons, when hormone replacement therapy is indicated for adrenal insufficiency, hypothyroidism, and hypogonadism, the doses needed to recapitulate physiologic homeostasis can be much higher than traditional replacement doses.

Patients on mitotane require routine monitoring for adverse effects. This includes laboratory evaluations for liver injury, blood counts, thyroid and adrenal hormone status, cholesterol, and periodically testosterone deficiency. In addition, patients should be seen every 3 months for history and examination and imaging surveillance of the abdomen and chest to assess for recurrence or progression. In the absence of recurrence or progression, mitotane therapy and monitoring should be continued for approximately 2 years. When recurrence is confirmed, intensification of therapy with alternative modalities (discussed later) should be considered.

Key Points for Mitotane Therapy

- Mitotane is a derivative of the insecticide DDT and is the most common adjuvant therapy.
- Adjuvant mitotane therapy is recommended for patients after complete surgical resection who have either stage III or stage IV disease and/or high-grade disease of any stage (Ki67 index >10%).
- Mitotane can induce a variety of gastrointestinal, hepatic, hematological, and neurologic complications in addition to multiple endocrinopathies.

ADJUVANT RADIATION THERAPY AND OTHER LOCAL THERAPEUTIC MEASURES

Because adrenal cortical carcinoma is a rare neoplasm, there are scant data on the use of adjuvant radiation therapy after surgical resection of the primary tumor. There are no randomized and controlled data to guide treatment recommendations. Data from retrospective cohort studies provide the highest level of evidence available. The largest of these series characterized outcomes for 20 patients compared with controls matched for stage, tumor grade, surgical margin status, and adjuvant mitotane use. Study results suggest a benefit among patients in local recurrence rate but no improvement in recurrence-free survival or overall survival.[28] Other smaller studies did not show benefit in clinical outcomes, but these studies were limited by the inclusion of patients with gross residual tumor (R2 resections) for whom therapy would not have been truly adjuvant, and patients who did not receive adjuvant mitotane.[29,30] The decision to proceed with adjuvant radiation must weigh the morbidity of treatment against the probability of tumor recurrence for a malignancy that is not likely to be cured if tumor recurs. Adjuvant radiation with mitotane, therefore, should be considered for patients with stage III R0 resection and on a case-by-case basis, for patients with any stage tumor with R1 or Rx resection or other high-risk features, including a high-grade, Ki67 greater than 10%, or intraoperative capsular rupture.

Because surgery is the only curative approach for primary adrenal cortical carcinoma, sequential surgical resections have an established role in the management of recurrent and metastatic tumor. For many patients, however, surgery may not be a therapeutic option due to comorbid disease or tumor location. Under these circumstances, local therapy with percutaneous ablation may play a role in disease control. Retrospective series provide the best evidence for using this approach, although available studies included very small sample sizes and many investigations include adrenal metastases from other primary tumor sites in addition to other primary adrenal tumors, such as pheochromocytoma. A variety of approaches have been published, including radiofrequency ablation, cryoablation, microwave ablation, and chemoembolization.[31–36] In aggregate, the data suggest that percutaneous ablation and chemoembolization can be performed safely and may provide a measure of local control for a subset of patients. Data from Wood and colleagues[36] showed that outcomes were better for tumors less than 5 cm. Although Ripley and colleagues[34] found 7 of 8 patients were free of disease at the site of their radiofrequency ablation of liver metastases, 5 of these patients developed extrahepatic metastases attesting to the need for systemic treatment.

Key Points for Radiation Therapy and Other Local Therapeutic Measures

- Adjuvant radiation therapy should be considered for patients with stage III R0 resection and on a case-by-case basis, for patients with any stage tumor with R1 or Rx resection or other high-risk features, including a high-grade, Ki67 greater than 10%, or intraoperative capsular rupture.
- Local therapy with percutaneous ablation and chemoembolization can be performed safely and can be considered on a case-by-case basis as an alternative to surgical therapy and/or systemic chemotherapy

CHEMOTHERAPY AND OTHER SYSTEMIC THERAPIES

First-line therapy for de novo metastatic or recurrent adrenal cortical carcinoma depends on a patient's performance status and tumor characteristics. Patients with more indolent tumors may be managed with mitotane alone. For those patients who can tolerate systemic chemotherapy who have aggressive tumor characteristics, the evidence dictating standard of care stems from the phase III randomized study FIRM-ACT trial (N = 304) that showed the superiority of the 4-drug regimen, etoposide, doxorubicin, and cisplatin with mitotane (EDP-M), over the alternative regimen, streptozocin-mitotane.[18] Fassnacht and colleagues[18] demonstrated a statistically significant improvement in progression-free survival for EDP-M compared with streptozocin-mitotane (5.3 months vs 2.0 months). Although there was a suggestion of an overall survival advantage for EDP-M, with a median survival 14.8 months versus 12 months, respectively, and the survival curves did not come together, the difference did not reach statistical significance. Patients were allowed to cross over to the alternative treatment at the time of progression; therefore, it is possible that the efficacy of EDP-M may have been underestimated. Another important realization is that despite the superiority of EDP-M, the mean survival was still dismal, highlighting the limitations of even the gold standard systemic treatment and underscoring the importance of using other treatment options when possible, such as targeted ablations, sequential surgical resections, and radiation. Patients with renal dysfunction or baseline neuropathy may not tolerate cisplatin, and doxorubicin is contraindicated in patients with poor cardiac function. Alternative first-line options include etoposide and cisplatin (or carboplatin for patients with renal dysfunction), but this combination has only phase II data to support its use.[37,38]

Well-studied second-line therapies after progression on EDP-M or etoposide, cisplatin with mitotane (EP-M) include streptozocin-mitotane and gemcitabine + capecitabine, with or without mitotane.[18,39,40] The response rates to second-line treatment are poor (<10%) although occasional complete responses have been documented. Tyrosine kinase inhibitors are among the other agents that have been tested, but response rates have not shown great potential; however, in at least 1 trial it was found that sunitinib levels may have been profoundly decreased due to mitotane-induced CYP3A4 activation, which may have influenced the results.[41] Immunotherapies offer an appealing treatment possibility based on the tumor agnostic responses that have been observed in other solid tumor malignancies. Initial results, however, from the JAVELIN study, a phase I open-label dose escalation study of avelumab (an anti–PD-L1 antibody) found a disappointing overall response rate of only 6%, with a median progression-free survival of less than 3 months.[42] Several clinical trials are currently under way using combined immune checkpoint blockade with anti-CTLA4 and anti–PD-L1 agents in addition to other novel combinations. Several approaches to target the receptors for insulinlike growth factor 1, vascular endothelial growth factor, and epidermal growth factor, as well as mammalian target of rapamycin (mTOR) inhibitors, have been tested without clear evidence of benefit.[43–49]

The quest for targeted and personalized therapies in ACC is ongoing. Molecular and genomic studies of ACC by the ENSAT and The Cancer Genome Atlas have revealed several molecular insights into ACC with the potential to improve risk stratification of ACC patients and basis for rationale targeted treatment strategies.[50–52] These insights, however, have not yet been translated to novel treatments or changes in clinical practice.

> ***Key Points***
> **FOR CHEMOTHERAPY AND OTHER SYSTEMIC THERAPIES**
>
> - EDP with mitotane is the first-line regimen for systemic chemotherapy.
> - Multiple clinical studies evaluating immunotherapies and other targeted therapies for ACC are in process.

SUMMARY

The treatment of ACC continues to be challenging. The mainstay of therapy remains surgery; a complete surgical resection of the primary tumor is desired for optimal survival and to reduce the burden of adrenal hormone excess. Whether subsequent surgical debulking, radiation, or targeted cytoreduction using ablations has long-term benefit is not yet known but is a common practice that is used on a case-by-case basis. There are only a limited number of systemic medical options used for ACC and they generally are comprised of older and established agents. Adjuvant mitotane is recommended particularly in high-grade and locoregional or metastatic disease. Platinum-based chemotherapy has been shown to be the most effective regimen for advanced ACC, especially when combined with mitotane. Many targeted therapeutics have failed to show benefit in ACC treatment; however, there are several ongoing studies, including many immunotherapy-based protocols, the results of which are with highly anticipated. Given the complexity and heterogeneity in ACC care, highly experienced and multidisciplinary teams are likely to provide the optimal care for such patients until more standardized and evidence-based approaches that can be easily disseminated are available. The future advancement of ACC research will similarly require large networks and collaborative research teams to maximize potential, such as the European Network for the Study of Adrenal Tumors (ENS@T) (http://www.ensat.org/) and the American Australian Asian Adrenal Alliance (https://adrenal-a5.org/).

REFERENCES

1. Fassnacht M, Dekkers OM, Else T, et al. European Society of Endocrinology Clinical Practice Guidelines on the management of adrenocortical carcinoma in adults, in collaboration with the European Network for the Study of Adrenal Tumors. Eur J Endocrinol 2018;179:G1–46.
2. Else T, Kim AC, Sabolch A, et al. Adrenocortical carcinoma. Endocr Rev 2014;35:282–326.
3. Kerkhofs TM, Verhoeven RH, Van der Zwan JM, et al. Adrenocortical carcinoma: a population-based study on incidence and survival in the Netherlands since 1993. Eur J Cancer 2013;49:2579–86.
4. Raymond VM, Everett JN, Furtado LV, et al. Adrenocortical carcinoma is a lynch syndrome-associated cancer. J Clin Oncol 2013;31:3012–8.
5. Wasserman JD, Novokmet A, Eichler-Jonsson C, et al. Prevalence and functional consequence of TP53 mutations in pediatric adrenocortical

carcinoma: a children's oncology group study. J Clin Oncol 2015;33:602–9.
6. Raymond VM, Else T, Everett JN, et al. Prevalence of germline TP53 mutations in a prospective series of unselected patients with adrenocortical carcinoma. J Clin Endocrinol Metab 2013;98:E119–25.
7. Vaidya A, Hamrahian AH, Bancos I, et al. The evaluation of incidentally discovered adrenal masses. Endocr Pract 2019;25:178–92.
8. Fassnacht M, Arlt W, Bancos I, et al. Management of adrenal incidentalomas: European Society of Endocrinology Clinical Practice Guideline in collaboration with the European Network for the Study of Adrenal Tumors. Eur J Endocrinol 2016;175:G1–34.
9. Arlt W, Biehl M, Taylor AE, et al. Urine steroid metabolomics as a biomarker tool for detecting malignancy in adrenal tumors. J Clin Endocrinol Metab 2011;96:3775–84.
10. Bancos I, Tamhane S, Shah M, et al. Diagnosis of endocrine disease: the diagnostic performance of adrenal biopsy: a systematic review and meta-analysis. Eur J Endocrinol 2016;175:R65–80.
11. Weiss LM, Medeiros LJ, Vickery AL Jr. Pathologic features of prognostic significance in adrenocortical carcinoma. Am J Surg Pathol 1989;13:202–6.
12. Weiss LM. Comparative histologic study of 43 metastasizing and nonmetastasizing adrenocortical tumors. The Am J Surg Pathol 1984;8:163–9.
13. Duregon E, Cappellesso R, Maffeis V, et al. Validation of the prognostic role of the "Helsinki Score" in 225 cases of adrenocortical carcinoma. Hum Pathol 2017;62:1–7.
14. Pennanen M, Heiskanen I, Sane T, et al. Helsinki score-a novel model for prediction of metastases in adrenocortical carcinomas. Hum Pathol 2015;46:404–10.
15. Duregon E, Fassina A, Volante M, et al. The reticulin algorithm for adrenocortical tumor diagnosis: a multicentric validation study on 245 unpublished cases. The Am J Surg Pathol 2013;37:1433–40.
16. Duregon E, Volante M, Cappia S, et al. Oncocytic adrenocortical tumors: diagnostic algorithm and mitochondrial DNA profile in 27 cases. Am J Surg Pathol 2011;35:1882–93.
17. Aubert S, Wacrenier A, Leroy X, et al. Weiss system revisited: a clinicopathologic and immunohistochemical study of 49 adrenocortical tumors. Am J Surg Pathol 2002;26:1612–9.
18. Fassnacht M, Terzolo M, Allolio B, et al. Combination chemotherapy in advanced adrenocortical carcinoma. N Engl J Med 2012;366:2189–97.
19. Autorino R, Bove P, De Sio M, et al. Open versus laparoscopic adrenalectomy for adrenocortical carcinoma: a meta-analysis of surgical and oncological outcomes. Ann Surg Oncol 2016;23:1195–202.
20. Lombardi CP, Raffaelli M, De Crea C, et al. Open versus endoscopic adrenalectomy in the treatment of localized (stage I/II) adrenocortical carcinoma: results of a multiinstitutional Italian survey. Surgery 2012;152:1158–64.
21. Dickson PV, Kim L, Yen TWF, et al. Evaluation, staging, and surgical management for adrenocortical carcinoma: an update from the SSO endocrine and head and neck disease site working group. Ann Surg Oncol 2018;25:3460–8.
22. Schteingart DE. Adjuvant mitotane therapy of adrenal cancer - use and controversy. N Engl J Med 2007;356:2415–8.
23. Sbiera S, Leich E, Liebisch G, et al. Mitotane inhibits Sterol-O-Acyl transferase 1 triggering lipid-mediated endoplasmic reticulum stress and apoptosis in adrenocortical carcinoma cells. Endocrinology 2015;156:3895–908.
24. Megerle F, Herrmann W, Schloetelburg W, et al. Mitotane monotherapy in patients with advanced adrenocortical carcinoma. J Clin Endocrinol Metab 2018;103:1686–95.
25. El Ghorayeb N, Rondeau G, Latour M, et al. Rapid and complete remission of metastatic adrenocortical carcinoma persisting 10 years after treatment with mitotane monotherapy: case report and review of the literature. Medicine (Baltimore) 2016;95:e3180.
26. Terzolo M, Angeli A, Fassnacht M, et al. Adjuvant mitotane treatment for adrenocortical carcinoma. N Engl J Med 2007;356:2372–80.
27. Kerkhofs TM, Baudin E, Terzolo M, et al. Comparison of two mitotane starting dose regimens in patients with advanced adrenocortical carcinoma. J Clin Endocrinol Metab 2013;98:4759–67.
28. Sabolch A, Else T, Griffith KA, et al. Adjuvant radiation therapy improves local control after surgical resection in patients with localized adrenocortical carcinoma. Int J Radiat Oncol Biol Phys 2015;92:252–9.
29. Fassnacht M, Hahner S, Polat B, et al. Efficacy of adjuvant radiotherapy of the tumor bed on local recurrence of adrenocortical carcinoma. J Clin Endocrinol Metab 2006;91:4501–4.
30. Habra MA, Ejaz S, Feng L, et al. A retrospective cohort analysis of the efficacy of adjuvant radiotherapy after primary surgical resection in patients with adrenocortical carcinoma. J Clin Endocrinol Metab 2013;98:192–7.
31. Cazejust J, De Baere T, Auperin A, et al. Transcatheter arterial chemoembolization for liver metastases in patients with adrenocortical carcinoma. J Vasc Interv Radiol 2010;21:1527–32.
32. Ethier MD, Beland MD, Mayo-Smith W. Image-guided ablation of adrenal tumors. Tech Vasc Interv Radiol 2013;16:262–8.
33. Li X, Fan W, Zhang L, et al. CT-guided percutaneous microwave ablation of adrenal malignant carcinoma: preliminary results. Cancer 2011;117:5182–8.

34. Ripley RT, Kemp CD, Davis JL, et al. Liver resection and ablation for metastatic adrenocortical carcinoma. Ann Surg Oncol 2011;18:1972–9.
35. Venkatesan AM, Locklin J, Dupuy DE, et al. Percutaneous ablation of adrenal tumors. Tech Vasc Interv Radiol 2010;13:89–99.
36. Wood BJ, Abraham J, Hvizda JL, et al. Radiofrequency ablation of adrenal tumors and adrenocortical carcinoma metastases. Cancer 2003;97:554–60.
37. Bonacci R, Gigliotti A, Baudin E, et al. Cytotoxic therapy with etoposide and cisplatin in advanced adrenocortical carcinoma. Br J Cancer 1998;78:546–9.
38. Williamson SK, Lew D, Miller GJ, et al. Phase II evaluation of cisplatin and etoposide followed by mitotane at disease progression in patients with locally advanced or metastatic adrenocortical carcinoma: a Southwest Oncology Group Study. Cancer 2000;88:1159–65.
39. Henning JEK, Deutschbein T, Altieri B, et al. Gemcitabine-based chemotherapy in adrenocortical carcinoma: a multicenter study of efficacy and predictive factors. J Clin Endocrinol Metab 2017;102:4323–32.
40. Sperone P, Ferrero A, Daffara F, et al. Gemcitabine plus metronomic 5-fluorouracil or capecitabine as a second-/third-line chemotherapy in advanced adrenocortical carcinoma: a multicenter phase II study. Endocr Relat Cancer 2010;17:445–53.
41. Kroiss M, Quinkler M, Johanssen S, et al. Sunitinib in refractory adrenocortical carcinoma: a phase II, single-arm, open-label trial. J Clin Endocrinol Metab 2012;97:3495–503.
42. Le Tourneau C, Hoimes C, Zarwan C, et al. Avelumab in patients with previously treated metastatic adrenocortical carcinoma: phase 1b results from the JAVELIN solid tumor trial. J Immunother Cancer 2018;6:111.
43. Fassnacht M, Berruti A, Baudin E, et al. Linsitinib (OSI-906) versus placebo for patients with locally advanced or metastatic adrenocortical carcinoma: a double-blind, randomised, phase 3 study. Lancet Oncol 2015;16:426–35.
44. Lerario AM, Worden FP, Ramm CA, et al. The combination of insulin-like growth factor receptor 1 (IGF1R) antibody cixutumumab and mitotane as a first-line therapy for patients with recurrent/metastatic adrenocortical carcinoma: a multi-institutional NCI-sponsored trial. Horm Cancer 2014;5:232–9.
45. Ganesan P, Piha-Paul S, Naing A, et al. Phase I clinical trial of lenalidomide in combination with temsirolimus in patients with advanced cancer. Invest New Drugs 2013;31:1505–13.
46. Naing A, Lorusso P, Fu S, et al. Insulin growth factor receptor (IGF-1R) antibody cixutumumab combined with the mTOR inhibitor temsirolimus in patients with metastatic adrenocortical carcinoma. Br J Cancer 2013;108:826–30.
47. Haluska P, Worden F, Olmos D, et al. Safety, tolerability, and pharmacokinetics of the anti-IGF-1R monoclonal antibody figitumumab in patients with refractory adrenocortical carcinoma. Cancer Chemother Pharmacol 2010;65:765–73.
48. Quinkler M, Hahner S, Wortmann S, et al. Treatment of advanced adrenocortical carcinoma with erlotinib plus gemcitabine. J Clin Endocrinol Metab 2008;93:2057–62.
49. Rosen LS. Inhibitors of the vascular endothelial growth factor receptor. Hematol Oncol Clin North Am 2002;16:1173–87.
50. Assie G, Letouze E, Fassnacht M, et al. Integrated genomic characterization of adrenocortical carcinoma. Nat Genet 2014;46:607–12.
51. Miller BS, Else T, Committee AAS. Personalized care of patients with adrenocortical carcinoma: a comprehensive approach. Endocr Pract 2017;23:705–15.
52. Zheng S, Cherniack AD, Dewal N, et al. Comprehensive pan-genomic characterization of adrenocortical carcinoma. Cancer Cell 2016;29:723–36.

Parathyroid Pathology

Julie Guilmette, MD[a], Peter M. Sadow, MD, PhD[b,*]

KEYWORDS

• Parathyroid • Primary hyperplasia • Parathyroid adenoma • Parathyroid carcinoma • Parafibromin

Key points

1. Proliferative parathyroid disorders represent the most common cause of hyperparathyroidism.
2. From 80% to 85% of primary hyperparathyroidism is caused by parathyroid adenoma, followed by primary parathyroid hyperplasia (15%) and parathyroid carcinoma (5%).
3. Parathyroid carcinoma key histologic features include vascular invasion, perineural invasion, invasion into adjacent structures, and metastatic disease.
4. Parathyroid carcinoma is typically sporadic but may arise as part of familial endocrine disorders: multiple endocrine neoplasia, hyperparathyroidism–jaw tumor syndrome, and familial isolated hyperparathyroidism.
5. Parafibromin immunohistochemistry may be a helpful diagnostic aid in distinguishing parathyroid carcinoma from parathyroid atypical adenoma.

ABSTRACT

Proliferative pathologic lesions of parathyroid glands encompass a spectrum of entities ranging from benign hyperplastic processes to malignant neoplasia. This review article outlines the pathophysiologic classification of parathyroid disorders and describes histologic, immunohistochemical, and molecular features that can be assessed to render accurate diagnoses.

OVERVIEW

Proliferative parathyroid disease is diagnostically challenging, because many disease entities within this group of disorders require supplementary clinical information and are not readily diagnosed with a light microscope and a good eye alone. In addition, for most pathologists, parathyroid specimens represent only a small percentage of case volume. Although the recognition and accurate diagnosis of the parathyroid lesions can be challenging because of limitations in conventional morphologic approaches, advances in radiological imaging techniques and rapid intraoperative parathyroid hormone assay combined with immunohistochemistry and molecular studies are progressively reducing diagnostic uncertainties and resolving diagnostic dilemmas.

EMBRYOLOGY AND ANATOMY OF THE PARATHYROID GLAND

Parathyroid glands develop as epithelial thickenings of the dorsal endoderm of the third and fourth branchial pouches around the fifth week of intrauterine life and are histologically visible only after 14 weeks.[1,2] The fourth pouch gives rise to the superior parathyroid glands, whereas the inferior parathyroid glands are derived from the third branchial pouch. By the end of their migration, approximately 80% of superior parathyroid glands are found near the posterior edge of the thyroid gland at the junction of the superior and central aspects

Conflict of interest: There are no conflicts of interest to report by any of the authors.
Ethical approval: This article does not contain any studies with human participants performed by the authors.

[a] Department of Pathology, Charles-Lemoyne Hospital, Sherbrooke University Affiliated Health Care Center, 3120 Boulevard Taschereau, Greenfield Park, Quebec J4V 2H1, Canada; [b] Departments of Pathology, Massachusetts General Hospital, Harvard Medical School, 55 Fruit Street, Boston, MA 02114-2696, USA
* Corresponding author.
E-mail address: psadow@mgh.harvard.edu

Surgical Pathology 12 (2019) 1007–1019
https://doi.org/10.1016/j.path.2019.08.006

of each thyroid lobe (**Fig. 1**).[3,4] The normal anatomic location of the inferior parathyroid glands is more variable than that of their superior counterparts. During embryogenesis and intrauterine development, the inferior parathyroid glands travel caudally in the neck and come to rest within 1 cm from the intersection of the inferior thyroid artery and the recurrent laryngeal nerve.[4]

Ectopic or variant locations of superior and inferior parathyroids are determined by migration routes. Ectopic superior parathyroid glands are uncommon but, when present, may be located in the central to posterior aspects of the mediastinum or as far as the developmental aortopulmonary window.[3,5] Larger glands may travel down in the tracheoesophageal groove and come to rest below the inferior parathyroid glands.[6] About 1% of the superior parathyroid glands may be observed in the paraesophageal or retroesophageal space.[6,7] In contrast, the end anatomic location of inferior parathyroid glands tends to be more variable because of their longer migratory route. It is estimated that 15% to 50% of inferior parathyroid glands descend to the thymus.[3,8] Additional unusual sites also include the skull base, angle of the mandible, or even above the superior parathyroid glands. The frequency of intrathyroidal glands is approximately 2% (**Fig. 2**).[3,4,9]

DISORDERS ARISING IN THE PARATHYROID GLAND

Abnormalities of the parathyroid glands are the most common causes of hypercalcemia. Pathologists facilitate the appropriate assessment and diagnosis of the underlying pathologic condition. The spectrum of parathyroid proliferative disorders includes parathyroid hyperplasia, parathyroid adenoma (PA), atypical PA, and parathyroid carcinoma (PC).

IMAGING

Normal parathyroid glands are small, with overall dimensions typically averaging 5 × 3 × 1 mm and weighing less than 50 mg, challenging radiologic detection.[5,10] Parathyroid proliferative disorders result in the enlargement of 1 or several glands, increasing the likelihood of lesional detection. The main purpose of imaging patients with hyperparathyroidism is to identify those who are suitable for minimally invasive surgery by correctly identifying the location of the enlarged gland or glands.[11,12]

Although several imaging modalities may be used preoperatively, dual-phase protocol 99mTc-sestamibi scintigraphy is currently the most widely used technique for visualization of parathyroid disease.[13–15] Sestamibi is a lipophilic cationic isonitrile derivative that accumulates in mitochondria-rich oxyphil cells, which are present in parathyroid tissue.[16] Sestamibi is washed out less rapidly from parathyroid tissue than from adjacent thyroid tissue. The scan sensitivity is limited in cases with atypical washout rates, such as rapid parathyroid washout or delayed thyroid washout. Rapid parathyroid washout is associated with parathyroid hyperplasia and other disorders.[11,16] Variation in the

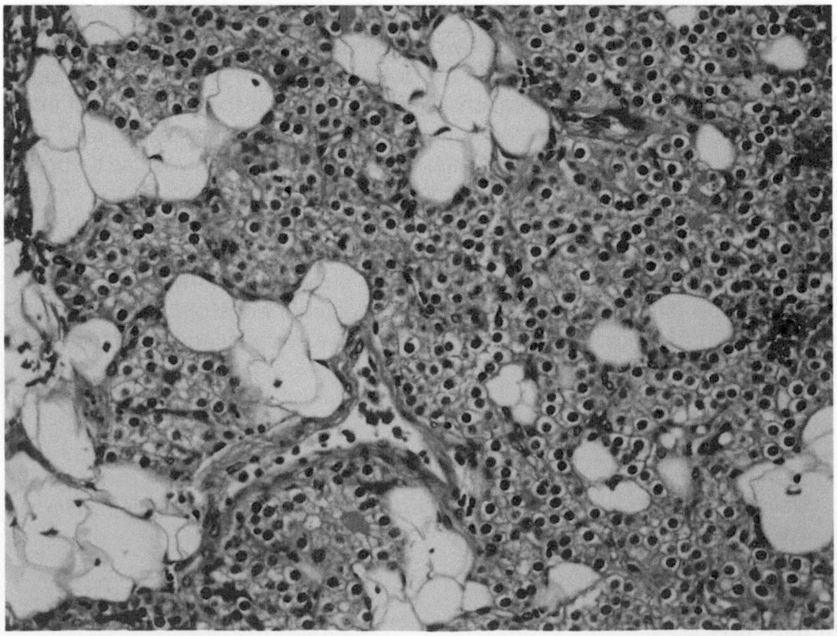

Fig. 1. Normal parathyroid gland composed mainly of chief cells and adipocytes with thin fibrous septa dividing gland into lobules (hematoxylin-eosin [H&E], original magnification ×400).

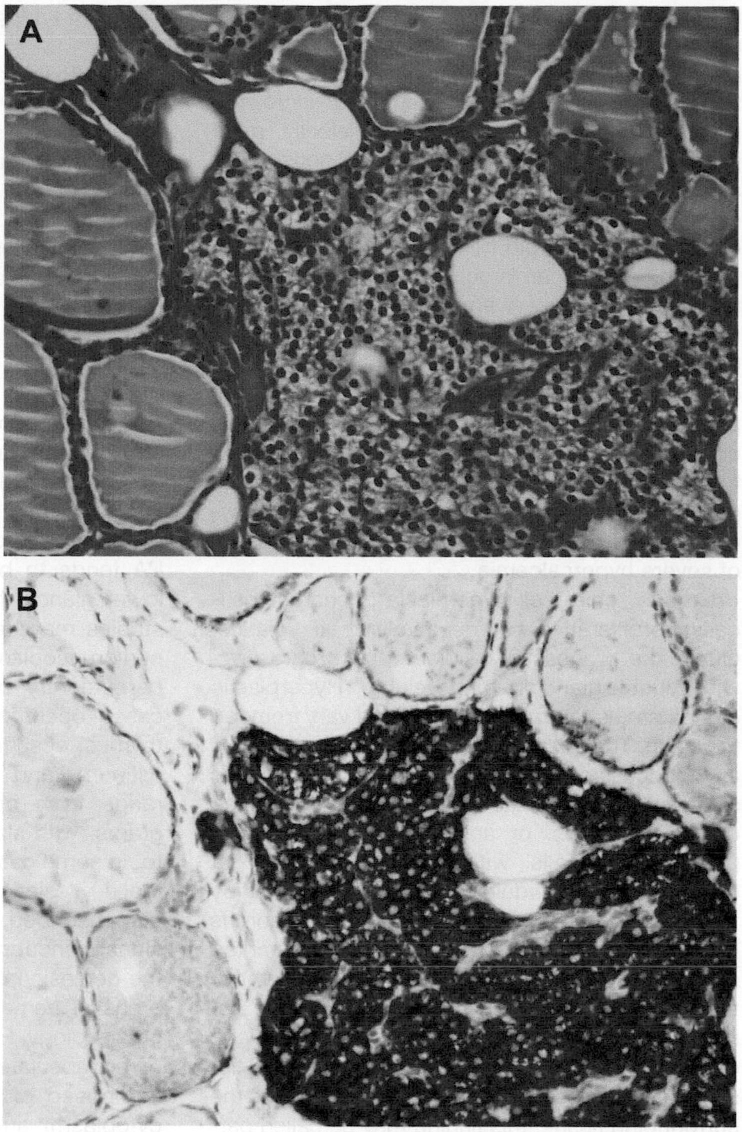

Fig. 2. (*A*) Incidental finding of ectopic intrathyroidal parathyroid tissue (H&E, original magnification ×400). (*B*) Parathyroid hormone (PTH) by immunohistochemistry highlights parathyroid chief cells, allowing proper identification (PTH, original magnification ×400).

scanning protocols makes the reported sensitivity of 99mTc-sestamibi scintigraphy range from 80% to 100%.[5,17] Other modalities, such as contrast-enhanced computed tomography (CT) and MRI, are less commonly used for preoperative localization but may be of benefit in cases of failed parathyroidectomy for the localization of ectopic glands.[11,18]

HYPERPLASIA AND HYPERPARATHYROIDISM

Parathyroid hyperplasia is defined as an absolute increase in parenchymal cell mass, which occurs from the proliferation of chief cells, oncocytes, and transitional oncocytes in multiple parathyroid glands.[10,19] In more than 50% of cases, the enlargement of glands is symmetric.[5] When asymmetric, the distinction between hyperplasia and adenoma may be challenging by standard morphologic criteria alone. Hyperparathyroidism is divided into primary, secondary, and tertiary hyperparathyroidism.

PRIMARY HYPERPARATHYROIDISM

From 80% to 85% of primary hyperparathyroidism is caused by PA, followed by primary parathyroid hyperplasia (15%) and PC (<5%).[12,20] Ectopic locations of hyperplastic parathyroid tissue have also been documented.[21] Patients with primary hyperparathyroidism have abnormal regulation of serum parathyroid hormone secretion. Primary hyperparathyroidism is characterized by increased serum calcium level in the setting of increased parathyroid hormone levels.[22,23] Clinically, most patients are asymptomatic or show nonspecific symptoms such as fatigue, mild depression, or cognitive impairment. It is with longstanding increased parathyroid hormone levels that symptomatic hypercalcemia occurs. In these cases, patients may present with a litany of associated comorbidities, from debilitating renal disorders (including nephrolithiasis and renal deficiency) to gastrointestinal issues (including nausea/vomiting, peptic ulcer disease, and pancreatitis) and skeletal complications (including bone pain, secondary fractures, and osteitis fibrosa cystica).[23–25] Neuropsychiatric disturbances, including lethargy, psychosis, and coma, may also arise in the setting of severe hypercalcemia.[24,26]

Grossly, chief cell hyperplasia is characteristically a proliferative disorder involving all 4 glands. Often, the process is insidious and progressive, with variable gland size and weight.[14] Hyperplastic glands are usually round to oval and vary from red to brown. The cut surface is usually homogeneous and occasionally slightly nodular. Histologic assessment reveals that each nodule is composed of sheets, cords, or an acinar arrangement of parenchymal cells with reduced stromal fat (**Fig. 3**). These nodules may be separated by fibrotic bands and septa, mimicking a fibrous capsule. The chief cells may reveal mild to marked nuclear pleomorphism and atypia. Degenerative features, including cystification, hemorrhage, hemosiderin deposition, and fibrosis, may be observed. When the hyperplastic parenchymal tissue lacks precise circumscription and involves the surrounding tissue, this finding may be called parathyromatosis, typically resulting from prior trauma.[27]

SECONDARY HYPERPARATHYROIDISM

Most parathyroid hyperplasia is the result of secondary hyperparathyroidism caused by chronic kidney disease (CKD), malabsorption syndrome, and chronic inadequate sunlight exposure. Impaired renal function leads to downregulation of the parathyroid vitamin D and calcium-sensing receptors, which negatively affect mineral metabolism and result in high serum phosphate level, low serum calcium level, and vitamin D deficiency.[28] Parathyroid hyperplasia, cardiovascular disease, and concomitant bone disorders are the most common clinical complications.[29]

TERTIARY HYPERPARATHYROIDISM

A significant proportion of patients with CKD and secondary hyperparathyroidism maintain increased levels of parathyroid hormone following kidney transplant. This state of hyperparathyroidism is known as tertiary hyperparathyroidism. Without appropriate management and treatment, tertiary hyperparathyroidism can lead to kidney allograft rejection and decreased patient survival.[30]

ADENOMA

PAs are responsible for approximately 85% of cases of primary hyperparathyroidism.[31] PA can occur among all age groups, with a peak incidence in the fifth and sixth decades and with a slight female predilection and a 2:1 female/male ratio.[19,32] PA tends to be located more frequently in the lower glands than in the upper glands, although studies may be conflicting.[33] Furthermore, these benign neoplasms may arise in any ectopic or supernumerary parathyroid gland, with described cases occurring in the retroesophageal space, thymus, vestigial aortopulmonary window, mediastinum, and thyroid gland.[3,34–39] PA weights range from approximately 300 mg to several grams, with sizes ranging from a few millimeters to, in some cases, more than 10 cm.[40,41] Grossly, these lesions are characterized as well-circumscribed, smooth, red-brown nodules, occasionally encapsulated. Larger lesions often replace the nonlesional parathyroid tissue and may show areas of hemorrhage and cystic degeneration.[42] On histology, PAs are typically well circumscribed or encapsulated by a thin, fibrous capsule and composed of chief cells (round nucleus, scant cytoplasm) arranged within a delicate capillary network. Lobules and nodules inside the adenoma can be observed, with some revealing oncocytic cell change, prominent pink cytoplasm of variable granularity. Adenomas composed entirely of oxyphilic or oncocytic cells occur and may be functional (**Fig. 4**).[43–46] This variant is uncommon and accounts for less than 6% of PA.[47] If not absent, stromal fat is usually sparse. A rim of normal or atrophic parathyroid tissue is typically identified adjacent to the adenoma in more than half of cases, but it may be harder or impossible to detect in larger lesions. The absence of a normocellular rim does not preclude the diagnosis of PA, because large adenomas may have outgrown the preexisting parathyroid or the rim may have simply been lost during sectioning.[3,41] In large tumors, areas of fibrosis, calcification, cholesterol clefts, and/or hemorrhage with hemosiderin deposition

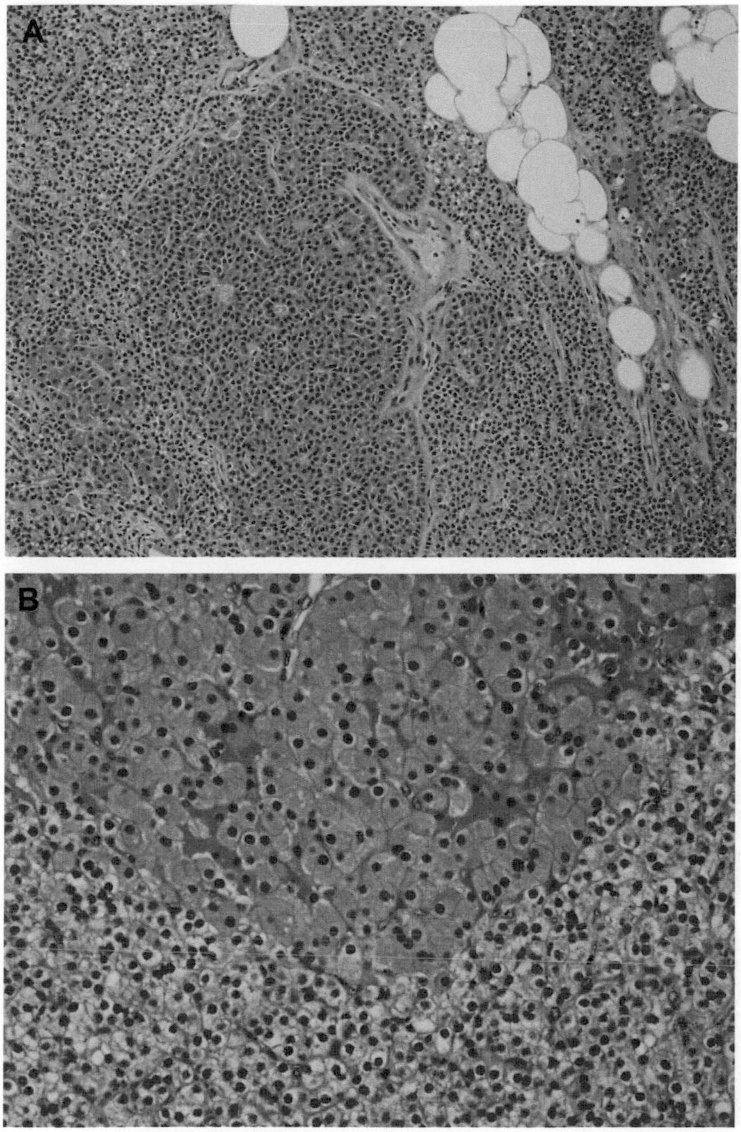

Fig. 3. (*A*) Parathyroid hyperplasia is characterized by chief cell proliferation involving all 4 glands (H&E, original magnification ×200). (*B*) Nodules of oncocytic cells are common (H&E, original magnification ×400).

may be seen. Most cells in PA are small, uniform, and bland with central, hyperchromatic nuclei. However, areas of marked endocrine nuclear atypia, including cells with enlarged, smudged, irregular nuclei or multiple nuclei, may be observed.[48] PA are not mitotically active but may be mildly proliferative, usually showing less than 1 mitosis per 10 high-power fields.[49] Increased mitotic activity and/or necrosis are worrisome features that should raise the possibility of malignancy.[50–53]

Other unusual variants of PA consist of lipoadenoma and water-clear cell adenoma. Parathyroid lipoadenomas are benign tumors made up of both stromal and parenchymal elements, with mature adipocytes comprising more than 50% of the tumor (**Fig. 5**).[54–56] Small nests of parathyroid parenchymal cells, mainly chief cells and infrequently chief and oncocytic cells, are found scattered throughout the tumor.[57] Lipoadenomas deviate from the typical distribution of fat noted in hyperplasia and neoplasia of the parathyroid. Water-clear cell adenomas are rare tumors with few cases reported in literature.[58–62] These adenomas are composed of intermediate to large cells with clear cytoplasm containing small vesicles and glycogen.[58,60] Lipoadenoma and water-clear cell adenoma are occasionally associated with primary hyperparathyroidism.[54,59,60,63,64]

Over the years, the diagnosis of double PA has lost favor among the medical community.[65] Many patients diagnosed with double PA eventually return with recurrent hyperparathyroidism

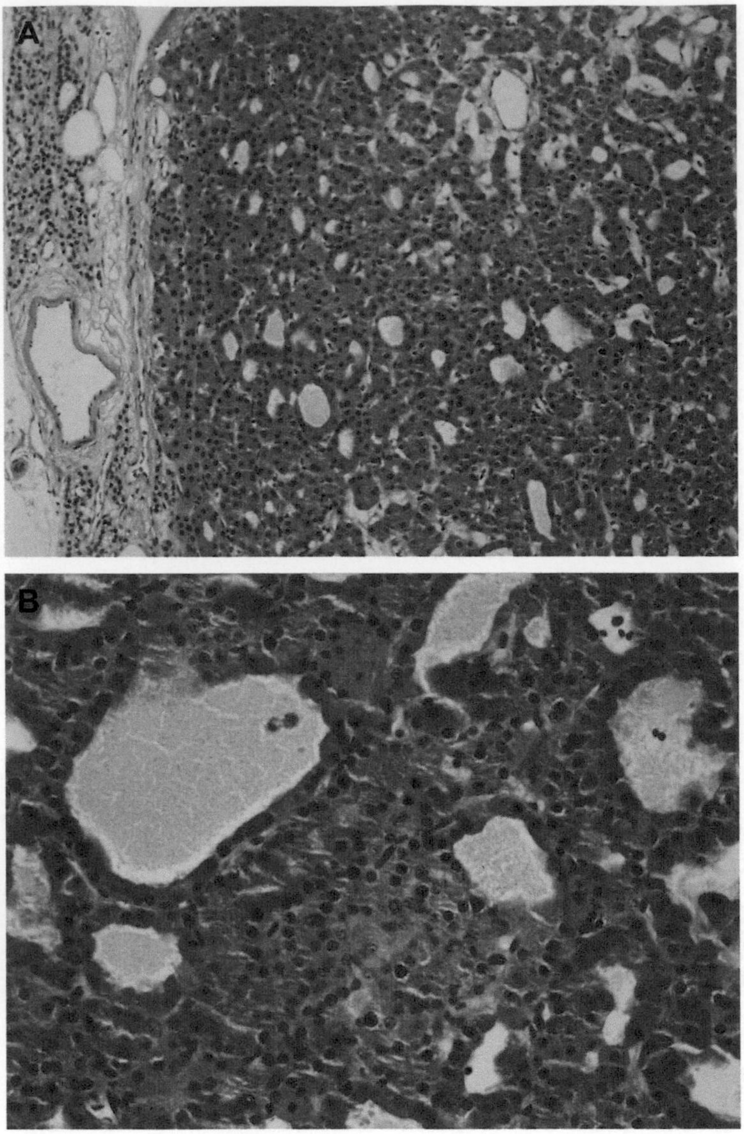

Fig. 4. (*A*) Oncocytic PA with residual normocellular parathyroid tissue identified outside the adenoma capsule (H&E, original magnification ×200). (*B*) Microcystic or cystic architecture may be observed inside the adenoma (H&E, original magnification ×400).

associated with residual glands. Nonetheless, the diagnosis of double adenoma requires the identification of certain criteria. Initially, the patient needs to present with 2 enlarged and histologically abnormal hypercellular parathyroid glands. The remaining 2 glands must be structurally and serologically normal. After the excision of both abnormal glands, long-term follow-up should remain uneventful because the patient should be cured from hyperparathyroidism. In addition, the patient should have a negative family history of parathyroid disease. With those stringent criteria, only a handful of definitive cases of double PA are described in the literature.[66–69]

A mutational genetic profile has been identified for PA that encompasses several tumor suppressors and oncogenes. Among others, mutations in CCND1, cyclin D1, multiple endocrine neoplasia (MEN) type 1, ZFX, EZH2, and many CDKN genes have been linked to the development of both sporadic and familial PA.[70–78]

ATYPICAL ADENOMA

Some parathyroid neoplasms show concerning features for malignancy, including broad bands of fibrosis, nuclear atypia, conspicuous mitotic figures, necrosis, and a desmoplastic stromal response. However, unequivocal features of malignancy, including direct infiltration of adjacent tissue, vascular invasion, or neural involvement, are not identified.[14,27,48,79–81] These borderline tumors

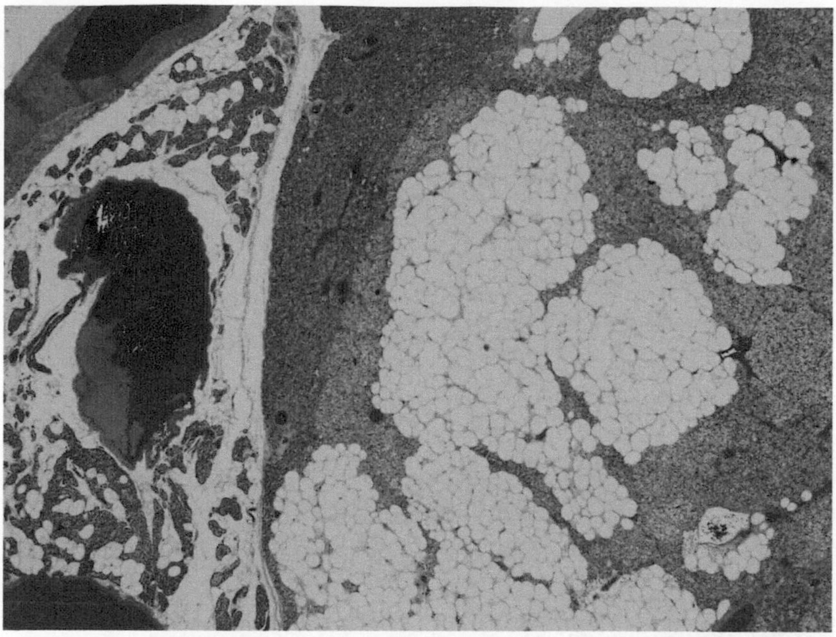

Fig. 5. Lipoadenoma is a rare variant of PA composed of mature adipose tissue and chief cells (H&E, original magnification ×200).

do not fulfill the histologic requirements for a diagnosis of carcinoma and are generally classified as atypical adenomas (AAs), tumors considered to be of uncertain malignant potential. Studies evaluating parafibromin immunoreactivity have proved valuable to predict the potential for recurrence in AAs.[82–86] Among the parafibromin (CDC73)-deficient group, 10% of AAs recurred, whereas none of the parafibromin (CDC73)-positive group did.[82] However, more long-term studies to assess for malignant biological potential and to determine the risk for metastatic disease among these lesions are needed.[27,87–89] In the meantime, patients with AA should benefit from close clinical follow-up. It is important not to make a diagnosis of carcinoma without unequivocal evidence of malignancy. Treatment (ie, surgery plus clinical follow-up) is often equivalent for AA and a localized PC, and, provided appropriate clinical follow-up, there is little need to emotionally traumatize the patient in borderline cases.

CARCINOMA

Carcinoma arising in a parathyroid gland is rare and accounts for less than 5% of primary hyperparathyroidism cases.[90–92] Unlike in PA and hyperplasia, the incidence of PC among women seems to predominate. Patients are typically young and almost always show symptoms related to increased serum calcium levels, which may reach as high as 15 mg/dL (normal typically 8.5–10.2 mg/dL). Most PC occurs in a sporadic setting, but cases in patients with familial endocrinopathies are well documented.[53,93–99]

PCs tend to be large, with an average weight of about 12 g (vs typical normal weight of 50 mg).[94] Preoperatively, carcinomas may show adherence to adjacent soft tissue, thyroid tissue, or even esophagus. Morphologically, there is a constellation of histologic findings to look for to confirm the diagnosis of PC. Per World Health Organization criteria, a diagnosis of PC requires unequivocal lymphovascular or perineural invasion, or invasion into adjacent structures, or metastatic disease. Characteristically, PC are hypercellular neoplasms with trabecular growth, thick fibrous bands, and a thick fibrous tumor capsule. Mitoses, virtually absent in both PA and hyperplasia, may be frequent and atypical in PC. Importantly, the presence of mitotic figures is not pathognomonic for malignancy but should at least lead to suspicion for malignancy in such neoplasms.[49] A similar concept applies to capsular invasion. Capsular invasion by neoplastic processes has been observed in PAs that have undergone hemorrhagic degeneration followed by fibrosis and entrapment of tumor cells within the capsule (**Fig. 6**).[100] Other features reported among PCs include tumor necrosis, tumor cell spindling, prominent macronucleoli, and atypical mitotic figures. Bondeson and colleagues[101] suggested that the histologic triad of macronucleoli, more than 5 mitoses per 50 high-power fields, and necrosis is associated

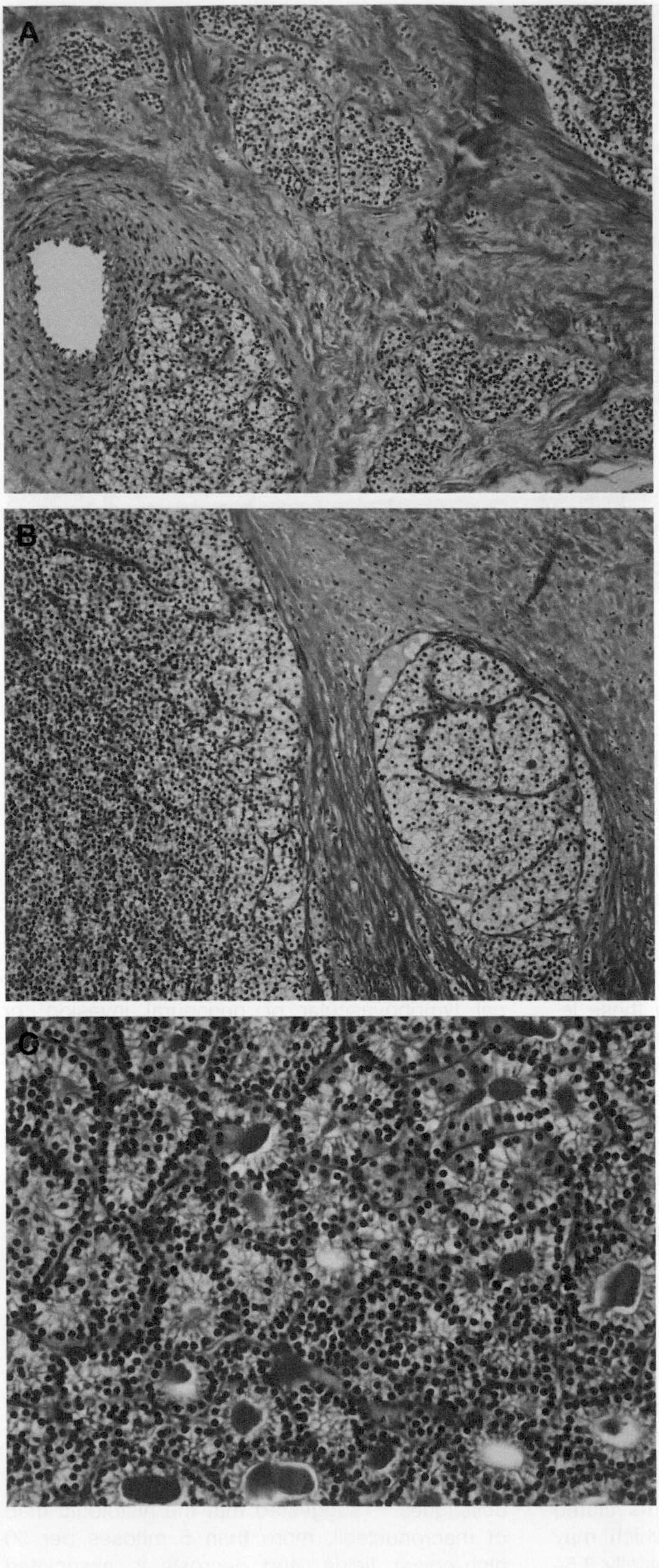

Fig. 6. (*A*) Thick fibrotic capsule with parathyroid cells infiltrating surrounding soft tissue associated with (*B*) true vascular invasion are key features of PC (H&E, original magnification ×200). (*C*) Microcystic growth pattern in PC with unremarkable bland cytologic features (H&E, original magnification ×400).

with recurrent disease, but this system is not widely used. The rarity of PCs has made it difficult to establish a definitive system to risk stratify these tumors.

The development of PC is usually a sporadic, 1-gland condition. PC arising in the setting of 4-gland hyperplasia or as part of secondary hyperparathyroidism is rare but has been documented.[102] Certain familial endocrine disorders related to CDC73 gene mutations, namely hyperparathyroidism–jaw tumor syndrome, familial isolated hyperparathyroidism, and sporadic PC with germline CDC73 mutations, are responsible for the occurrence of some PCs.[94,95,103–105] As a result, genetic counseling should be considered for patients with PC. CDC73, also known as HRPT2, is a tumor suppressor gene located on chromosome 1q31.2, which has been documented as a driver in both familial and sporadic PC. In its normal state, CDC73 protein, parafibromin, regulates both gene expression and transcription, inhibiting cell proliferation and maintaining the cellular structural framework. Its inactivation, whether resulting from sporadic or germline mutation, drives tumorigenesis, although the complex mechanisms of action are not well understood.[70,85,106] Next-generation sequencing of several PCs has confirmed the presence of additional candidates as putative drivers of parathyroid carcinogenesis, including CCND1, PRUNE2, PIK3CA, HMT2D, ADCK1, MTOR, THRAP3, and CDKN2C, although, again, the mechanisms of action are not well documented because of the rarity of mutations and low incidence of PC.[40,78,107]

Although metastases are unusual at the time of diagnosis, metastatic disease has been reported in more than 30% of cases and is commonly found in regional lymph nodes, bone, lung, and liver. In advanced metastatic disease, the severity of symptoms is directly proportional to tumor burden, which is concordant with parathyroid hormone levels produced. The overall prognosis for such disease is usually favorable, with an estimated 5-year overall survival of 78% to 85%.[91] It is common for patients to experience multiple disease recurrence over a course of 15 to 20 years.[91,100,108–112]

IMMUNOHISTOCHEMISTRY

In general, immunohistochemical studies are not needed for the diagnosis of parathyroid disease. Parathyroid tissue, whether as part of a normal gland or abnormal hyperplastic or neoplastic process, is immunoreactive with antibodies to chromogranin and parathyroid hormone, often useful when attempting to differentiate parathyroid tissue from thyroid tissue, a common conundrum. Use of MIB1 Immunohisochemical use of the Ki-67 proliferative index to distinguish PA from hyperplasia has been attempted, but has had limited success.[68] The primary role for immunohistochemistry is for identification of parathyroid tissue. Secondarily, immunohistochemistry has been used to attempt differentiation between adenoma, AA, and PC. In some circumstances, parathyroid neoplasms have histologic features suspicious for malignancy, but the full spectrum of findings needed to make the diagnosis are not present. For these problematic cases, some studies have suggested the use of a broad panel of immunohistochemical markers, including bcl-1, Ki-67, and p27,[48,113] although most laboratories do not have several of these markers, and their diagnostic utility, as a panel, is modest at best. Importantly, the protein product of CDC73, parafibromin, is expressed in the nuclei of benign parathyroid tissue, adenomas, and some AAs, except for those arising in the setting of hyperparathyroidism–jaw tumor syndrome.[14,114] Studies have further shown that loss of nuclear expression of parafibromin may be seen in atypical PAs and carcinomas. However, this immunostain is notoriously difficult to properly titrate and, because it is in such infrequent use clinically, it is not very helpful as a validated marker for malignancy.[14]

MULTIPLE ENDOCRINE NEOPLASIA SYNDROMES

MEN type 1 and 2 are hereditary cancer syndromes. They are characterized by the emergence of various benign and malignant neoplasms. MEN1 is associated mainly with parathyroid, pituitary, and pancreatic tumors, whereas MEN2 is more likely associated with medullary thyroid carcinoma, pheochromocytoma, and parathyroid disorders.[14,115] Although parathyroid tumors are found in both MEN1 and MEN2, patients with MEN1 most commonly have parathyroid proliferative disorder as part of their syndrome, with nearly 90% of them diagnosed with parathyroid hyperplasia.[40] PA and carcinoma can also be seen as part of these syndromes. The possibility of MEN syndrome should always be kept in mind when evaluating these patients.

SUMMARY

The parathyroid glands are unique organs responsible for maintaining calcium homeostasis through parathyroid hormone secretion and end-organ/tissue response. Parathyroid dysfunction alters this fragile homeostasis, primarily through hyperparathyroidism, a common endocrine disorder. Primary hyperparathyroidism includes a wide spectrum of parathyroid proliferative lesions, such as parathyroid hyperplasia, PA, atypical PA, and PC. Proper classification of the pathologic spectrum of parathyroid disease is essential for effective clinical management and facilitating appropriate patient discussions regarding morbidity and long-term prognosis.

REFERENCES

1. Mallik S, Aggarwal P, Singh I, et al. A study on development and morphogenesis of parathyroid gland in the developing human embryo. J Med Soc 2017;31(3):195–200.
2. Grevellec A, Tucker AS. The pharyngeal pouches and clefts: development, evolution, structure and derivatives. Semin Cell Dev Biol 2010;21(3): 325–32.
3. Akerström G, Malmaeus J, Bergström R. Surgical anatomy of human parathyroid glands. Surgery 1984;95(1):14–21.
4. Fancy T, Gallagher D, Hornig JD. Surgical anatomy of the thyroid and parathyroid glands. Otolaryngol Clin North Am 2010;43(2):221–7.
5. Åkerström G, Rudberg C, Grimelius L, et al. Histologic parathyroid abnormalities in an autopsy series. Hum Pathol 1986;17(5):520–7.
6. Phitayakorn R, McHenry CR. Incidence and location of ectopic abnormal parathyroid glands. Am J Surg 2006;191(3):418–23.
7. LoPinto M, Rubio GA, Khan ZF, et al. Location of abnormal parathyroid glands: lessons from 810 parathyroidectomies. J Surg Res 2017;20(7): 22–6.
8. Uno N, Tominaga Y, Matsuoka S, et al. Incidence of parathyroid glands located in thymus in patients with renal hyperparathyroidism. World J Surg 2008;32(11):2516–9.
9. Goodman A, Politz D, Lopez J, et al. Intrathyroid parathyroid adenoma: Incidence and location - The case against thyroid lobectomy. Otolaryngol Head Neck Surg 2011;144(6):867–71.
10. MacKenzie-Feder J, Sirrs S, Anderson D, et al. Primary hyperparathyroidism: an overview. Int J Endocrinol 2011;2011(1):1–8.
11. Patel CN, Salahudeen HM, Lansdown M, et al. Clinical utility of ultrasound and99mTc sestamibi SPECT/CT for preoperative localization of parathyroid adenoma in patients with primary hyperparathyroidism. Clin Radiol 2010;65(4):278–87.
12. Ruda JM, Hollenbeak CS, Stack BC. A systematic review of the diagnosis and treatment of primary hyperparathyroidism from 1995 to 2003. Otolaryngol - Head Neck Surg 2005; 132(3):359–72.
13. Piciucchi S, Barone D, Dubini A, et al. Primary hyperparathyroidism: imaging to pathology. J Clin Imaging Sci 2012;2(1):59–63.
14. Delellis RA. Parathyroid tumors and related disorders. Mod Pathol 2011;24(Suppl 2):S78–93.
15. Elgazzar A, Alenezi S, Asa'ad S. Scintigraphic parathyroid imaging: concepts and new developments. Res Rep Nucl Med 2015;2015(5):9–18.
16. O'Doherty MJ, Kettle AG, Wells P, et al. Parathyroid imaging with technetium-99m-sestamibi: preoperative localization and tissue uptake studies. J Nucl Med 1992;33(3):313–8.
17. Mitchell BK, Merrell RC, Kinder BK. Localization studies in patients with hyperparathyroidism. Surg Clin North Am 1995;75(3):483–98.
18. Beland MD, Mayo-Smith WW, Grand DJ, et al. Dynamic MDCT for localization of occult parathyroid adenomas in 26 patients with primary hyperparathyroidism. Am J Roentgenol 2011;196(1): 61–5.
19. Silva BC, Cusano NE, Bilezikian JP. Primary hyperparathyroidism. Best Pract Res Clin Endocrinol Metab 2018;32(5):593–607.
20. Molinari AS, Irvin GL, Deriso GT, et al. Incidence of multiglandular disease in primary hyperparathyroidism determined by parathyroid hormone secretion. Surgery 1996;120(6):934–6.
21. Souza ÉRV, Scrignoli JA, Bezerra FC, et al. Devastating skeletal effects of delayed diagnosis of complicated primary hyperparathyroidism because of ectopic adenoma. J Clin Rheumatol 2008;14(5):281–4.
22. Khan AA, Hanley DA, Rizzoli R, et al. Primary hyperparathyroidism: review and recommendations on evaluation, diagnosis, and management. A Canadian and international consensus. Osteoporos Int 2017;28(1):1–19.
23. Pallan S, Khan A. Primary hyperparathyroidism: Update on presentation, diagnosis, and management in primary care. Can Fam Physician 2011; 57(2):184–9.
24. Carroll MF, Schade DS. A practical approach to hypercalcemia. Am Fam Physician 2003;67(9): 1959–66.
25. Barakat MT, Ashrafian H, Todd JF, et al. Severe hypercalcaemia from secretion of parathyroid hormone-related peptide. Lancet Oncol 2004; 5(10):633–5.
26. Metzger R, Milas M. Inherited cancer syndromes and the thyroid: An update. Curr Opin Oncol 2014;26(1):51–61.
27. Fernandez-Ranvier GG, Khanafshar E, Jensen K, et al. Parathyroid carcinoma, atypical parathyroid adenoma, or parathyromatosis? Cancer 2007; 110(2):255–64.
28. Cunningham J, Locatelli F, Rodriguez M. Secondary hyperparathyroidism: Pathogenesis, disease

progression, and therapeutic options. Clin J Am Soc Nephrol 2011;6(4):913–21.
29. Tomasello S. Secondary hyperparathyroidism and chronic kidney disease. Diabetes Spectr 2008; 21(1):19–25.
30. Dulfer RR, Franssen GJH, Hesselink DA, et al. Systematic review of surgical and medical treatment for tertiary hyperparathyroidism. Br J Surg 2017; 104(7):804–13.
31. Marcocci C, Cetani F. Clinical practice. Primary hyperparathyroidism. N Engl J Med 2011;365(25): 2389–97.
32. Fraser W. Hyperparathyroidism. Lancet 2009; 374(9684):145–58.
33. Debruyne F, Ostyn F, Delaere P. Distribution of the solitary adenoma over the parathyroid glands. J Laryngol Otol 1997;111(5):459–60.
34. Birdas TJ, Keenan RJ. Mediastinal parathyroid adenoma [8]. Ann Thorac Surg 2005;97(4):259–61.
35. Iihara M, Suzuki R, Kawamata A, et al. Thoracoscopic removal of mediastinal parathyroid lesions: Selection of surgical approach and pitfalls of preoperative and intraoperative localization. World J Surg 2012;36(6):1327–34.
36. Pawlik TM, Richards M, Giordano TJ, et al. Identification and management of intravagal parathyroid adenoma. World J Surg 2001;25(4):419–23.
37. Arnault V, Beaulieu A, Lifante JC, et al. Multicenter study of 19 aortopulmonary window parathyroid tumors: the challenge of embryologic origin. World J Surg 2010;34(9):2211–6.
38. Spinelli C, Liserre J, Pucci V, et al. Primary hyperparathyroidism: fifth parathyroid intrathymic adenoma in a young patient. J Pediatr Endocrinol Metab 2012;25(7):781–4.
39. Stalberg P, Grodski S, Sidhu S, et al. Cervical thymectomy for intrathymic parathyroid adenomas during minimally invasive parathyroidectomy. Surgery 2007;141(5):626–9.
40. Wieneke JA, Smith A. Parathyroid adenoma. Head Neck Pathol 2008;2(4):305–8.
41. Summers GW. Parathyroid update: a review of 220 cases. Ear Nose Throat J 1996;75(7):434–9.
42. Van der Walt J. Pathology of the parathyroid glands. Diagn Histopathol 2012;18(6):221–33.
43. Giorgadze T, Stratton B, Baloch ZW, et al. Oncocytic parathyroid adenoma: Problem in cytological diagnosis. Diagn Cytopathol 2004;31(4):276–80.
44. Erickson L, Jin L, Papotti M. Oxyphil parathyroid carcinomas: a clinicopathological and immunohistochemical study of 10 cases. Am J Surg Pathol 2002;26(3):344–9.
45. Paul A, Villepelet A, Lefèvre M, et al. Oncocytic parathyroid adenoma. Eur Ann Otorhinolaryngol Head Neck Dis 2015;132(5):301–3.
46. Paker I, Yilmazer D, Yandakci K, et al. Intrathyroidal oncocytic parathyroid adenoma: a diagnostic pitfall on fine-needle aspiration. Diagn Cytopathol 2010; 38(11):833–6.
47. Howson P, Kruijff S, Aniss A, et al. Oxyphil cell parathyroid adenomas causing primary hyperparathyroidism: a clinico-pathological correlation. Endocr Pathol 2015;26(3):250–4.
48. Stojadinovic A, Hoos A, Nissan A, et al. Parathyroid neoplasms: Clinical, histopathological, and tissue microarray-based molecular analysis. Hum Pathol 2003;34(1):54–64.
49. Snover D, Foucar K. Mitotic activity in benign parathyroid disease. Am J Clin Pathol 1981;75(2): 345–7.
50. Chang YJ, Mittal V, Remine S, et al. Correlation between clinical and histological findings in parathyroid tumors suspicious for carcinoma. Am Surg 2006;72(5):419–26.
51. Szender B, Farid P, Vegso G. Apoptosis and P53, Bcl-2 and Bax gene expression in parathyroid glands of patients with hyperparathyroidism. Pathol Oncol Res 2004;10(1):98–103.
52. DeLellis RA, Mazzaglia P, Mangray S. Primary hyperparathyroidism: a current perspective. Arch Pathol Lab Med 2008;132(8):1251–62.
53. DeLellis RA. Parathyroid carcinoma: an overview. Adv Anat Pathol 2005;12(2):53–61.
54. Chow L, Erickson L, Abu-Lebdeh H, et al. Parathyroid lipoadenomas: a rare cause of primary hyperparathyroidism. Endocr Pract 2006;12(2):131–6.
55. Johnson N, Serpell JW, Johnson WR, et al. Parathyroid lipoadenoma. ANZ J Surg 2015;85(6):489–90.
56. Hyrcza MD, Sargın P, Mete O. Parathyroid Lipoadenoma: a clinicopathological diagnosis and possible trap for the unaware pathologist. Endocr Pathol 2016;27(1):34–41.
57. Cetani F, Torregrossa L, Marcocci C. A large functioning parathyroid lipoadenoma. Endocrine 2016; 53(2):615–6.
58. Murakami K, Watanabe M, Nakashima N, et al. Water-clear cell adenoma associated with primary hyperparathyroidism: report of a case. Surg Today 2014;44(4):773–7.
59. Kodama H, Iihara M, Okamoto T, et al. Water-clear cell parathyroid adenoma causing primary hyperparathyroidism in a patient with neurofibromatosis type 1:Report of a case. Surg Today 2007;37(10): 884–7.
60. Piggott RP, Waters PS, Ashraf J, et al. Water-clear cell adenoma: a rare form of hyperparathyroidism. Int J Surg Case Rep 2013;4(10):911–3.
61. Arik D, Dündar E, Yilmaz E, et al. Water-clear cell adenoma of the mediastinal parathyroid gland. Turk Patoloji Derg 2017;1(1):1–5.
62. Chou YH, Jhuang JY, Hsieh MS. Water-clear cell parathyroid adenoma in a patient with acute pancreatitis. J Formos Med Assoc 2014;113(11): 872–3.

63. Bansal R, Trivedi P, Sarin J, et al. Lipoadenoma of the parathyroid gland - a rare cause of hyperparathyroidism. Gulf J Oncolog 2012;3(11):63–5.
64. Özden S, Güreşci S, Saylam B, et al. A rare cause of primary hyperparathyroidism: Parathyroid lipoadenoma. Auris Nasus Larynx 2018;45(6):1245–8.
65. Harness J, Ramsburg S, Nishiyama R. Multiple adenomas of the parathyroid: do they exist? Arch Surg 1979;114(5):468–74.
66. Tezelman S, Shen W, Shaver J. Double parathyroid adenomas. Clinical and biochemical characteristics before and after parathyroidectomy. Ann Surg 1993;218(3):300–7.
67. Zhou W, Katz MH, Deftos LJ, et al. Metachronous double parathyroid adenomas involving two different cell types: chief cell and oxyphil cell. Endocr Pract 2003;9(6):522–5.
68. Bergson EJ, Heller KS. The clinical significance and anatomic distribution of parathyroid double adenomas. J Am Coll Surg 2004;198(2):185–9.
69. Ogus M, Mayir B, Dinckan A. Mediastinal, cystic and functional parathyroid adenoma in patients with double parathyroid adenomas: a case report. Acta Chir Belg 2006;106(10):736–8.
70. Costa-Guda J, Arnold A. Genetic and epigenetic changes in sporadic endocrine tumors: Parathyroid tumors. Mol Cell Endocrinol 2014;386(1–2):46–54.
71. Costa-Guda J, Soong CP, Parekh VI, et al. germline and somatic mutations in cyclin-dependent kinase inhibitor genes CDKN1A, CDKN2B, and CDKN2C in sporadic parathyroid adenomas. Horm Cancer 2013;4(5):301–7.
72. Imanishi Y, Hosokawa Y, Yoshimoto K, et al. Primary hyperparathyroidism caused by parathyroid-targeted overexpression of cyclin d1 in transgenic mice. J Clin Invest 2001;107(9):1093–102.
73. Chandrasekharappa SC, Guru SC, Manickam P, et al. Positional cloning of the gene for multiple endocrine neoplasia-type 1. Science 1997; 276(5311):404–7.
74. Pellegata NS, Quintanilla-Martinez L, Siggelkow H, et al. Germ-line mutations in p27Kip1 cause a multiple endocrine neoplasia syndrome in rats and humans. Proc Natl Acad Sci U S A 2006;103(42): 15558–63.
75. Cromer MK, Starker LF, Choi M, et al. Identification of somatic mutations in parathyroid tumors using whole-exome sequencing. J Clin Endocrinol Metab 2012;97(9):E1774–81.
76. Soong C-P, Arnold A. Recurrent ZFX mutations in human sporadic parathyroid adenomas. Oncoscience 2014;1(5):360–6.
77. Iolascon A, Faienza MF, Coppola B, et al. Analysis of cyclin-dependent kinase inhibitor genes (CDKN2A, CDKN2B, andCDKN2C) in childhood rhabdomyosarcoma. Genes Chromosomes Cancer 1996;15(4):217–22.
78. Pandya C, Uzilov AV, Bellizzi J, et al. Genomic profiling reveals mutational landscape in parathyroid carcinomas. JCI Insight 2017;2(6):61–5.
79. Guiter G, Delellis R. Risk of recurrence or metastasis in atypical parathyroid adenoma. Mod Pathol 2002;15(1):115A.
80. Ippolito G, Palazzo FF, Sebag F, et al. Intraoperative diagnosis and treatment of parathyroid cancer and atypical parathyroid adenoma. Br J Surg 2007; 94(5):566–70.
81. Levin KE, Galante M, Clark OH. Parathyroid carcinoma versus parathyroid adenoma in patients with profound hypercalcemia. Surgery 1987; 101(6):649–60.
82. Kruijff S, Sidhu SB, Sywak MS, et al. Negative parafibromin staining predicts malignant behavior in atypical parathyroid adenomas. Ann Surg Oncol 2014;21(2):426–33.
83. Tan MH, Morrison C, Wang P, et al. Loss of parafibromin immunoreactivity is a distinguishing feature of parathyroid carcinoma. Clin Cancer Res 2004; 10(19):6629–37.
84. Cetani F, Ambrogini E, Viacava P, et al. Should parafibromin staining replace HRTP2 gene analysis as an additional tool for histologic diagnosis of parathyroid carcinoma? Eur J Endocrinol 2007;156(5): 547–54.
85. Newey PJ, Bowl MR, Thakker RV. Parafibromin - functional insights. J Intern Med 2009;266(1): 84–98.
86. Kim HK, Oh YL, Kim SH, et al. Parafibromin immunohistochemical staining to differentiate parathyroid carcinoma from parathyroid adenoma. Head Neck 2012;34(2):201–6.
87. Goshen O, Aviel-Ronen S, Dori S, et al. Brown tumour of hyperparathyroidism in the mandible associated with atypical parathyroid adenoma. J Laryngol Otol 2000;114(4):302–4.
88. Wani S, Hao Z. Atypical cystic adenoma of the parathyroid gland: case report and review of literature. Endocr Pract 2005;11(2):389–93.
89. Yener S, Saklamaz A, Demir T. Primary hyperparathyroidism due to atypical parathyroid adenoma presenting with peroneus brevis tendon rupture. J Endocrinol Invest 2007;30(5):442–4.
90. Duan K, Mete Ö. Parathyroid carcinoma: diagnosis and clinical implications. Turk Patoloji Derg 2015; 31(Suppl 1):80–97.
91. Asare EA, Sturgeon C, Winchester DJ, et al. Parathyroid carcinoma: an update on treatment outcomes and prognostic factors from the national cancer data base (NCDB). Ann Surg Oncol 2015; 22(12):3990–5.
92. Kassahun WT, Jonas S. Focus on parathyroid carcinoma. Int J Surg 2011;9(1):13–9.
93. Centani F, Pardi E, Marcocci C. Parathyroid Carcinoma. Front Horm Res 2019;51:63–76.

94. Vaswani N. The parathyroids: basic and clinical concepts. JAMA 1995;273(9):753–62.
95. Howell VM, Haven CJ, Kahnoski K, et al. HRPT2 mutations are associated with malignancy in sporadic parathyroid tumours. J Med Genet 2003; 40(9):657–63.
96. Betea D, Potorac I, Beckers A. Parathyroid carcinoma: challenges in diagnosis and treatment. Ann Endocrinol (Paris) 2015;26(6):1221–38.
97. Wei CH, Harari A. Parathyroid carcinoma: update and guidelines for management. Curr Treat Options Oncol 2012;13(1):11–23.
98. Gill AJ. Understanding the genetic basis of parathyroid carcinoma. Endocr Pathol 2014;25(1):30–4.
99. Adam MA, Untch BR, Olson JA Jr. Parathyroid carcinoma: current understanding and new insights into gene expression and intraoperative parathyroid hormone kinetics. Oncologist 2010;15(1):61–72.
100. Kameyama M, Fujii H, Konishi M. Parathyroid carcinomas: can clinical outcomes for parathyroid carcinomas be determined by histologic evaluation alone? Endocr Pathol 2002;13(1):135–9.
101. Bondeson L, Sandelin K, Grimelius L. Histopathological variables and DNA cytometry in parathyroid carcinoma. Am J Surg Pathol 1993;17(8):820–9.
102. Nasrallah MP, Fraker DL, LiVolsi VA. Parathyroid carcinoma in the setting of tertiary hyperparathyroidism after renal transplant. Endocr Pathol 2014;25(4):433–5.
103. Shattuck TM, Välimäki S, Obara T, et al. Somatic and germ line mutations of the *HRPT2* gene in sporadic parathyroid carcinoma. N Engl J Med 2003; 349(18):1722–9.
104. Bradley KJ, Cavaco BM, Bowl MR, et al. Parafibromin mutations in hereditary hyperparathyroidism syndromes and parathyroid tumours. Clin Endocrinol 2006;64(3):299–306.
105. Bricaire L, Odou MF, Cardot-Bauters C, et al. Frequent large germline HRPT2 deletions in a french national cohort of patients with primary hyperparathyroidism. J Clin Endocrinol Metab 2013. https://doi.org/10.1210/jc.2012-2789.
106. Costa AG, Bilezikian JP. Bone turnover markers in hyperparathyroidism. J Clin Densitom 2013;16(1): 22–7.
107. Kasaian K, Wiseman SM, Thiessen N, et al. Complete genomic landscape of a recurring sporadic parathyroid carcinoma. J Pathol 2013;230(3): 249–60.
108. Kebebew E, Arici C, Duh QY, et al. Localization and reoperation results for persistent and recurrent parathyroid carcinoma. Arch Surg 2001;136(8): 878–85.
109. Brown J, Mohamed H, Williams-Smith L. Primary hyperparathyroidism secondary to simultaneous bilateral parathyroid carcinoma. Ear Nose Throat J 2002;2(2):393–8.
110. Wiseman SM, Rigual NR, Hicks WL, et al. Parathyroid carcinoma: a multicenter review of clinicopathologic features and treatment outcomes. Ear Nose Throat J 2004;83(7):491–4.
111. Busaidy NL, Jimenez C, Habra MA, et al. Parathyroid carcinoma: a 22-year experience. Head Neck 2004;26(8):716–26.
112. Harari A, Waring A, Fernandez-Ranvier G, et al. Parathyroid carcinoma: a 43-year outcome and survival analysis. J Clin Endocrinol Metab 2011; 96(12):3679–86.
113. Vargas MP, Vargas HI, Kleiner DE, et al. The role of prognostic markers (MiB-1, RB, and bcl-2) in the diagnosis of parathyroid tumors. Mod Pathol 1997;10(1):12–7.
114. Howell VM, Gill A, Clarkson A, et al. Accuracy of combined protein gene product 9.5 and parafibromin markers for immunohistochemical diagnosis of parathyroid carcinoma. J Clin Endocrinol Metab 2009;94(2):434–41.
115. Pacheco MC. Multiple endocrine neoplasia: a genetically diverse group of familial tumor syndromes. J Pediatr Genet 2016;5(2):89–97.

Neuroendocrine Tumors of the Gastrointestinal Tract and Pancreas

Natalie Patel, MD[a], Andrea Barbieri, MD[b], Joanna Gibson, MD, PhD[c,*]

KEYWORDS

• Well-differentiated neuroendocrine tumor • Ki-67 • Poorly differentiated neuroendocrine carcinoma • WHO classification and grade

Key points

- Nomenclature and classification of neuroendocrine neoplasms of the gastrointestinal tract and pancreas have undergone significant changes in the last decade.
- Diagnosis of neuroendocrine neoplasms of the gastrointestinal tract and pancreas requires accurate determination of differentiation and World Health Organization (WHO) grade classification.
- Well-differentiated neuroendocrine tumors are classified as grade 1, 2, or 3 based on the mitotic rate and Ki-67 proliferative index according to WHO guidelines.
- Poorly differentiated neuroendocrine carcinomas are, by definition, WHO grade 3 tumors with a very poor prognosis.

ABSTRACT

Neuroendocrine neoplasms (NENs) of the gastrointestinal (GI) tract and pancreas are a rare and heterogeneous group of neoplasms characterized by common cellular features as well as unique site-specific traits. GI and pancreatic NENs are much rarer than the more common adenocarcinomas arising at these sites. However, the incidences of GI and pancreatic NENs have increased significantly, particularly in the stomach and common site, followed by rectum, appendix, colon, and stomach. Pancreatic NENs are also uncommon, with fewer than 1 per 100,000, accounting for 1% to 2% of all pancreatic neoplasms.

OVERVIEW

Neuroendocrine cells are differentiated epithelial cells found throughout the gastrointestinal (GI) tract and pancreas that secrete a variety of peptides and other hormones, depending on the organ in which they are found (**Fig. 1**).[1–4] Neuroendocrine cells are derived from adult GI stem cells, rather than the neurocrest.[5] Neuroendocrine cells store the peptides within

Disclosure: The authors have no relevant relationship with a commercial company that has a direct financial interest in the subject matter or material discussed in this article or with a company making a competing product.

[a] Gastrointestinal and Pancreaticobiliary Pathology, Department of Pathology, Yale School of Medicine, Yale New Haven Hospital, 20 York Street, New Haven, CT 06510, USA; [b] Department of Pathology, Yale School of Medicine, Yale New Haven Hospital, 20 York Street, EP2-608, New Haven, CT 06510, USA; [c] Department of Pathology, Yale School of Medicine, Yale New Haven Hospital, 20 York Street, EP2-610, New Haven, CT 06510, USA
* Corresponding author.
E-mail address: joanna.gibson@yale.edu

Surgical Pathology 12 (2019) 1021–1044
https://doi.org/10.1016/j.path.2019.08.007

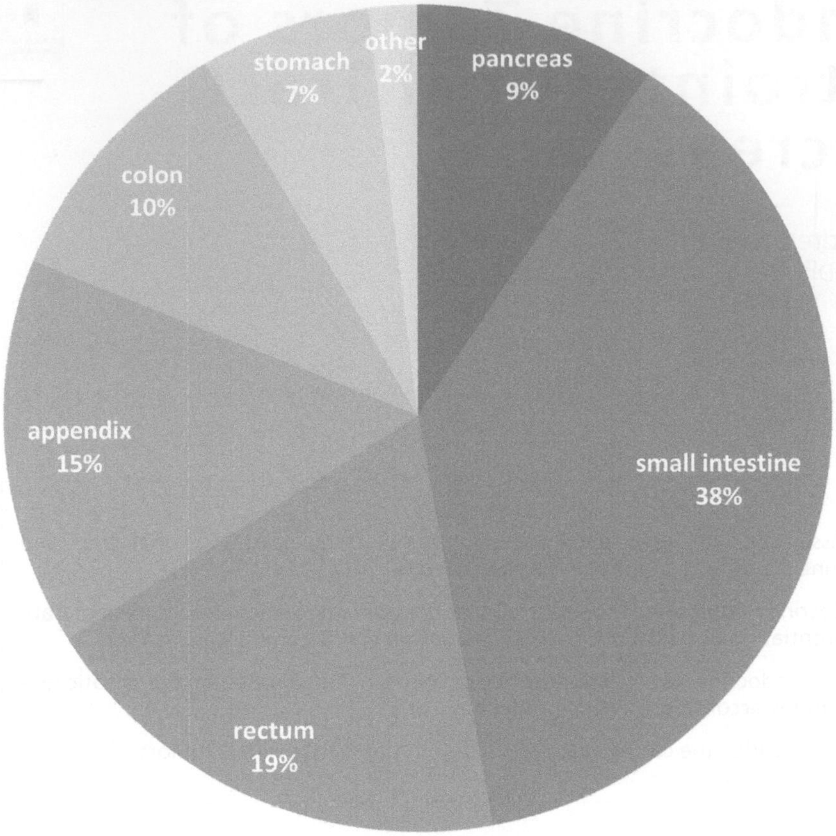

Fig. 1. Distribution of gastroenteropancreatic neuroendocrine neoplasms (NENs) according to Surveillance, Epidemiology, and End Results (SEER) data and World Health Organization (WHO) information. Because small appendiceal tumors are often not reported to SEER, the percentage of appendiceal NENs is likely considerably higher than shown. (*Data from* references 1-4).

synapticlike secretory vesicles, which also contain the proteins chromogranin A and synaptophysin, markers of neuroendocrine cell differentiation.[6] Epithelial tumors with neuroendocrine cell differentiation (ie, neuroendocrine cell neoplasms [NENs]) share the cellular features of neuroendocrine cells to varying extent, depending on the organ involved.

Classification and terminology of GI and pancreatic NENs has evolved significantly in recent decades. Many early classification schemes were based on specific organs in which tumors arose or the association of neuroendocrine tumors (NETs) with specific secreted peptides and functional syndromes, which resulted in clinically confusing terminologies. Older terms for GI or pancreatic NETs included carcinoid tumor and pancreatic islet cell tumor. Although these older terms have fallen out of favor in the current World Health Organization (WHO) terminology, many clinicians still use the older terms colloquially. The last 2 to 3 decades have experienced significant changes in how GI and pancreatic NENs are detected, diagnosed, and managed. Two major categories of NENs in the GI tract and pancreas have emerged: well-differentiated NETs (WDNETs) and poorly differentiated neuroendocrine carcinomas (PDNECs) (**Table 1**).

WELL-DIFFERENTIATED NEUROENDOCRINE TUMORS OF THE GASTROINTESTINAL TRACT AND PANCREAS

Grossly, WDNETs of the GI tract and pancreas are well-circumscribed firm lesions with a uniform tan to yellow cut surface (**Fig. 2**). The tumor borders are typically well delineated, with a pushing-type invasion of adjacent tissue. Occasionally, hemorrhagic areas may be present and, rarely, NETs may appear cystic because of central degeneration (see **Fig. 2**). On histologic examination, well-differentiated NETs are typically cellular tumors characterized by a proliferation of uniform round to ovoid cells with enlarged nuclei and ample amphophilic or lightly eosinophilic cytoplasm (**Fig. 3**). Tumor cells can also have a plasmacytoid appearance with eccentric nuclei and moderate amounts of cytoplasm. The chromatin is most often described as having a stippled salt-and-pepper–type pattern, but this characteristic depends on fixation and other preanalytical factors. Tumor

Table 1
Key histologic findings of gastroenteric and pancreatic neuroendocrine neoplasm

	WDNET	PDNEC
Tumor Border	Well circumscribed with pushing type invasion	Infiltrative, poorly circumscribed
Growth Patterns	• Solid • Trabecular • Nested • Gyriform • Pseudoglandular	• Solid • Sheetlike
Cytology	• Uniform round cells • Ample amphophilic to eosinophilic cytoplasm • Centrally located nuclei with inconspicuous nucleoli • Coarse salt-and-pepper chromatin • Rarely, pleomorphic or clear cell changes	Small cell type • Small cell • Scant cytoplasm • Inconspicuous nuclei • Nuclear molding Large cell type • Polygonal cells • Moderate cytoplasm • Prominent nucleoli

cells grow in a variety of patterns, including nested, solid, trabecular, pseudoglandular, and gyriform (see **Fig. 3**). Rarely, WDNETs can have a spindled cytoplasmic appearance.

The stroma of WDNETs shows fibrosis and, in some cases, hyalinization (see **Fig. 3**; **Fig. 4**). There is usually a rich vascular network, which can make assessment of lymphovascular invasion difficult if nests of tumor are abutting vessels. In cases with suspected lymphovascular invasion, vascular markers such as cluster of differentiation (CD) 34, CD31, or D2-40 can be helpful in confirming its presence. Amyloid deposition is also rarely observed, particularly in cases of WDNETs that secrete insulin (see **Fig. 4**).[7] The presence of amyloid can be confirmed with Congo red staining and apple green birefringence on polarization. The amyloid is derived from islet amyloid polypeptide and is not associated with systemic amyloidosis.[8]

Well-differentiated tumors contain secretory vesicles, as shown by diffuse staining with neuroendocrine cell markers (such as chromogranin and synaptophysin) (**Fig. 5**). The secretory vesicles can also be shown on electron microscopic examination as numerous intracellular round cytoplasmic densities, although electron microscopy is rarely used for diagnostic purposes currently.

POORLY DIFFERENTIATED NEUROENDOCRINE CARCINOMA

PDNECs of the GI tract or pancreas are high-grade carcinomas that resemble neuroendocrine carcinoma (NEC)of the lung. Grossly, GI or pancreatic PDNECs are typically large tumors with invasion into and destruction of surrounding normal tissue. The tumor borders are infiltrative, although, compared with ductal adenocarcinoma, the tumors are better demarcated. Necrosis and hemorrhage are common. Morphologically, PDNECs are classified as either small cell carcinoma or large cell NEC (**Fig. 6**). In general, progression from NET to NEC does not occur; however, very rarely, WDNETs can be associated with a PDNEC component.[9] PDNECs of the GI tract and pancreas are discussed later.

FUNCTIONAL CLASSIFICATION

In addition to the morphologic classification outlined earlier, GI and pancreatic WDNETs are also classified as functioning or nonfunctioning, based on the presence of a clinical syndrome caused by tumor hormone secretion. NETs are known to secrete as many as 40 different peptides or other compounds.[10] The functional status of NETs may affect the nomenclature of NETs. In general, functioning GI and pancreatic WDNETs are named after the predominant hormone secreted by the tumor and resulting clinical syndrome (eg, insulinoma). Detection of a hormone by immunohistochemical staining of the WDNET is insufficient for a diagnosis of a functioning NET. For example, if the tumor stains positively with insulin but the patient does not have hypoglycemia, the tumor should not be considered an insulinoma. In contrast, a functioning WDNET associated with clinical syndromes of insulin overexpression may show weak, faint, focal, or even negative staining with insulin immunohistochemistry (IHC).

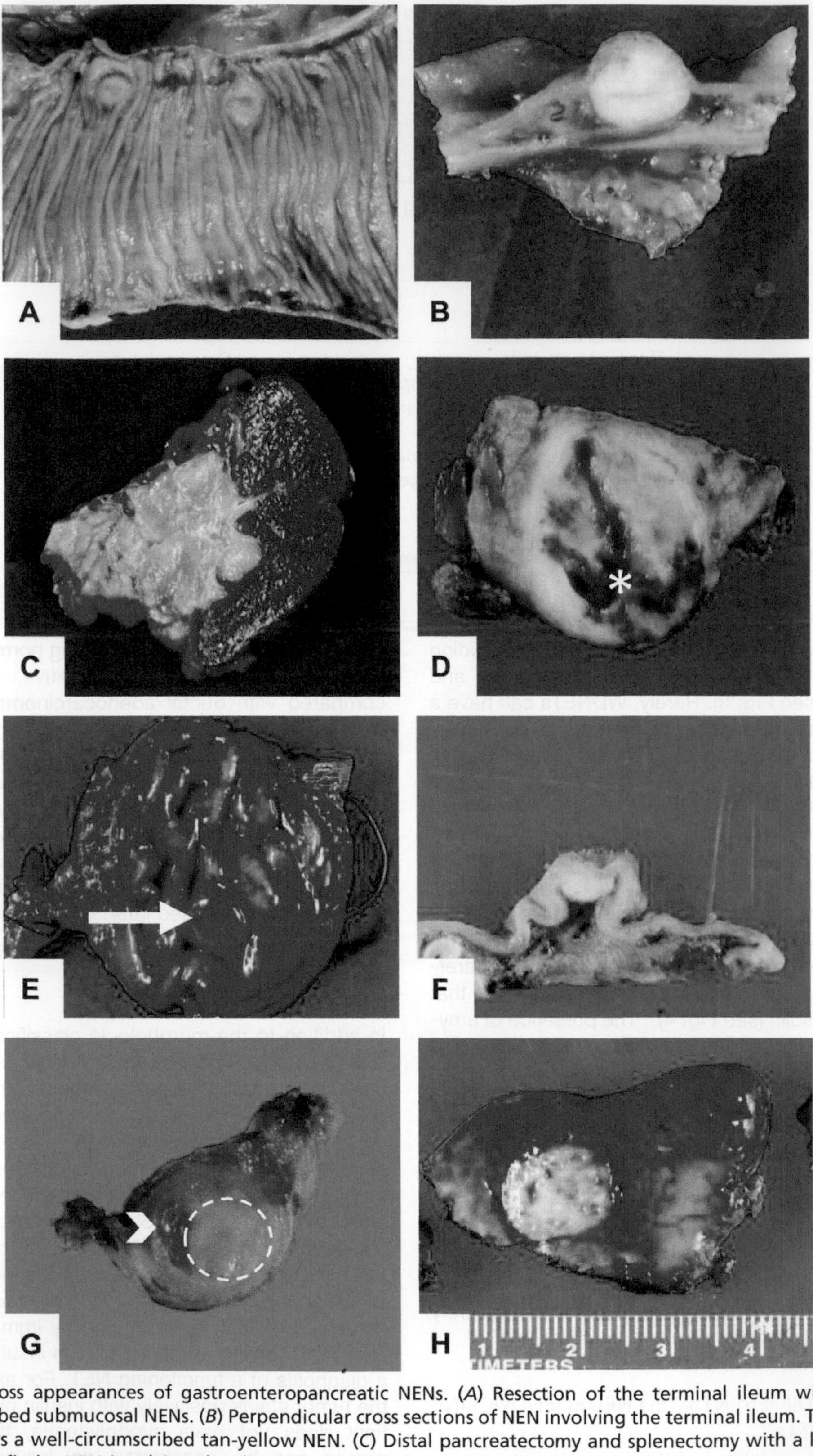

Fig. 2. Gross appearances of gastroenteropancreatic NENs. (*A*) Resection of the terminal ileum with 2 well-circumscribed submucosal NENs. (*B*) Perpendicular cross sections of NEN involving the terminal ileum. The cut surface shows a well-circumscribed tan-yellow NEN. (*C*) Distal pancreatectomy and splenectomy with a large lobulated tan, fleshy NEN involving the distal pancreas and extending into the splenic hilum. (*D*) Cross sections of pancreatic NEN shows a tumor with a partially circumferential fibrous pseudocapsule and a tan-yellow cut surface with cystic change (*asterisk*). (*E*) Partial gastrectomy with a tan-pink polypoid submucosal nodule (*arrow*). (*F*) Cut section of mucosal folds shows a yellow cut surface limited to the submucosa. (*G*) Cross section of appendix with an incidental NEN (*dotted circle*). The appendiceal lumen is distended and obstructed by NEN (*arrowhead*). (*H*) A liver wedge resection containing a well-delineated tan-yellow metastatic NEN from a terminal ileum primary.

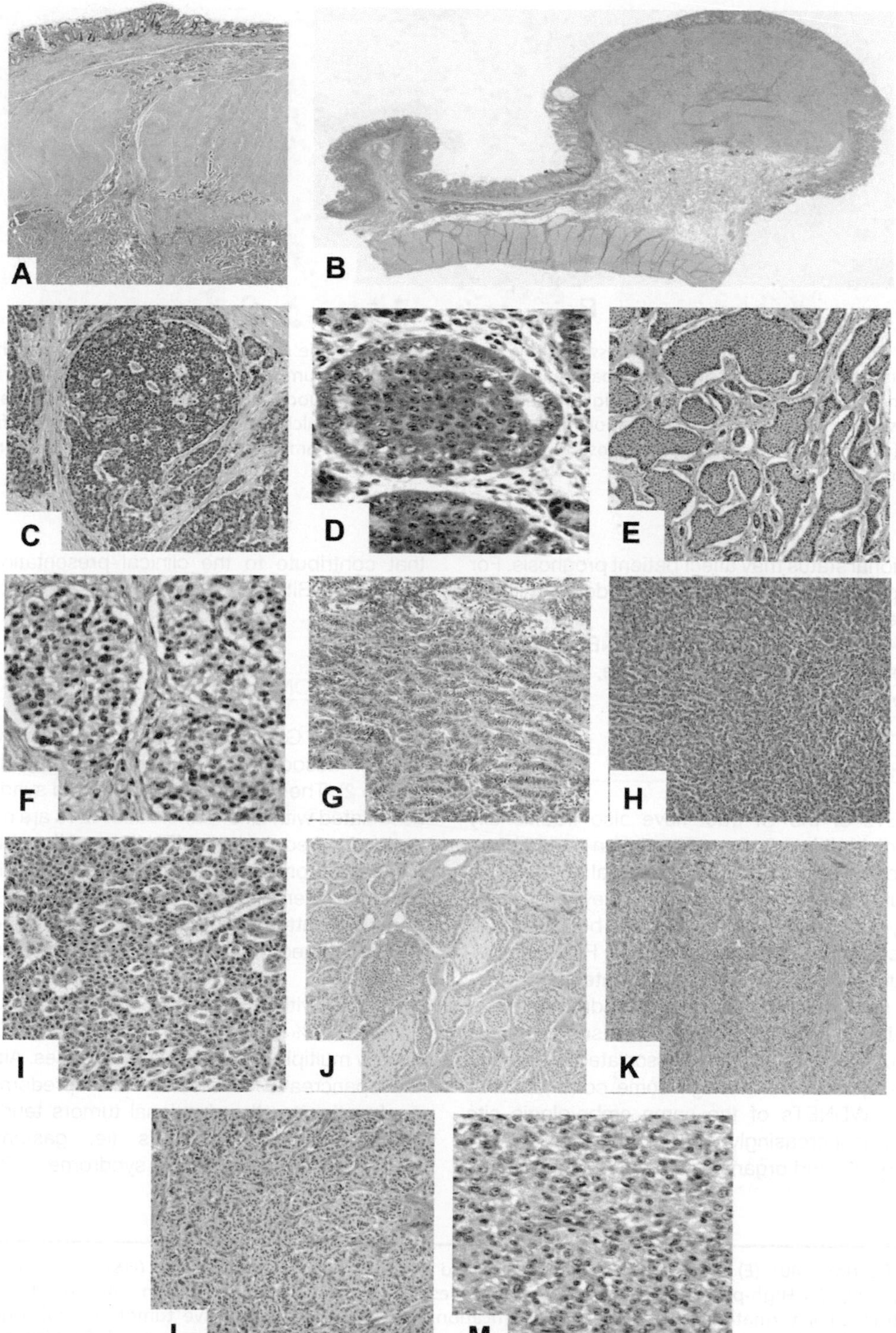

Fig. 3. Histologic appearances of gastroenteropancreatic NENs. (*A*) Low-power view of terminal ileum well-differentiated NET with deeply invasive infiltrative pseudoglands and nests of tumor cells through the muscularis propria into the subserosa (hematoxylin-eosin [H&E], original magnification ×2). (*B*) Gastric well-differentiated NET forming a polypoid mucosal mass. Tumor cells involve the mucosa and submucosa without infiltrative deep invasion (H&E, original magnification ×1). (*C*) Well-differentiated NET with rosette pattern of growth (H&E, original magnification ×20). (*D*) High-power view of rosette formation with prominent intracytoplasmic granules at the periphery of the nests. These granules are characteristic of WDNET of midgut origin (H&E, original

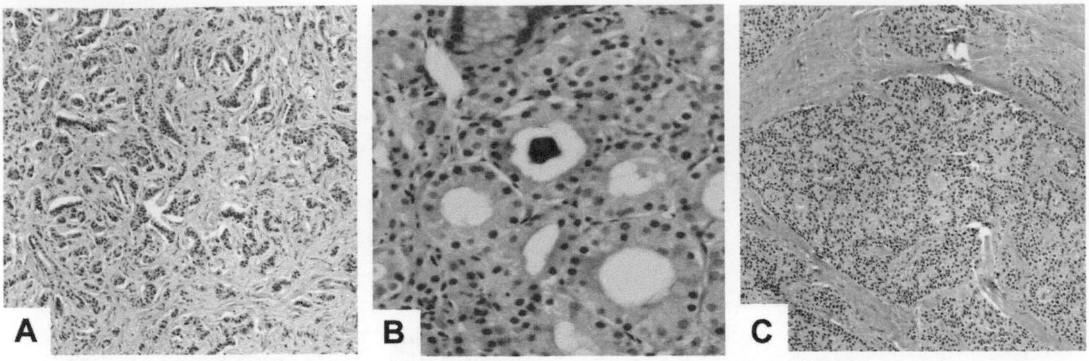

Fig. 4. There are some characteristic associations between the hormone expressed and the tumor morphology. (*A*) Functional WDNET of the distal pancreas producing glucagon. Tumor cells have a cordlike pattern with prominent hyalinized stroma (H&E, original magnification ×20). (*B*) Duodenal somatostatinoma with characteristic pseudoglandular/tubular formation and psammomatous-type calcification (H&E, original magnification ×40). (*C*) Pancreatic insulinoma with rosette pattern and eosinophilic amyloidlike stroma (H&E, original magnification ×20).

Functional status may affect patient prognosis. For example, insulinomas have an indolent clinical course.[11] However, the biology and clinical behavior of most functioning NETs remains defined by the grade and stage, just as for nonfunctioning NETs.

EMBRYOLOGIC ORIGIN

WDNETs of the GI tract have also traditionally been divided into 3 groups based on the embryologic origin of the portion of the tubal gut (foregut, midgut, and hindgut) in which they arise. The embryologic origin of WDNETs may be associated with certain tumor characteristics. For example, midgut WDNETs tend to be associated with serotonin secretion and carcinoid syndrome (especially in the setting of liver metastases), whereas hindgut WDNETs are rarely associated with a hormonal syndrome. Although some commonalities among WDNETs of the same embryologic site exist, it is increasingly evident that each specific primary site and organ has unique clinical features that contribute to the clinical presentation and prognosis. Site-specific WDNETs are discussed later.

ASSOCIATION WITH INHERITED SYNDROMES

Importantly, GI and pancreatic WDNETs have significant associations with inherited syndromes (**Table 2**). The most common inherited syndromes associated with GI or pancreatic NETs are multiple endocrine neoplasia 1 (MEN1), von Hippel-Lindau (VHL) syndrome, neurofibromatosis 1 (NF1), and tuberous sclerosis, all of which have an autosomal dominant pattern of inheritance.[12] The association with inherited syndromes does not include PDNECs.

Patients with MEN1 have pancreatic WDNETs in 30% to 75% of cases and duodenal WDNETs, usually multiple, in 50% to 80% of cases. Although the pancreatic WDNETs are predominantly nonfunctioning, the duodenal tumors tend to be gastrin-producing WDNETs (ie, gastrinomas), leading to Zollinger-Ellison syndrome.[13] Patients

magnification ×40). (*E*) Tumor cells growing in a nested and ribbonlike growth pattern (H&E, original magnification ×20). (*F*) High-power view of tumor cells in nests (H&E, original magnification ×40). (*G*) Tumor cells with trabecular formation (H&E, original magnification ×20). (*H*) Loosely cohesive tumor cells with gyriform growth and focal pseudoglandular formation (H&E, original magnification ×20). (*I*) Tumor cells forming pseudoacinar structures (H&E, original magnification ×40). (*J*) Grade 1, WDNET with extensive perineural invasion (H&E, original magnification ×20). (*K*) Grade 2 pancreatic WDNET with nests of tumor cells embedded in a fibrous stroma (H&E, original magnification ×10). (*L*) WDNET tumor cells show enlarged bizarre pleomorphic nuclei and occasional multinucleated cells, characteristic of endocrine-type atypia often seen in NETs of the GI tract and pancreas (H&E, original magnification ×20). (*M*) Sheetlike growth of well-differentiated tumor cells. Neoplastic cells have rounded nuclei with stippled chromatin, occasional inconspicuous nucleoli, and abundant amphophilic cytoplasm (H&E, original magnification ×40).

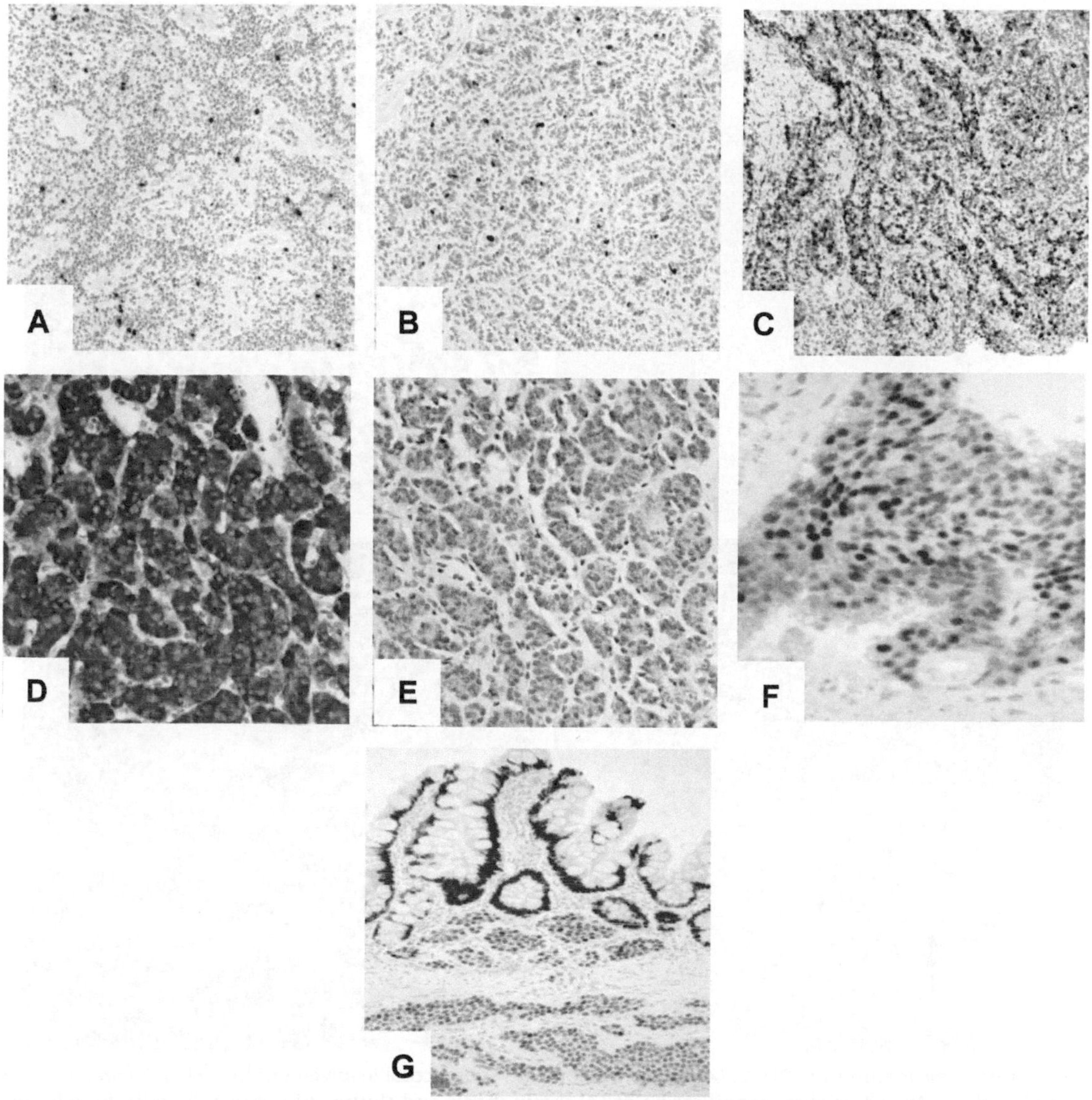

Fig. 5. Immunohistochemistry of WDNETs. (*A*) Ki-67 immunohistochemical stain showing nuclear staining of occasional tumor cells, consistent with WHO grade 1, Ki-67 proliferative index (PI) of 1.1% (original magnification ×20). (*B*) WHO grade 2, Ki-67 PI of 5.1% (original magnification ×20). (*C*) Ki-67 immunostain highlights a significant proportion of well-differentiated NET cells and is consistent with WHO grade 3, Ki-67 PI of 40% (original magnification ×20). (*D*) Strong, diffuse cytoplasmic staining of WDNET with synaptophysin immunostain (original magnification ×40). (*E*) Chromogranin immunostain with granular cytoplasmic staining of tumor cells (original magnification ×40). (*F*) WDNET with metastatic spread to a lymph node. PDX-1 immunostain shows strong nuclear staining, suggesting spread from a pancreatic or gastric primary (original magnification ×40). (*G*) CDX-2 immunostain with strong nuclear staining of tumor cells, consistent with jejunoileal (or appendiceal) primary (original magnification ×20).

with MEN1 who have gastrinomas also often have small gastric WDNETs and enterochromaffinlike (ECL) hyperplasia.

Pancreatic WDNETs occur in approximately 15% of patients with VHL syndrome.[14,15] Most are nonfunctioning. In approximately 50% of patients, multiple WDNETs are seen. VHL-associated WDNETs have distinctive morphologic features, including marked hypervascularity, marked nuclear atypia, and cellular clearing.[16] Microadenomatosis can also be seen. Prognosis seems to be better than for patients who have sporadic WDNETs. NETs outside the pancreas have been rarely reported.[17]

Patients with NF1 develop somatostatin-producing WDNETs of the duodenum, although

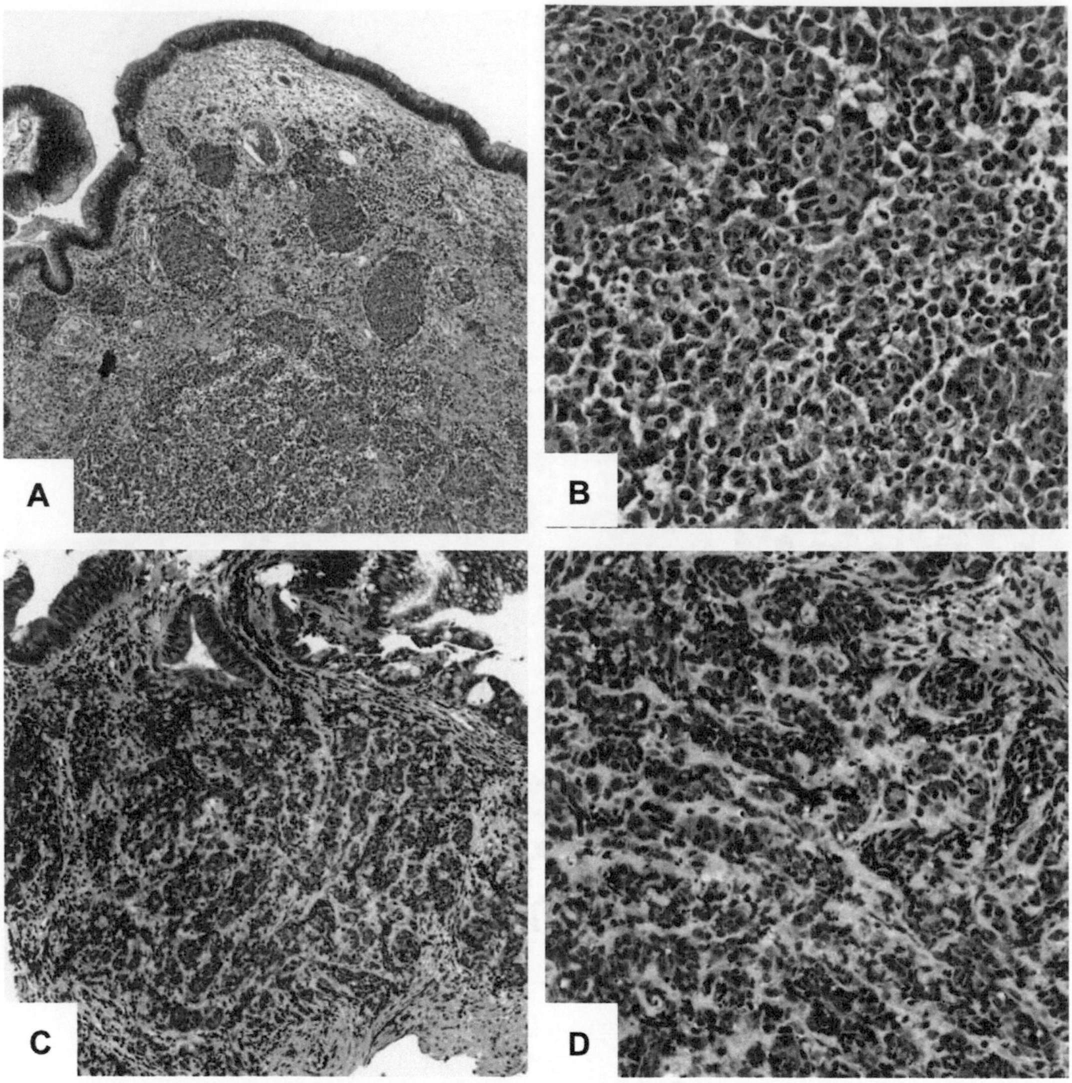

Fig. 6. Histologic features of PDNEC. (*A*) Sigmoid colon with submucosal involvement by a PDNEC (H&E, original magnification ×10). (*B*) Higher magnification of (*A*) shows sheets and clusters of tumor cells with irregular nuclear contours, conspicuous nucleoli, mitotic figures, and apoptotic bodies, consistent with large cell NEC (H&E, original magnification ×40). (*C*) Colon with submucosal involvement by nests of poorly differentiated tumor cells with crush artifact (H&E, original magnification ×20). (*D*) Higher magnification of (*C*) reveals tumor cells with high N/C ratio, nuclear molding, mitosis, and apoptotic debris, compatible with small cell NEC (H&E, original magnification ×40).

the syndrome of somatostatinoma is rare among these patients (ie, most are nonfunctioning). Studies have shown that up to 30% of patients with somatostatin-producing NETs of the duodenum are associated with NF1.[18] Somatostatin-producing NETs have characteristic tubular/glandular growth pattern with psammomatous calcification in two-thirds of patients (see **Fig. 4**). Although less frequent, patients with NF1 can also have WDNETs of the pancreas.

Glucagon cell hyperplasia and neoplasia (GCHN) is an extremely rare disorder caused by mutations of the GCGR gene, with fewer than 10 cases reported. Patients with GCHN show pancreatic hypertrophic islets, as well as numerous microadenomas.[19,20]

HISTOLOGIC GRADING OF WELL-DIFFERENTIATED NEUROENDOCRINE TUMORS

The WHO grading of GI and pancreas NETs is based on assessment of proliferative activity in the tumor. Current protocols require assessment

Table 2
Key points: methods of grading of neuroendocrine neoplasms

Ki-67 Proliferative Index	Mitotic Index
Percentage of tumor cells staining with Ki-67	Number of mitoses in 2 mm²/10 HPF
Recommended Methods	
• Manual count of 500–2000 cells using printed images • Digital imaging analysis	• Count mitoses in 50 HPF and average per 2 mm²/10 HPF

Abbreviation: HPF, high-power fields.

of both the mitotic count and the Ki-67 proliferative index (see **Table 2**).[21] Both should be assessed in tumor hotspots, the region of tumor that has most activity as observed based on scanning the tumor at intermediate magnification (see **Fig. 5**; **Fig. 7**).[22] The grading scheme can be applied to all GI and pancreas NETs. The WHO grade is assigned as follows in WDNETs of the GI tract and pancreas: grade 1 (G1) tumors have fewer than 2 mitoses per 10 high-power fields (HPF) and Ki-67 index of less than 3%, and grade 2 (G2) tumors have 2 to 20 mitoses per 10 HPFs and Ki-67 index of 3% to 20%. In the pancreas, grade 3 (G3) WDNETs have more than 20 mitoses per 10 HPFs and Ki-67 index of greater than 20% (see **Fig. 5**, **Table 3**). All PDNECs by definition are grade 3 as well. In case of discordance between the mitotic grade versus the Ki-67 index, the higher value is used to assign the final grade. In general, it is usually the Ki-67 proliferative index that is of the higher grade in cases in which there is discordance with the mitotic count.[22] This discordance can occur in part because of the delays in fixation that have been shown to decrease mitotic activity as much as 50%.[23] On rare occasions, the Ki-67 proliferative index may be surprisingly high and can hint at an unexpected WDNET mimic, such as acinar cell carcinoma.[24]

MITOTIC COUNT

The number of mitoses is reported per 2-mm² field, which approximates 10 HPF using a 40× objective, depending on the microscope and objective being used. A minimum of 50 HPF should be examined to obtain an accurate number.[25] The total number of tumor cells in a 2-mm² field varies in different tumors. Mitotic figures should be well delineated. Avoidance of mitotic figure mimics can be difficult. Degenerating/pyknotic nuclei, apoptotic bodies, as well as nuclei of nontumor cells, are known pitfalls that can lead to overestimation of the grade. Mitotic count has been reported to have poor reproducibility between observers.[26] Voss and colleagues[25] reported the use of the phosphohistone H3 immunohistochemical stain as an alternative to morphologic mitotic analysis. In their study of 63 cases, phosphohistone H3 immunohistochemical staining had reduced time and improved

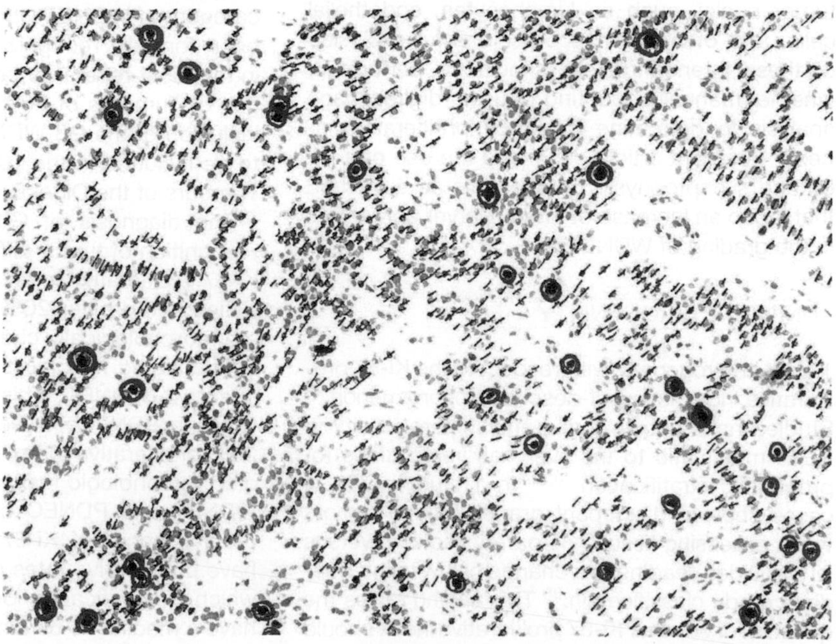

Fig. 7. Ki-67 counting method. A printed color image of Ki-67 immunostain taken at hot spots of a WDNET. Manual cell count completed by crossing off the Ki-67–negative tumor cells (*black lines*) and circling the Ki-67–positive cells (*circled in pink*) (original magnification ×20).

Table 3
Key points: World Health Organization classification and grading neuroendocrine tumors

	Mitotic Index	Ki-67 Proliferation Index (%)
WHO 2010 (GI)		
WDNET, Grade 1	<2	<3
WDNET, Grade 2	2–20	3–20
PDNEC, Grade 3	>20	>20
WHO 2017 (Pancreas)		
WDNET, Grade 1	<2	<3
WDNET, Grade 2	2–20	3–20
WDNET, Grade 3	>20	>20
PDNEC, Grade 3	>20	>20

interobserver reproducibility in mitotic rate assessment and grade assignment.

KI-67 PROLIFERATION INDEX

To determine the Ki-67 proliferative index, the WHO/European Neuroendocrine Tumor Society (ENETS) recommends counting 2000 tumor nuclei manually and calculating the percentage of positively staining nuclei (see **Fig. 7**).[27] In some instances, counting as few as 500 cells may be sufficient for grading. Digital imaging analysis is also an acceptable method that has been shown to be comparable with manual counting.[22] Eyeball estimation methods are not reliable and lack precision, and are therefore not recommended.[22]

One of the challenges to Ki-67 proliferative index quantitation is the interference of proliferating nontumor nuclei, such as lymphocytes, endothelial cells, and other stromal cells. Careful exclusion of these interfering cells should be performed, whether manually counting or using digital image analysis to determine the Ki-67 proliferative index.[22] A recent article described the use of a Ki-67 and synaptophysin double stain as a method that led to an increase of interobserver agreement in the grading of WDNETs.[28]

TUMOR HETEROGENEITY

Tumor heterogeneity with respect to the Ki-67 proliferative index is a well-described phenomenon.[29] Studies have shown that tumor heterogeneity in NETs metastatic to the liver has implications for prognostic stratification.[30,31] In 1 study, 47% of cases showed discrepant grades among tumors when assessing tissue microarray sections versus whole slides, leading to a change of low to intermediate grade classification.[30] This finding raises the question of whether Ki-67 proliferative index should be assessed on preoperative biopsies, resection specimens, or metastatic disease. However, grading of core biopsies or even fine-needle aspiration specimens remains prognostic and is therefore recommended. However, given the inherent heterogeneity, repeating Ki-67 counts on subsequent specimens may be helpful, especially in cases in which a tumor was initially graded as WHO grade 1.

EMERGENCE OF THE GRADE 3 WELL-DIFFERENTIATED NEUROENDOCRINE TUMOR CATEGORY

Rarely, WDNETs have proliferative activity that corresponds to grade 3 based on Ki-67 index. This rare group of NETs seems to have a worse prognosis than grade 2 WDNETs, but a better prognosis than poorly differentiated NEC.[8,24] The category of WDNET with grade 3 Ki-67 index has been formally recognized in the pancreas NETs in the most recent update of the WHO Classification of Tumours of Endocrine Organs.[32] A similar inclusion of the G3 WDNET category is expected to be included in the 2019 WHO Classification of Tumours of the Digestive System.

The diagnosis of G3 WDNET hinges on the recognition of tumor differentiation, as well as the Ki-67 proliferative index. The G3 WDNET tumors, defined as greater 20% Ki-67 proliferative index, are morphologically characterized as having well-differentiated histologic features, similar to grade 1 and 2 WDNET. This definition is in contrast with the PDNECs, which also have greater than 20% proliferative index but have poorly differentiated morphologic features. Although both the G3 WDNET and PDNEC categories are defined by greater than 20% Ki-67 rates, most G3 WDNETs have proliferative rates in the 20% to 55% range, which is significantly lower than PDNECs, which have a median Ki-67 index of 80%.[33]

The difference between G3 WDNET and PDNEC extends to the molecular changes. Tang and colleagues[9] found that loss of TP53 and Rb1 is seen in PDNEC, whereas G3 WDNET are associated with DAXX and ATRX2 loss. In a follow-up study, Sigel and colleagues[34] found that some G3 WDNET can show nonplasmacytoid morphology, pleomorphic nuclei, and abundant cytoplasm, which can be challenging for well-differentiated classification, and it is recommended to use ancillary mutational analysis and/or immunohistochemical staining as an adjunct in diagnosis. The incidence of G3 WDNETs has been increasing because of greater recognition of this subset of tumors.[35,36] G3 WDNETs are reportedly most common in the pancreas.[33,37] Furthermore, G3 WDNETs that have Ki-67 proliferative indices less than 55% do not respond to platinum-based chemotherapy like PDNECs.[38]

PROGNOSIS AND STAGING OF NEUROENDOCRINE NEOPLASMS

The prognosis of GI and pancreatic NENs depends on tumor stage, margin status, WHO grade, histologic differentiation, and site of origin. In general, PDNECs confer a poor prognosis and have a rapid clinical course, with survival beyond 1 year being rare.[37] In contrast, WDNETs generally have a much better prognosis, with an overall 5-year survival of 67%.[9] However, there is a lot of variability in the prognosis among the WDNET group. Surgery remains the mainstay of treatment of localized WDNETs, and the extent of surgical resection depends on the tumor size and organ involved. The current eighth edition of the American Joint Committee on Cancer (AJCC) staging manual has tumor, node, metastasis (TNM) staging systems outlined for WDNETs of the duodenum (including ampulla of Vater), appendix, colon, jejunum and ileum, pancreas, and stomach.[39] PDNECs are staged using the same staging system as adenocarcinoma of the corresponding organ of involvement. Additional data on prognosis, staging, and surgical management of WDNETs are discussed later for each organ-specific site, where applicable.

IMMUNOHISTOCHEMISTRY OF WELL-DIFFERENTIATED NEUROENDOCRINE TUMORS

MARKERS OF NEUROENDOCRINE DIFFERENTIATION

WDNETs express markers of neuroendocrine differentiation, including synaptophysin and chromogranin A. The pattern of expression of synaptophysin is most commonly diffuse and strong, whereas chromogranin expression may be more variable, showing diffuse, apical, and sometimes less intense positivity (see **Fig. 5**). CD56, CD57, and neuron-specific enolase are also expressed in NETs, but are not considered specific enough to show neuroendocrine differentiation when used in isolation.[40,41] Although the general neuroendocrine markers such as synaptophysin and chromogranin A can confirm the presence of neuroendocrine differentiation in NETs, particularly if there is doubt based on unusual or variant morphologic features, these markers do not have the ability to discriminate between sites of origin of NETs.

Recently, Insulinoma associated 1 (INSM1) was proposed as a general marker of neuroendocrine cell differentiation.[42] INSM1 is a nuclear transcription factor that has been reported to be a sensitive marker of neuroendocrine differentiation in a variety of neoplasms, both well and poorly differentiated, including tumors in the lung,[43,44] pancreas,[45] head, and neck,[46] and Merkel cell carcinoma.[42,47] However, the data are insufficient at this time to support the use of INSM1 as a stand-alone specific marker of neuroendocrine differentiation, particularly in poorly differentiated neoplasms.

PRIMARY SITE-SPECIFIC IMMUNOHISTOCHEMISTRY: CDX2, PAX8, PDX1, ISL-1

GI and pancreatic NETs share morphologic features with NETs of other sites. In the setting of liver metastasis, determining the site of origin is important, because it increasingly has implications for treatment and prognosis. If the site of origin cannot be determined from the clinical history, physical examination, and/or radiographic studies, several lineage-specific immunohistochemical markers can be used to investigate the site of origin. Numerous research articles have been published examining the use of lineage-specific markers to assign primary site in the setting of metastatic WDNET to the liver.[48–53]

In many studies, panels that include Thyroid transcription factor 1 (TTF1), Caudal Type Homeobox 2 (CDX2), ISL LIM Homeobox 1 (ISL-1), Pax8, and pancreatic and duodenal homeobox 1 (PDX1), among other markers, can be used to distinguish WDNETs of the lung, gut, and pancreas (see **Fig. 5, Table 4**). In a recent study of 85 WDNETs, Yang and colleagues[50] found that a 3-marker panel of TTF1, CDX2, and ISL1 had sensitivities of 81%, 89%, and 63% and specificities of

Table 4
Site-specific immunohistochemical markers

Site of Primary	Approximate % of Cases Positive (Roughly Similar in Primaries and Metastases)				
	CDX2	PAX8	Isl-1	PDX1	NKX2.2
Jejunoileal	90[a]	Rare	Rare	Rare	92
Pancreatic	20[b]	70	80	55	71
Duodenal	30[b]	80	80	85	100
Gastric	15[b]	15	15	60	17
Rectal	30[b]	60	60	15	100
Appendiceal	90[a]	15	15	40	100
Pulmonary	Rare	Rare	Rare	5	0

Approximate percentage of positive staining abstracted from several sources: Refs.[53–59]
[a] Usually strongly positive.
[b] Usually weak, patchy staining.

100%, 94%, and 100% in separating metastatic NETs into 3 major primary sites: lung, small intestine, and pancreas/rectum. More recently, Yang and colleagues[51] reported in 2018 the addition of NK2 homeobox 2 (NKX2.2) as part of a panel for assessment of primary site. NKX2.2 showed more sensitivity than CDX2 and PDX1 in determining the origin of GI and pancreatic WDNETs in a cohort of 98 tumors.[51]

In some cases, despite a combination clinical investigation and IHC analysis, the primary site of WDNET cannot be determined.[54] In 1 study of 1340 cases, 14% of NENs, including 448 WDNETs and 44 PDNECs, the primary site could not be assigned.[55]

PEPTIDE HORMONE IMMUNOHISTOCHEMISTRY

At present, there is no guideline or requirement to confirm the presence of a hormone using IHC within the tumor in patients with a clinical functional syndrome. Of note, if a patient has a clinically functional syndrome and multiple WDNETs, performing peptide IHC may be useful for determination of metastasis versus second primary tumor.[56]

Peptide hormone expression can also be detected in clinically nonfunctioning tumors, a finding of no clinical significance, and should not be used to suggest a possible diagnosis of a functional syndrome. It has been reported that 40% of WDNETs can express multiple hormones with glucagon (see **Fig. 4**), somatostatin, and pancreatic polypeptides being the most common hormones detected.[57] In some cases, characteristic associations between the hormone expressed and the morphologic features may occur. For example, glucagon-expressing tumors frequently show cystic changes.[58] Somatostatin-positive tumors often show pseudoglandular architecture with numerous psammoma bodies (see **Fig. 4**).[59] Tumors that have serotonin expression tend to have prominent trabecular growth.[60]

SITE-SPECIFIC FEATURES OF WELL-DIFFERENTIATED NEUROENDOCRINE TUMORS

STOMACH (ASSOCIATION WITH AUTOIMMUNE GASTRITIS AND MULTIPLE ENDOCRINE NEOPLASIA SYNDROME/ ZOLLINGER-ELLISON, SPORADIC)

In the stomach, 3 categories of NETs are recognized.[61] Type 1 gastric NETs account for most gastric NETs, up to 80%. Type 1 NETs arise in the setting of autoimmune atrophic gastritis and are more common in women and in older patients.[62,63] In general, if a gastric NET is detected, it is important to assess the background gastric mucosa for the possibility of autoimmune atrophic gastritis as a possible cause, if the diagnosis is not already known.

Type 1 gastric NETs tend to be small, less than 1 cm, and often are multiple (**Fig. 8**). Patients with autoimmune atrophic gastritis develop hypergastrinemia, which results from the autoimmune destruction of parietal cells (see **Fig. 8**) leading to a compensatory stimulation of gastrin-producing G cells in the stomach antrum. Type 1 gastric NETs in these patients are thought to arise from chronic gastrin-mediated stimulation of ECL cells within the atrophic mucosa of the stomach body. Type 1 NETs of the stomach are generally very indolent clinically. In 2 studies examining 167 patients in total, most type 1 gastric NETs were grade 1 and most were stage 1, with no mortality after prolonged follow-up[64,65] In 1 study, more than half (55.6%) had multifocal NETs.[65] Metastatic disease in type 1 gastric NETs occurs in a small percentage of patients; however, the overall prognosis remains favorable. In a study of 20 patients with type 1 gastric NETs who had metastasis with an average Ki-67 index of 6.8%, either to lymph nodes or liver, all 20 patients remained alive during the 83-month mean follow-up period.[66] Given the indolent and multifocal disease process in patients with type 1 gastric NETs, the utility of the Ki-67 proliferative rate (or rates if multiple tumors are detected) remains unclear and seems to have limited clinical value compared with other

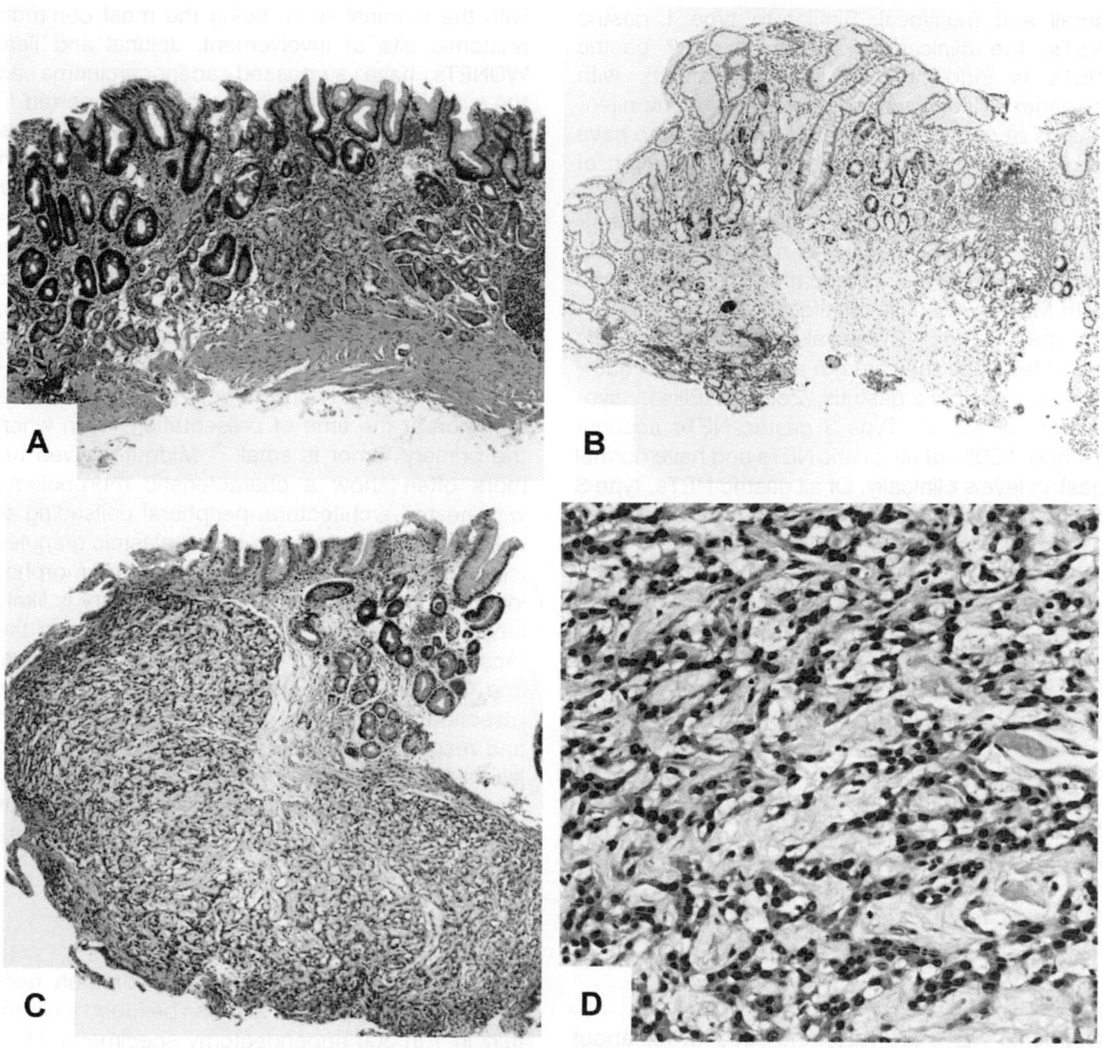

Fig. 8. Gastric NET arising in the setting of autoimmune atrophic gastritis. (*A*) Low-power view of gastric body with complete oxyntic gland atrophy, lymphoplasmacytic infiltrate within the lamina propria, and focal intestinal metaplasia (H&E, original magnification ×10). (*B*) Chromogranin immunohistochemical stain highlights enterochromaffin cell hyperplasia of the atrophic gastric body (original magnification ×10). (*C*) Gastric body with WDNETs, measuring approximately 2 mm in a background of atrophic gastric mucosa (H&E, original magnification ×10). (*D*) High-power view of WDNET with cordlike pattern and myxoid stroma (H&E, original magnification ×40).

gut NET sites and clinical contexts. In general, patients with type 1 NETs of the stomach can be managed with endoscopic removal of visible lesions.[65] Some patients benefit from long-acting somatostatin analogues.[64] Antrectomy, to remove the gastrin-containing portion of the stomach, can also be considered in certain cases.[67]

Type 2 gastric NETs occur in the setting of Zollinger-Ellison syndrome, some of which may be associated with MEN1. Type 2 gastric NETs account for 5% or less of all gastric NETs.[68] Zollinger-Ellison syndrome is characterized by duodenal or pancreatic NETs that produce gastrin (ie, gastrinomas). Patients with MEN1 syndrome typically have small duodenal gastrinomas, whereas patients with sporadic gastrinomas tend to have larger tumors within the pancreas.[69] As a result, patients with Zollinger-Ellison have hypergastrinemia and develop severe peptic ulcer disease. Similar to type 1 gastric NETs, chronic gastrin overexpression leading to stimulation of ECL cells is thought to enable the growth of gastric NETs in patients with gastrinomas. However, the background stomach mucosa in these patients does not show atrophy or other features of autoimmune gastritis. Type 2 gastric NETs tend to be small and multifocal. Similar to type 1 gastric NETs, the clinical behavior of type 2 gastric NETs is indolent. The goal in patients with Zollinger-Ellison syndrome is to treat the manifestations of peptic ulcer disease. Patients who have sporadic gastrinoma leading to the formation of type 2 gastric NETs, without metastatic disease, should be offered surgical resection of the gastrinoma, which is curative in most patients.[70] In contrast, surgery is not recommended for patients with MEN1 who have multifocal gastrinomas.

Type 3 gastric NETs are also known as sporadic NETs because they are not associated with autoimmune atrophic gastritis, Zollinger-Ellison syndrome, or MEN1. Type 3 gastric NETs account for about 20% of all gastric NETs and have normal gastrin levels clinically. Of all gastric NETs, type 3 NETs have the most aggressive clinical course, with metastasis in up to 65% of patients.[68,71]

INTESTINAL

The incidence of small bowel NETs is increasing, in part because of increased accessibility of endoscopy and imaging.[72] Small bowel WDNETs are the most common WDNETs of the GI tract.[73] In contrast with foregut and hindgut WDNETs, in which adenocarcinoma is more common than NENs, in the small bowel/midgut, WDNETs are more common than adenocarcinoma of this site.[74] In addition, distal small bowel NETs within 60 cm of the ileocecal valve are more common than those arising in the duodenum.

Duodenum and Ampulla of Vater

Duodenal NETs are rare, and account for about 11% of small bowel NETs. Typically, duodenal NETs are found in the first or second portion of the duodenum, with about 20% occurring near the ampulla of Vater. Most duodenal NETs are nonfunctioning and incidentally detected. Duodenal gastrinomas are the most common and are either sporadic or associated with MEN1 syndrome. Somatostatin-producing tumors account for about 15% of duodenal NETs and these are almost exclusively located near the ampulla of Vater. There is an association with NF1 in 20% to 30% of somatostatin-producing duodenal tumors.[18] Ampullary WDNETs are very rare and may be associated with biliary obstruction. Ampullary WDNETs also have a higher likelihood of lymph node metastases than other duodenal sites.[75]

Jejunum and Ileum

Jejunal and ileal NETs account for almost 50% of all gut WDNETs and most small bowel WDNETs, with the terminal ileum being the most common anatomic site of involvement. Jejunal and ileal WDNETs have surpassed adenocarcinoma as the most common small bowel tumors reported.[74] Almost one-third of jejunal and ileal NETs are multifocal, with 2 or more tumors detected in 25% of patients at the time of diagnosis.[72] Liver metastasis at the time of presentation is also common.[76,77] Clinical presentation is variable, with abdominal pain being most common. Abdominal pain has been attributed to intussusception, obstruction/mass effect, or mesenteric ischemia caused by bulky mesenteric adenopathy. Metastases to regional lymph nodes or to the liver are common at the time of presentation, even when the primary tumor is small.[76] Midgut-derived tumors often show a characteristic morphology, with nested architecture, peripheral palisading of cells, and bright eosinophilic cytoplasmic granules (see **Fig. 3**). If a tumor metastasis has this morphologic pattern, it suggests that the primary is likely located in the small bowel, with ileum being the most common site of origin. Patients with jejunal and ileal WDNETs should be offered surgical resection, with careful attention to identification and resection of multifocal disease. Prognosis in jejunal/ileal WDNETs depends on the stage. With distant metastases, the 5-year survival rate ranges from 40% to 85%, and 10-year survival rates are 40% to 60%.[78,79]

APPENDIX

Appendiceal NETs are the most common neoplasms of the appendix, and can be found incidentally in 1 in 300 appendectomy specimens. Most appendiceal NETs are submucosal and most are found in the appendiceal tip (see **Fig. 2**). However, 10% of appendiceal NETs are found at the base, where tumors can cause obstruction and appendicitis. Typically, appendiceal WDNETs have a good prognosis.[80] Lymph node metastases occur infrequently and, even when present, 10-year survival approaches 100%.[81–83] Tumor size is the most established prognostic factor, but, in recent years, mesoappendiceal invasion, tumor grade, and lymphovascular invasion have also been implicated as risk factor in predicting higher risk of metastasis. In general, follow-up of tumors that are less than 2 cm is not needed and appendectomy alone is curative. Right hemicolectomy can be considered for tumors greater than 2 cm or for tumors 1 to 2 cm if other risk factors are present.[84]

Of note, a rare tumor of the appendix, commonly referred to as goblet cell carcinoid, is not considered to be part of the GI NET tumors, despite the term carcinoid in its name. Goblet cell carcinoid is a unique malignant tumor with a clinical behavior and prognosis closer to those of adenocarcinoma rather than NETs. Goblet cell carcinoids are often associated with a signet ring cell carcinoma or adenocarcinoma, which is not a feature of typical NETs.[85,86] Patient outcome studies support renaming and reclassifying goblet cell carcinoid as goblet cell adenocarcinoma.[87,88]

COLON

Primary colonic WDNETs are rare and include midgut tumors of the right colon (cecum and ascending colon) and hindgut tumors of the left colon (transverse, descending, and sigmoid colon). Most patients with colonic WDNETs present with advanced disease and many of these patients present with metastasis, with outcomes similar to the jejunal/ileal WDNETs.[89]

RECTUM

Rectal WDNETs are the second most common WDNETs of the GI tract, after small bowel WDNETs.[73] Rectal WDNETs are almost always asymptomatic and are detected during colonoscopy that is performed for other reasons. Because of this association, most rectal WDNETs are detected in patients greater than 50 years of age and most rectal NETs are also localized at the time of diagnosis.[90] They are solitary and often have a polypoid subepithelial appearance endoscopically. The color of the lesion is frequently described as yellow, and this feature can cause WDNETs to be confused for lipomas.

The prognosis of rectal WDNETs is correlated with tumor size, depth of invasion, lymphovascular invasion, and mitotic rate.[91] Tumors that are smaller than 1 cm, have no muscularis propria involvement or lymphovascular invasion, and have mitotic indices less than 2 per 10 HPF show metastatic disease in less than 2% of patients. In contrast, rectal WDNETs greater than 2 cm have 50% to 80% risk of metastatic disease.[92,93] Tumors between 1 and 1.9 cm have an intermediate risk of metastases. Surgical options for rectal WDNETs include local excision (including polypectomy or endoscopic mucosal resection), as well as surgical resection (including low anterior resection and abdominoperineal resection).[94]

GALLBLADDER, BILIARY TRACT, AND LIVER

Primary WDNETs of the biliary tract (including gallbladder) and liver are very rare. Metastasis from elsewhere in the GI tract should be considered before making a diagnosis of primary WDNET in one of these sites. Gallbladder and biliary tree WDNETs probably represent less than 1% of all GI WDNETs.[95] Making a diagnosis of primary liver WDNET is also difficult, because metastatic disease to the liver is much more common. Immunohistochemical staining may be helpful in diagnosing metastatic disease (discussed earlier). However, the definitive distinction between primary versus metastatic disease at these sites requires careful correlation with the clinical and radiologic findings, if immunohistochemical stains prove unhelpful.[96] When considering neuroendocrine neoplasm of any grade that involves the biliary tree or gallbladder, PDNECs are more frequent than WDNETs.[97]

PANCREAS

Pancreatic NETs are generally slow-growing tumors that affect both genders equally and can occur over a wide age range. They are the second most common tumor of the pancreas after ductal adenocarcinoma and account for about 3% of all pancreatic neoplasms. Two-thirds of pancreatic NETs arise in the head of the pancreas, whereas the remainder are in the body and tail. Most WDNETs of the pancreas are sporadic, and approximately 10% of pancreatic tumors are associated with a hereditary syndrome, MEN1 being most common.[98] It is reported that nonfunctioning WDNETs account most, 60% to 90% depending on the study, of all pancreatic WDNETs.[99] Although most of the tumors are clinically nonfunctioning, any pancreatic NET may secrete peptides, hormones, or biogenic substances such as pancreatic polypeptide or chromogranin, which can be detected and measured in the serum or by immunohistochemical stains, but at levels too low for syndromic clinical effects. Nonfunctioning tumors present at more advanced stages, thought to occur because of the slow-growing nature of tumors and lack of associated symptoms to trigger a diagnostic work-up, such as is also the case for tumors in the tail of the pancreas. However, nonfunctioning tumors in the head of the pancreas may present with obstruction of the bile duct and cause associated biliary symptoms, thereby leading to earlier detection. Involvement of the bile duct is also associated with serotonin-secreting tumors.[50] Overall, there is an increase in the detection of pancreatic WDNETs caused by the increasing use of abdominal imaging techniques.[100]

Grossly, tumors are well circumscribed, white to yellow, with well-delineated borders. Occasionally, tumors are cystic or show central degeneration (see **Fig. 2**). Tumors less than 5 mm, if nonfunctioning and not associated with a syndrome, are called neuroendocrine microadenomas and are benign. Microadenomas can be identified on macroscopic or microscopic examination. Autopsy series suggest that the prevalence of microadenomas is 1% to 10% of the population.[101] The presence of multiple pancreatic microadenomas, referred to microadenomatosis, is associated with MEN1 syndrome.[56]

Microscopically, pancreatic WDNETs have features similar to WDNETs of other sites, although the range in morphology is more varied than that seen for ileal WDNETs. Rare morphologic variants of WDNETs include clear cell, oncocytic, or pleomorphic. Clear cell variants of WDNETs are particularly associated with VHL syndrome. Oncocytic WDNETs have abundant granular eosinophilic cytoplasm, a feature reminiscent of hepatocellular carcinoma, which can lead to a challenging differential diagnosis when evaluating liver metastases. Some studies have found that oncocytic WDNETs have a more aggressive behavior. For example, in 1 study of 11 patients with oncocytic nonfunctioning WDNETs, nearly 50% of patients had liver or lymph node metastasis at the time of diagnosis.[102] Pleomorphism in pancreatic WDNETs, characterized by bizarre large nuclei in more than 20% of cells, does not seem to affect clinical behavior, but can lead to a mistaken diagnosis of ductal adenocarcinoma (see **Fig. 3**).[103] Immunohistochemical staining, as well as Ki-67 assessment, can help in this differential diagnosis. Serotonin-producing tumors are associated with a prominent trabecular architecture and stromal fibrosis.[50]

The eighth edition of the AJCC manual now features a separate section for the staging of WDNETs of the pancreas, different from the staging protocols for ductal adenocarcinoma and PDNECs.[33] WHO grade classification is performed based on mitotic count and Ki-67 proliferative index, as for other WDNETs. In 2017, the WHO updated classification of pancreatic WDNETs to include grade 3 WDNETs, distinguishing them from PDNECs. Studies estimate that G3 WDNETs comprise around 10% of all pancreatic NENs and have Ki-67 proliferative indices in the range of 20% to 50%.[28,99] The clinical behavior of G3 WDNETs of the pancreas is more aggressive than grade 1 and 2 WDNETs, but not as aggressive as PDNECs.[37,104] Overall survival in pancreatic WDNETs is 33% at 5 years, 17% at 10 years, and 10% at 20 years.[105] Of the functioning tumors, insulin-secreting WDNETs have the best prognosis, whereas tumors producing gastrin, glucagon, or somatostatin behave more aggressively.[106] The main prognostic markers for nonfunctioning tumors are similar to those of other WDNETs, and include tumor stage, size, lymphovascular invasion, and mitotic rate/Ki-67 proliferative index. Surgical resection improves patient survival. Techniques and extent of resection vary depending on the anatomic location of the tumor. In certain clinical circumstances, nonoperative management may be appropriate when high-quality imaging indicates minimal growth and no suspicious features of metastasis.[100] More recently, everolimus, an oral inhibitor targeting the mammalian target of rapamycin (mTor) pathway, has been approved for and shown efficacy in the treatment of advanced pancreatic WDNETs.[107,108]

POORLY DIFFERENTIATED NEUROENDOCRINE CARCINOMA OF THE GASTROINTESTINAL TRACT AND PANCREAS

The WHO recognizes 2 general types of PDNEC: small cell carcinoma and large cell carcinoma. These 2 categories show a morphology, clinical behavior, and chemotherapy responsiveness that is similar to the lung NEC counterparts.[109] After exclusion of lung small cell carcinoma, the GI tract and pancreas are the most common sites of PDNEC, although overall these carcinomas are rare.[110] The incidence of PDNEC is difficult to establish because of the rarity of the tumor. In a study based on a Norwegian population, the incidence of high-grade pancreatic PDNEC was 0.4 per 100,000,[111] and colorectal PDNEC was 0.2 per 100,000 in a US population.[112] The most common sites of PDNEC within the GI tract are esophagus, stomach, pancreas, and colon/rectum.[113] Large cell NEC of the GI tract accounts for about 60% of the cases. Patient clinical presentation is highly variable depending on the primary site of the PDNEC. Metastatic disease is common at the time of presentation. PDNECs are nonsecretory tumors and are not associated with a functional or hereditary syndrome.

POORLY DIFFERENTIATED NEUROENDOCRINE CARCINOMA: MICROSCOPIC FEATURES AND IMMUNOHISTOCHEMISTRY FINDINGS

Poorly differentiated NECs are typically classified as large cell NEC or small cell carcinoma, similar to the lung high-grade NECs. The tumor growth pattern tends to be sheetlike or diffuse in architecture, with rare areas of rosetting, trabeculae, or nesting. PDNEC tumors cells are small to large, depending on the subtype. Small cell–type PDNEC tumor cells have scant cytoplasm with high nuclear/cytoplasmic ratio, fine chromatin, inconspicuous nucleoli, and nuclear molding (see **Fig. 6**). Large cell–type PDNEC tumor cells are polygonal, with moderate amounts of cytoplasm, prominent nucleoli, and coarse chromatin (see **Fig. 6**). Mitoses are readily appreciated, as well as single cell apoptosis. Tumor necrosis is also common and can be extensive. The stromal reaction tends to be sparse. In the colon, a surface adenomatous component can be present.[114]

Immunohistochemical confirmation of neuroendocrine differentiation in PDNEC is an important diagnostic step. Synaptophysin is positive in nearly all cases. However, the intensity and extent of staining can vary. Chromogranin can be scant or even negative in some cases of PDNEC. Although CD56 is not a specific neuroendocrine marker, in combination with synaptophysin, it can contribute to the recognition of PDNECs. Site-specific markers, such as TTF1, CDX2, and ISL1, are not helpful, because these can be expressed in PDNECs of any site.[38,115] Although, by definition, the Ki-67 index in PDNEC is greater than 20%, in most cases the index is greater than 50%.[38]

POORLY DIFFERENTIATED NEUROENDOCRINE CARCINOMA: DIFFERENTIAL DIAGNOSIS

The differential diagnosis of PDNEC can be challenging and varies depending on the anatomic site of involvement. The main differential diagnosis in the pancreas is acinar cell carcinoma. Acinar cell carcinoma is a solid and cellular tumor of the pancreas characterized by large neoplastic cells arranged in acinar, cribriform, or solid growth patterns. Immunostains of acinar cell differentiation, including trypsin, chymotrypsin, BCL10, and beta-catenin (nuclear), can help with this differential.[37] The Ki-67 proliferative index of acinar cell carcinoma is typically lower than in PDNEC. Other possible differential diagnoses in the pancreas include solid pseudopapillary neoplasm, pancreatoblastoma, and solid variants of ductal adenocarcinoma. Use of additional markers, such as vimentin, keratins, and alpha fetoprotein, may be helpful in characterizing the tumor differentiation. Medullary carcinoma and poorly differentiated adenocarcinoma are the main differential diagnostic considerations in the GI tract. It is best to use a combination of immunohistochemical markers and a high index of suspicion when considering the possible diagnosis of PDNEC or possible differential diagnoses. In difficult cases, molecular analysis is emerging as an adjunct diagnostic aid.

MANEC is very rare category of mixed carcinomas; the MANEC abbreviation has been used to refer to both mixed acinar-NEC of the pancreas and mixed adenocarcinoma-NEC of the colon or stomach (**Fig. 9**).[116] In general, greater than 30% of each component has been used for the diagnosis of MANEC. In the most recent 2017 WHO Classification of Tumours of Endocrine Organs, the category of mixed neuroendocrine-nonneuroendocrine neoplasm (MiNEN) was introduced as an alternative term for MANEC, to reflect that both ductal and acinar carcinomas can be seen in combination with either WDNET or PDNEC in the pancreas. The presence of scattered neuroendocrine cells within an otherwise typical adenocarcinoma is seen in up to 40% of cases and is not sufficient for a diagnosis of a mixed tumor.[117]

POORLY DIFFERENTIATED NEUROENDOCRINE CARCINOMA: PROGNOSIS AND TREATMENT

PDNETs have an aggressive clinical course, with frequent early distant metastases. Median survival is less than 1 year, and 5-year survival rates in the single digits.[118] There does not seem to be a difference between the large and small cell types of NEC and prognosis. Chemotherapy is the treatment of choice in unresectable or metastatic PDNECs, usually in combination with platinum-containing compounds.[38,119] Combination BRAF-MEK targeted therapy has been suggested as a novel therapeutic approach and is under investigation in patients with advanced PDNECs.[120]

MOLECULAR CHARACTERISTICS OF NEUROENDOCRINE TUMORS AND NEUROENDOCRINE CARCINOMAS

Although WDNETs and PDNECs share neuroendocrine differentiation and some histologic features, these 2 groups seem to have distinct histogenic and molecular characteristics (**Table 5**). The difference between the molecular features of WDNETs and PDNECs has been best characterized in the pancreas. In a landmark study by Jiao and colleagues[121] in 2011, the investigators examined the exomic sequence of 18,000 protein coding genes in a set of 10 well-characterized pancreatic WDNETs. Specifically, pancreatic WDNETs showed inactivation of the tumor suppressor gene MEN1 in 45% of cases or mutations of DAXX or ATRX in 45% of pancreatic NETs. In a smaller percentage of pancreatic WDNETs, genes in the mTOR pathway (PTEN, PIK3CA, TSC2) are mutated. A later study by Scarpa and colleagues[122] expanded on the molecular features in pancreatic WDNETs by examining whole-exome sequencing of 102 clinically sporadic

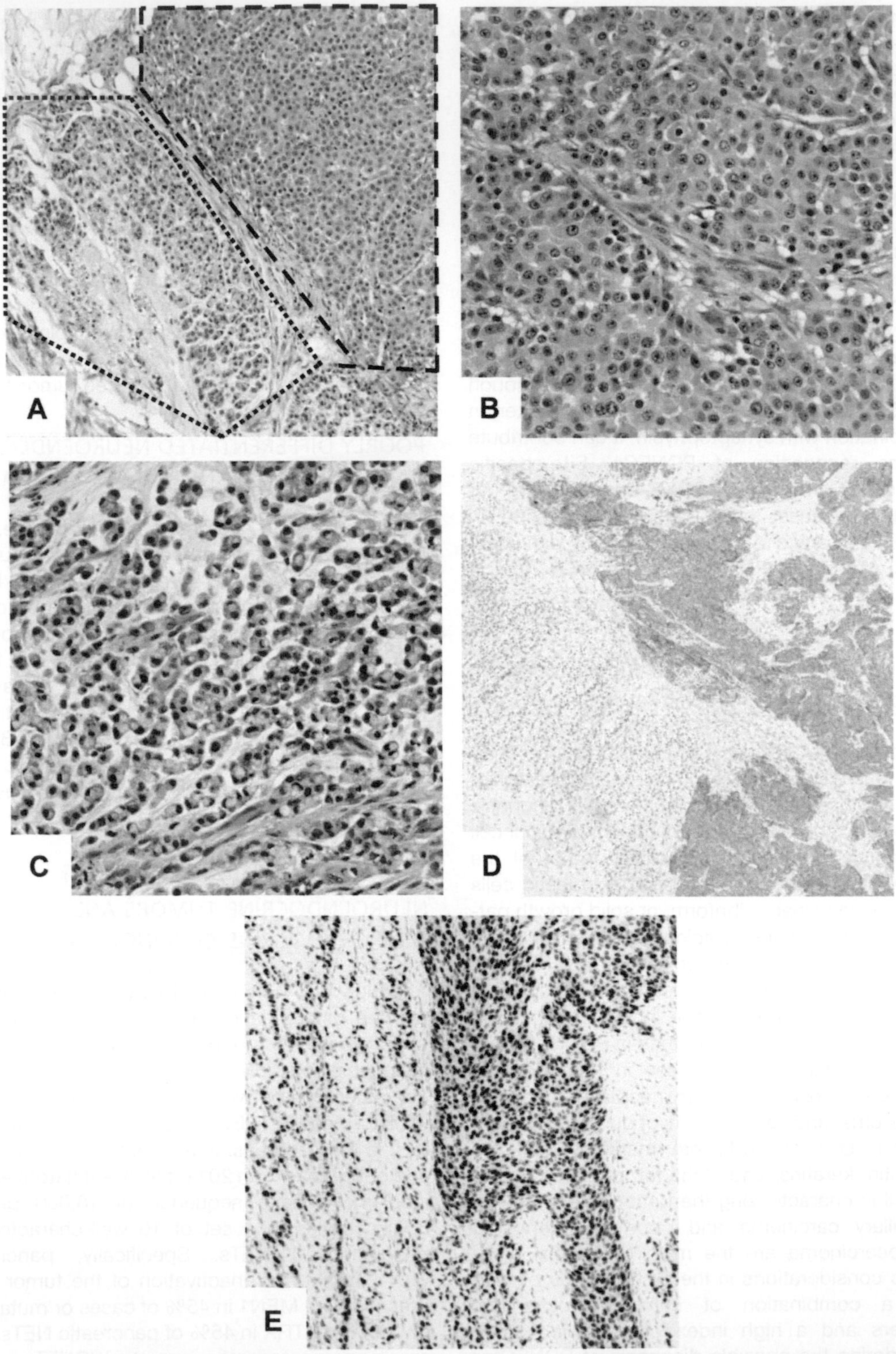

Fig. 9. Histologic features of MANEC. (*A*) Colon resection with MANEC. The left lower quadrant (*dotted line*) is composed of signet ring cell adenocarcinoma and the right upper quadrant (*dashed line*) is composed of a PDNEC (H&E, original magnification ×20). (*B*) PDNEC with sheetlike growth, and greater than 20% Ki-67 (*E*) (H&E, original magnification ×40). (*C*) Signet ring cell adenocarcinoma in (*E*) (H&E, original magnification ×40). (*D*) Synaptophysin immunostain highlighting PDNEC in the right upper corner (original magnification ×20). (*E*) Ki-67 immunostain showing a proliferation index of 90% in both the poorly differentiated adenocarcinoma and PDNEC (original magnification ×40).

Table 5
Key immunohistochemical and molecular features of gastroenteric and pancreatic neuroendocrine neoplasm

	WDNET	Small Cell/Large Cell NECs
Immunohistochemical Characteristics		
Endocrine Differentiation	• Synaptophysin and chromogranin (strong, diffuse)	• Synaptophysin, variable intensity • Variable to absent chromogranin • CD56
Site Specific	• Helpful to determine site of origin; see **Table 4** for details	• Not useful
Hormones	• Variable expression	• Not useful
Molecular Changes (Point Mutations, Deletions, Insertions)		
Genes	• DAXX/ATRX • Inactivation of MEN1 • mTOR pathway alterations (including TSC2, PTEN, PIK3CA)	• TP53 • RB1 • CDKN2A

tumors. The investigators found DNA damage repair defects in a subset of tumors, including mutations of MUTYH, CHEK2, and BRCA2.

The most frequent molecular alteration found in PDNEC involves the p53 gene. Mutations of p53 were observed in 50% to 100% of cases.[123] Other commonly found alterations in PDNEC include mutations of KRAS, p16, Rb1, and cyclin D1.[124] Microsatellite instability (MSI) can be detected in PDNECs, and in many cases MSI is associated with MANEC. In 1 study of 89 patients with PDNEC and/or MANEC, MSI was observed in 12.4% of cases, including 7 intestinal and 4 gastric tumors.[125] Most of these cases had MLH1 methylation. BRAF V600E mutations have also been detected in a minority of PDNEC cases.[126] Importantly, Klempner and colleagues[120] reported 2 patients with BRAF-mutated PDNEC who showed rapid and durable response to BRAF-MEK inhibition.

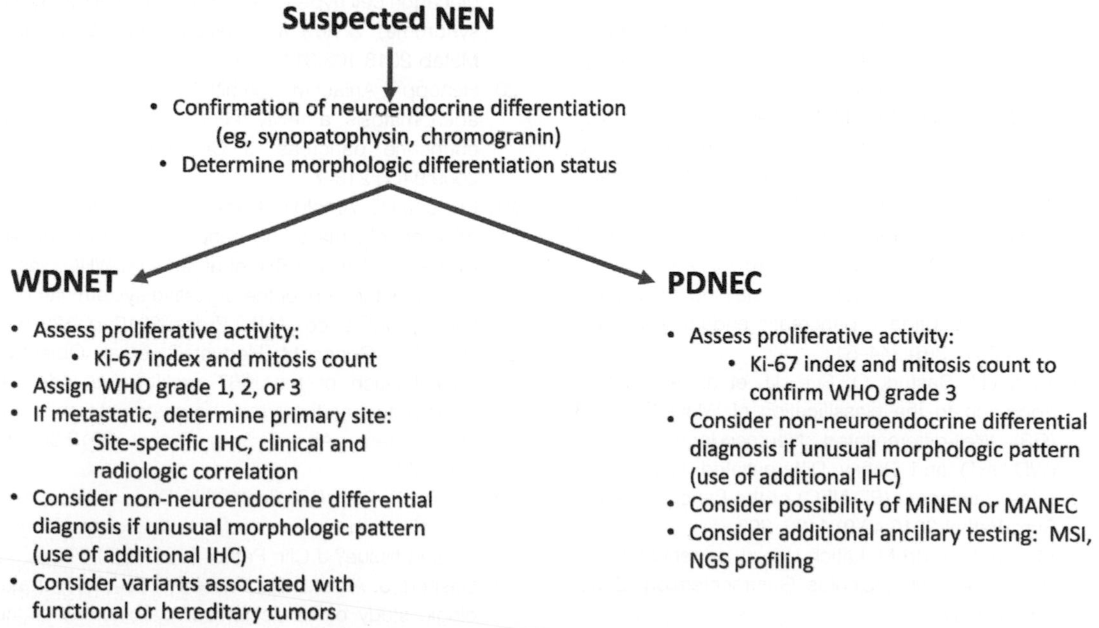
Suspected NEN
• Confirmation of neuroendocrine differentiation (eg, synopatophysin, chromogranin)
• Determine morphologic differentiation status
WDNET
• Assess proliferative activity:
• Ki-67 index and mitosis count
• Assign WHO grade 1, 2, or 3
• If metastatic, determine primary site:
• Site-specific IHC, clinical and radiologic correlation
• Consider non-neuroendocrine differential diagnosis if unusual morphologic pattern (use of additional IHC)
• Consider variants associated with functional or hereditary tumors
PDNEC
• Assess proliferative activity:
• Ki-67 index and mitosis count to confirm WHO grade 3
• Consider non-neuroendocrine differential diagnosis if unusual morphologic pattern (use of additional IHC)
• Consider possibility of MiNEN or MANEC
• Consider additional ancillary testing: MSI, NGS profiling

Fig. 10. Diagnostic algorithm to approach neuroendocrine tumors based on histology and degree of differentiation. NGS, next-generation sequencing.

SUMMARY

NENs of the GI tract and pancreas comprise 2 broad groups: WDNETs and PDNECs. The diagnostic algorithm begins with confirmation of neuroendocrine differentiation and determination of degree of histologic differentiation to differentiate these 2 groups (Fig. 10). The Ki-67 proliferative index is endorsed widely to grade WDNETs and PDNECs according to WHO criteria. These 2 categories of tumors have different morphologic, immunophenotypic, molecular, and clinical features. The prognosis of WDNETs varies widely depending on the organ of origin, functional status, hereditary association, AJCC tumor stage, and WHO proliferative grading, whereas PDNECs uniformly have a poor prognosis.

REFERENCES

1. Maggard MA, O'Connell JB, Ko CY. Updated population-based review of carcinoid tumors. Ann Surg 2004;240(1):117–22.
2. Fesinmeyer MD, Austin MA, Li CI, et al. Differences in survival by histologic type of pancreatic cancer. Cancer Epidemiol Biomarkers Prev 2005;14(7):1766–73.
3. Mocellin S, Nitti D. Gastrointestinal carcinoid: epidemiological and survival evidence from a large population-based study (n = 25 531). Ann Oncol 2013;24(12):3040–4.
4. Rehfeld JF. The new biology of gastrointestinal hormones. Physiol Rev 1998;78(4):1087–108.
5. Pearse AG. The cytochemistry and ultrastructure of polypeptide hormone-producing cells of the APUD series and the embryologic, physiologic and pathologic implications of the concept. J Histochem Cytochem 1969;17(5):303–13.
6. Wiedenmann B, John M, Riecken E-O, et al. Molecular and cell biological aspects of neuroendocrine tumors of the gastroenteropancreatic system. J Mol Med (Berl) 1998;76(9):637–47.
7. Callacondo D, Arenas JL, Ganoza AJ, et al. Giant insulinoma. Pancreas 2013;42(8):1323–32.
8. Tomita T. Immunocytochemical staining for islet amyloid polypeptide in pancreatic endocrine tumors. Islets 2011;3(6):344–51.
9. Tang LH, Basturk O, Sue JJ, et al. A practical approach to the classification of WHO Grade 3 (G3) Well-differentiated Neuroendocrine Tumor (WD-NET) and Poorly Differentiated Neuroendocrine Carcinoma (PD-NEC) of the Pancreas. Am J Surg Pathol 2016;40(9):1192–202.
10. Modlin IM, Kidd M, Latich I, et al. current status of gastrointestinal carcinoids. Gastroenterology 2005;128(6):1717–51.
11. Peltola E, Hannula P, Huhtala H, et al. Characteristics and outcomes of 79 patients with an insulinoma: a nationwide retrospective study in Finland. Int J Endocrinol 2018;2018(Sd 16):1–10.
12. Jensen RT, Berna MJ, Bingham DB, et al. Inherited pancreatic endocrine tumor syndromes: advances in molecular pathogenesis, diagnosis, management, and controversies. Cancer 2008;113(7 Suppl):1807–43.
13. Gumbs AA, Moore PS, Falconi M, et al. Review of the clinical, histological, and molecular aspects of pancreatic endocrine neoplasms. J Surg Oncol 2002;81(1):45–53.
14. Blansfield JA, Choyke L, Morita SY, et al. Clinical, genetic and radiographic analysis of 108 patients with von Hippel-Lindau disease (VHL) manifested by pancreatic neuroendocrine neoplasms (PNETs). Surgery 2007;142(6):814–8, [discussion: 818.e1-2].
15. Richard S, Gardie B, Couvé S, et al. Von Hippel-Lindau: how a rare disease illuminates cancer biology. Semin Cancer Biol 2013;23:26–37.
16. Gucer H, Szentgyorgyi E, Ezzat S, et al. Inhibin-expressing clear cell neuroendocrine tumor of the ampulla: an unusual presentation of von Hippel-Lindau disease. Virchows Arch 2013;463(4):593–7.
17. Fellows IW, Leach IH, Smith PG, et al. Carcinoid tumour of the common bile duct-a novel complication of von Hippel-Lindau syndrome. Gut 1990;31:728–9.
18. Relles D, Baek J, Witkiewicz A, et al. Periampullary and duodenal neoplasms in neurofibromatosis type 1: two cases and an updated 20-year review of the literature yielding 76 cases. J Gastrointest Surg 2010;14(6):1052–61.
19. Gild ML, Tsang V, Samra J, et al. Hypercalcemia in glucagon cell hyperplasia and neoplasia (Mahvash syndrome): a new association. J Clin Endocrinol Metab 2018;103:3119–23.
20. Henopp T, Anlauf M, Schmitt A, et al. Glucagon cell adenomatosis: a newly recognized disease of the endocrine pancreas. J Clin Endocrinol Metab 2009;94(1):213–7.
21. Klimstra DS, Arnold R, Capella C, et al. Neuroendocrine neoplasms of the pancreas. In: Bosman TF, Carneiro F, Hruban RH, et al, editors. WHO classification of tumours of the digestive system. 4th edition. Lyon (France): IARC Press; 2010. p. 322–6.
22. Tang LH, Gonen M, Hedvat C, et al. Objective quantification of the Ki67 proliferative index in neuroendocrine tumors of the gastroenteropancreatic system. Am J Surg Pathol 2012;36(12):1761–70.
23. Cross SS, Start RD, Smith JHF. Does delay in fixation affect the number of mitotic figures in processed tissue? J Clin Pathol 1990;43(7):597–9.
24. Casnedi S, Albarello L, Sessa F, et al. Clinicopathologic study of 62 acinar cell carcinomas of the pancreas. Am J Surg Pathol 2012;36(12):1782–95.

25. Voss SM, Riley MP, Lokhandwala PM, et al. Mitotic count by phosphohistone h3 immunohistochemical staining predicts survival and improves interobserver reproducibility in well-differentiated neuroendocrine tumors of the pancreas. Am J Surg Pathol 2015;39(1):13–24.
26. Yang Z, Tang LH, Klimstra DS. Gastroenteropancreatic neuroendocrine neoplasms: historical context and current issues. Semin Diagn Pathol 2013;30(3):186–96.
27. Rindi G, Arnold R, Bosman FT, et al. Nomenclature and classification of neuroendocrine neoplasms of the digestive system. In: Bosman TF, Carneiro F, Hruban RH, et al, editors. WHO classification of tumours of the digestive system. 4th edition. Lyon (France): IARC Press; 2010. p. 13–4.
28. Matsukuma K, Olson KA, Gui D, et al. Synaptophysin-Ki67 double stain: a novel technique that improves interobserver agreement in the grading of well-differentiated gastrointestinal neuroendocrine tumors. Mod Pathol 2017;30:620–9.
29. Yang Z, Tang LH, Klimstra DS. Effect of tumor heterogeneity on the assessment of Ki67 labeling index in well-differentiated neuroendocrine tumors metastatic to the liver. Am J Surg Pathol 2011; 35(6):853–60.
30. Couvelard A, Deschamps L, Ravaud P, et al. Heterogeneity of tumor prognostic markers: a reproducibility study applied to liver metastases of pancreatic endocrine tumors. Mod Pathol 2009;22:273–81.
31. Coriat R, Walter T, Beno B, et al. Gastroentero pancreatic well-differentiated grade 3 neuroendocrine tumors: review and position statement. Oncologist 2016;21(10):1191–9.
32. Klopperl G, Couvelard A, Hruban RH, et al. WHO classification of neoplasms of the neuroendocrine pancreas. In: Lloyd RV, Osamura RY, Kloppel G, et al, editors. WHO classification of tumours of endocrine organs. 4th edition. Lyon (France): IARC Press; 2017. p. 209–14.
33. Heetfeld M, Chougnet CN, Olsen IH, et al. Characteristics and treatment of patients with G3 gastroenteropancreatic neuroendocrine neoplasms. Endocr Relat Cancer 2015;22(4):657–64.
34. Sigel CS, Krauss Silva VW, Reid MD, et al. Well differentiated grade 3 pancreatic neuroendocrine tumors compared with related neoplasms: a morphologic study. Cancer Cytopathol 2018; 126(5):326–35.
35. Dasari A, Shen C, Halperin D, et al. Trends in the incidence, prevalence, and survival outcomes in patients with neuroendocrine tumors in the United States. JAMA Oncol 2017;3(10):1335–42.
36. Leoncini E, Boffetta P, Shafir M, et al. Increased incidence trend of low-grade and high-grade neuroendocrine neoplasms. Endocrine 2017; 58(2):368–79.
37. Basturk O, Yang Z, Tang LH, et al. The high-grade (WHO G3) pancreatic neuroendocrine tumor category is morphologically and biologically heterogenous and includes both well differentiated and poorly differentiated neoplasms. Am J Surg Pathol 2015;39(5):683–90.
38. Sorbye H, Welin S, Langer SW, et al. Predictive and prognostic factors for treatment and survival in 305 patients with advanced gastrointestinal neuroendocrine carcinoma (WHO G3): the NORDIC NEC study. Ann Oncol 2013;24(1):152–60.
39. Amin MB, Edge S, Greene F, et al, editors. AJCC cancer staging manual. 8th edition. AG Switzerland: Springer International Publishing; 2017.
40. Lloyd RV, Mervak T, Schmidt K, et al. Immunohistochemical detection of chromogranin and neuron-specific enolase in pancreatic endocrine neoplasms. Am J Surg Pathol 1984;8(8):607–14.
41. Shi C, Klimstra DS. Pancreatic neuroendocrine tumors: pathologic and molecular characteristics. Semin Diagn Pathol 2014;31(6):498–511.
42. Rosenbaum JN, Guo Z, Baus RM, et al. INSM1: a novel immunohistochemical and molecular marker for neuroendocrine and neuroepithelial neoplasms. Am J Clin Pathol 2015;144:579–91.
43. Rooper LM, Sharma R, Li QK, et al. INSM1 demonstrates superior performance to the individual and combined use of synaptophysin, chromogranin and CD56 for diagnosing neuroendocrine tumors of the thoracic cavity. Am J Surg Pathol 2017;41(11):1561–9.
44. Mukhopadhyay S, Dermawan JK, Lanigan CP, et al. Insulinoma-associated protein 1 (INSM1) is a sensitive and highly specific marker of neuroendocrine differentiation in primary lung neoplasms: an immunohistochemical study of 345 cases, including 292 whole-tissue sections. Mod Pathol 2019;32(1): 100–9.
45. Tanigawa M, Nakayama M, Taira T, et al. Insulinoma-associated protein 1 (INSM1) is a useful marker for pancreatic neuroendocrine tumor. Med Mol Morphol 2018;51(1):32–40.
46. Rooper LM, Bishop JA, Westra WH. INSM1 is a sensitive and specific marker of neuroendocrine differentiation in head and neck tumors. Am J Surg Pathol 2018;42(5):665–71.
47. Rush PS, Rosenbaum JN, Roy M, et al. Insulinoma-associated 1: a novel nuclear marker in Merkel cell carcinoma (cutaneous neuroendocrine carcinoma). J Cutan Pathol 2018;45(2):129–35.
48. Chan ES, Alexander J, Swanson PE, et al. PDX-1, CDX-2, TTF-1, and CK7. Am J Surg Pathol 2012; 36(5):737–43.
49. Srivastava A, Hornick JL. Immunohistochemical staining for CDX-2, PDX-1, NESP-55, and TTF-1 can help distinguish gastrointestinal carcinoid tumors from pancreatic endocrine and pulmonary carcinoid tumors. Am J Surg Pathol 2009;33(4):626–32.

50. Yang Z, Klimstra DS, Hruban RH, et al. Immunohistochemical characterization of the origins of metastatic well-differentiated neuroendocrine tumors to the liver. Am J Surg Pathol 2017;41(7):915–22.
51. Yang MX, Coates RF, Ambaye A, et al. NKX2.2, PDX-1 and CDX-2 as potential biomarkers to differentiate well-differentiated neuroendocrine tumors. Biomark Res 2018;6(1):15.
52. Long KB, Srivastava A, Hirsch MS, et al. PAX8 expression in well-differentiated pancreatic endocrine tumors: correlation with clinicopathologic features and comparison with gastrointestinal and pulmonary carcinoid tumors. Am J Surg Pathol 2010;34(5):723–9.
53. Mertens RB, Koo J, Dhall D, et al. Value of islet 1 and PAX8 in identifying metastatic neuroendocrine tumors of pancreatic origin. Mod Pathol 2012;25(6):893–901.
54. Yao JC, Hassan M, Phan A, et al. One hundred years after "carcinoid": epidemiology of and prognostic factors for neuroendocrine tumors in 35,825 cases in the United States. J Clin Oncol 2008;26(18):3063–72.
55. Scoazec J-Y, Couvelard A, Monges G, et al. Professional practices and diagnostic issues in neuroendocrine tumour pathology: results of a prospective one-year survey among French pathologists (the PRONET Study). Neuroendocrinology 2016;105(1):67–76.
56. Anlauf M, Schlenger R, Perren A, et al. Microadenomatosis of the endocrine pancreas in patients with and without the multiple endocrine neoplasia type 1 syndrome. Am J Surg Pathol 2006;30(5):560–74.
57. Kapran Y, Bauersfeld J, Anlauf M, et al. Multihormonality and entrapment of islets in pancreatic endocrine tumors. Virchows Arch 2006;448(4):394–8.
58. Konukiewitz B, Enosawa T, Klöppel G. Glucagon expression in cystic pancreatic neuroendocrine neoplasms: an immunohistochemical analysis. Virchows Arch 2011;458(1):47–53.
59. Garbrecht N, Anlauf M, Schmitt A, et al. Somatostatin-producing neuroendocrine tumors of the duodenum and pancreas: incidence, types, biological behavior, association with inherited syndromes, and functional activity. Endocr Relat Cancer 2008;15(1):229–41.
60. McCall CM, Shi C, Klein AP, et al. Serotonin expression in pancreatic neuroendocrine tumors correlates with a trabecular histologic pattern and large duct involvement. Hum Pathol 2012;43(8):1169–76.
61. Borch K, Ahrén B, Ahlman H, et al. Gastric carcinoids: biologic behavior and prognosis after differentiated treatment in relation to type. Ann Surg 2005;242(1):64–73.
62. Sculco D, Bilgrami S. Pernicious anemia and gastric carcinoid tumor: case report and review. Am J Gastroenterol 1997;92(8):1378–80.
63. Thomas RM, Baybick JH, Elsayed AM, et al. Gastric carcinoids. An immunohistochemical and clinicopathologic study of 104 patients. Cancer 1994;73(8):2053–8.
64. Thomas D, Tsolakis AV, Grozinsky-Glasberg S, et al. Long-term follow-up of a large series of patients with type 1 gastric carcinoid tumors: data from a multicenter study. Eur J Endocrinol 2013;168(2):185–93.
65. Chen WC, Warner RRP, Ward SC, et al. Management and disease outcome of type I gastric neuroendocrine tumors: the Mount Sinai experience. Dig Dis Sci 2015;60:996–1003.
66. Grozinsky-Glasberg S, Thomas D, Strosberg JR, et al. Metastatic type 1 gastric carcinoid: a real threat or just a myth? World J Gastroenterol 2013;19(46):8687–95.
67. Gladdy RA, Strong VE, Coit D, et al. Defining surgical indications for type I gastric carcinoid tumor. Ann Surg Oncol 2009;16(11):3154–60.
68. Gilligan CJ, Lawton GP, Tang LH, et al. Gastric carcinoid tumors: the biology and therapy of an enigmatic and controversial lesion. Am J Gastroenterol 1995;90(3):338–52.
69. Epelboym I, Mazeh H. Zollinger-Ellison syndrome: classical considerations and current controversies. Oncologist 2014;19(1):44–50.
70. Norton JA, Fraker DL, Alexander HR, et al. Surgery increases survival in patients with gastrinoma. Ann Surg 2006;244(3):410–8.
71. Bordi C. Endocrine tumours of the stomach. Pathol Res Pract 1995;191(4):373–80.
72. Modlin IM, Champaneria MC, Chan AKC, et al. A three-decade analysis of 3,911 small intestinal neuroendocrine tumors: the rapid pace of no progress. Am J Gastroenterol 2007;102(7):1464–73.
73. Tsikitis VL, Wertheim BC, Guerrero MA. Trends of incidence and survival of gastrointestinal neuroendocrine tumors in the United States: a seer analysis. J Cancer 2012;3:292–302.
74. Bilimoria KY, Bentrem DJ, Wayne JD, et al. Small bowel cancer in the United States: changes in epidemiology, treatment, and survival over the last 20 years. Ann Surg 2009;249(1):63–71.
75. Carter J, Grenert J, Rubenstein L, et al. Neuroendocrine tumors of the ampulla of vater: biological behavior and surgical management. Arch Surg 2009;144(6):527–31.
76. Burke AP, Thomas RM, Elsayed AM, et al. Carcinoids of the jejunum and ileum: an immunohistochemical and clinicopathologic study of 167 cases. Cancer 1997;79(6):1086–93.
77. Loftus JP, van Heerden JA. Surgical management of gastrointestinal carcinoid tumors. Adv Surg 1995;28:317–36.

78. Kim MK, Warner RRP, Roayaie S, et al. Revised staging classification improves outcome prediction for small intestinal neuroendocrine tumors. J Clin Oncol 2013;31(30):3776–81.
79. Strosberg J, Gardner N, Kvols L. Survival and prognostic factor analysis of 146 metastatic neuroendocrine tumors of the mid-gut. Neuroendocrinology 2009;89(4):471–6.
80. Rorstad O. Prognostic indicators for carcinoid neuroendocrine tumors of the gastrointestinal tract. J Surg Oncol 2005;89(3):151–60.
81. Pawa N, Clift AK, Osmani H, et al. Surgical management of patients with neuroendocrine neoplasms of the appendix: appendectomy or more. Neuroendocrinology 2018;106(3):242–51.
82. Groth SS, Virnig BA, Al-Refaie WB, et al. Appendiceal carcinoid tumors: predictors of lymph node metastasis and the impact of right hemicolectomy on survival. J Surg Oncol 2011;103(1):39–45.
83. Mullen JT, Savarese DMF. Carcinoid tumors of the appendix: a population-based study. J Surg Oncol 2011;104(1):41–4.
84. Toumpanakis C, Fazio N, Tiensuu Janson E, et al. Unmet needs in appendiceal neuroendocrine neoplasms. Neuroendocrinology 2019;108(1):37–44.
85. Burke AP, Sobin LH, Federspiel BH, et al. Goblet cell carcinoids and related tumors of the vermiform appendix. Am J Clin Pathol 1990;94(1):27–35.
86. Tang LH, Shia J, Soslow RA, et al. Pathologic classification and clinical behavior of the spectrum of goblet cell carcinoid tumors of the appendix. Am J Surg Pathol 2008;32(10):1429–43.
87. Yozu M, Johncilla ME, Srivastava A, et al. Histologic and outcome study supports reclassifying appendiceal goblet cell carcinoids as goblet cell adenocarcinomas, and grading and staging similarly to colonic adenocarcinomas. Am J Surg Pathol 2018;42(7):898–910.
88. Lee MdLH, Mcconnell YJ, Tsang E, et al. Simplified 2-tier histologic grading system accurately predicts outcomes in goblet cell carcinoid of the appendix. Hum Pathol 2015;46:1881–9.
89. Ballantyne GH, Savoca PE, Flannery JT, et al. Incidence and mortality of carcinoids of the colon. Data from the connecticut tumor registry. Cancer 1992;69(10):2400–5.
90. Caplin M, Sundin A, Nillson O, et al. ENETS consensus guidelines for the management of patients with digestive neuroendocrine neoplasms: colorectal neuroendocrine neoplasms. Neuroendocrinology 2012;95(2):88–97.
91. Fahy BN, Tang LH, Klimstra D, et al. Carcinoid of the Rectum Risk Stratification (CaRRs): a strategy for preoperative outcome assessment. Ann Surg Oncol 2007;14(5):1735–43.
92. Landry CS, Brock G, Scoggins CR, et al. A proposed staging system for rectal carcinoid tumors based on an analysis of 4701 patients. Surgery 2008;144(3):460–6.
93. de Mestier L, Brixi H, Gincul R, et al. Updating the management of patients with rectal neuroendocrine tumors. Endoscopy 2013;45(12):1039–46.
94. Byrne RM, Pommier RF. Small bowel and colorectal carcinoids. Clin Colon Rectal Surg 2018;31(5):301–8.
95. Lee KJ, Cho JH, Lee SH, et al. Clinicopathological characteristics of biliary neuroendocrine neoplasms: a multicenter study. Scand J Gastroenterol 2017;52(4):437–41.
96. Chen R-W, Qiu M-J, Chen Y, et al. Analysis of the clinicopathological features and prognostic factors of primary hepatic neuroendocrine tumors. Oncol Lett 2018;15(6):8604–10.
97. Michalopoulos N, Papavramidis TS, Karayannopoulou G, et al. neuroendocrine tumors of extrahepatic biliary tract. Pathol Oncol Res 2014;20(4):765–75.
98. Esposito I, Segler A, Steiger K, et al. Pathology, genetics and precursors of human and experimental pancreatic neoplasms: an update. Pancreatology 2015;15(6):598–610.
99. Falconi M, Bartsch DK, Eriksson B, et al. ENETS consensus guidelines for the management of patients with digestive neuroendocrine neoplasms of the digestive system: well-differentiated pancreatic non-functioning tumors. Neuroendocrinology 2012; 95(2):120–34.
100. Lee LC, Grant CS, Salomao DR, et al. Small, nonfunctioning, asymptomatic pancreatic neuroendocrine tumors (PNETs): role for nonoperative management. Surgery 2012;152(6):965–74.
101. Kimura W, Kuroda A, Morioka Y. clinical pathology of endocrine tumors of the pancreas. analysis of autopsy cases. Dig Dis Sci 1991;36(7):933–42.
102. Volante M, La Rosa S, Castellano I, et al. Clinicopathological features of a series of 11 oncocytic endocrine tumours of the pancreas. Virchows Arch 2006;448(5):545–51.
103. Zee SY, Hochwald SN, Conlon KC, et al. Pleomorphic pancreatic endocrine neoplasms: a variant commonly confused with adenocarcinoma. Am J Surg Pathol 2005;29(9):1194–200.
104. Yachida S, Vakiani E, White CM, et al. Small cell and large cell neuroendocrine carcinomas of the pancreas are genetically similar and distinct from well-differentiated pancreatic neuroendocrine tumors. Am J Surg Pathol 2012;36(2):173–84.
105. Franko J, Feng W, Yip L, et al. Non-functional neuroendocrine carcinoma of the pancreas: incidence, tumor biology, and outcomes in 2,158 patients. J Gastrointest Surg 2010;14(3):541–8.
106. Kim JY, Kim MS, Kim KS, et al. Clinicopathologic and prognostic significance of multiple hormone expression in pancreatic neuroendocrine tumors. Am J Surg Pathol 2015;39(5):592–601.

107. Yao JC, Shah MH, Ito T, et al. Everolimus for advanced pancreatic neuroendocrine tumors. N Engl J Med 2011;364(6):514–23.
108. Panzuto F, Rinzivillo M, Spada F, et al. Everolimus in pancreatic neuroendocrine carcinomas G3. Pancreas 2017;46(3):302–5.
109. Walenkamp AME, Sonke GS, Sleijfer DT. Clinical and therapeutic aspects of extrapulmonary small cell carcinoma. Cancer Treat Rev 2009;35(3): 228–36.
110. Korse CM, Taal BG, Van Velthuysen MLF, et al. Incidence and survival of neuroendocrine tumours in the Netherlands according to histological grade: experience of two decades of cancer registry. Eur J Cancer 2013;49(8):1975–83.
111. Cetinkaya RB, Aagnes B, Thiis-Evensen E, et al. Trends in incidence of neuroendocrine neoplasms in Norway: a report of 16,075 cases from 1993 through 2010. Neuroendocrinology 2016;104(1): 1–10.
112. Kang H, O'Connell JB, Leonardi MJ, et al. Rare tumors of the colon and rectum: a national review. Int J Colorectal Dis 2007;22(2):183–9.
113. Dasari A, Mehta K, Byers LA, et al. Comparative study of lung and extrapulmonary poorly differentiated neuroendocrine carcinomas: a SEER database analysis of 162,983 cases. Cancer 2018; 124(4):807–15.
114. Woischke C, Schaaf CW, Yang H-M, et al. In-depth mutational analyses of colorectal neuroendocrine carcinomas with adenoma or adenocarcinoma components. Mod Pathol 2017;30(1): 95–103.
115. Verset L, Arvanitakis M, Loi P, et al. TTF-1 positive small cell cancers: don't think they're always primary pulmonary! World J Gastrointest Oncol 2011;3(10):144.
116. Ohike N, Adsay NV, La Rosa S, et al. Mixed neuroendocrine-non-neuroendocrine neoplasms. In: Lloyd RV, Osamura RY, Kloppel G, et al, editors. WHO classification of tumours of endocrine organs. 4th edition. Lyon (France): IARC Press; 2017. p. 238.
117. Yao GY, Zhou JL, Lai M De, et al. Neuroendocrine markers in adenocarcinomas: an investigation of 356 cases. World J Gastroenterol 2003;9(4): 858–61.
118. Strosberg JR, Cheema A, Weber J, et al. Prognostic validity of a Novel American Joint Committee on Cancer staging classification for pancreatic neuroendocrine tumors. J Clin Oncol 2011;29(22): 3044–9.
119. Alese OB, Jiang R, Shaib W, et al. High-grade gastrointestinal neuroendocrine carcinoma management and outcomes: a national cancer database study. Oncologist 2019;24(7):911–20.
120. Klempner SJ, Gershenhorn B, Tran P, et al. BRAFV600E mutations in high-grade colorectal neuroendocrine tumors may predict responsiveness to BRAF-MEK combination therapy. Cancer Discov 2016;6(6):594–600.
121. Jiao Y, Shi C, Edil BH, et al. DAXX/ATRX, MEN1, and mTOR Pathway Genes Are Frequently Altered in Pancreatic Neuroendocrine Tumors. Science 2011;331(6021):1199–203.
122. Scarpa A, Chang DK, Nones K, et al. Whole-genome landscape of pancreatic neuroendocrine tumours. Nature 2017;543(7643):65–71.
123. Girardi DM, Silva ACB, Rêgo JFM, et al. Unraveling molecular pathways of poorly differentiated neuroendocrine carcinomas of the gastroenteropancreatic system: a systematic review. Cancer Treat Rev 2017;56:28–35.
124. Takizawa N, Ohishi Y, Hirahashi M, et al. Molecular characteristics of colorectal neuroendocrine carcinoma; Similarities with adenocarcinoma rather than neuroendocrine tumor. Hum Pathol 2015; 46(12):1890–900.
125. Sahnane N, Furlan D, Monti M, et al. Microsatellite unstable gastrointestinal neuroendocrine carcinomas: a new clinicopathologic entity. Endocr Relat Cancer 2015;22(1):35–45.
126. Idrees K, Padmanabhan C, Liu E, et al. Frequent BRAF mutations suggest a novel oncogenic driver in colonic neuroendocrine carcinoma. J Surg Oncol 2018;117(2):284–9.

Treatment of Gastroenteropancreatic Neuroendocrine Tumors

Kimberly Perez, MD*, Jennifer Chan, MD, MPH

KEYWORDS

• Neuroendocrine tumors • Gastroenteropancreatic • Neuroendocrine system • Gastrointestinal tract

ABSTRACT

Neuroendocrine tumors (NETs) represent a group of biologically and clinically heterogeneous neoplasms arising from the diffuse neuroendocrine system. Although NETs may develop in almost any organ, they commonly arise in the gastrointestinal tract and pancreas and are referred to as gastroenteropancreatic (GEP)-NETs when they arise from these sites. In recent years, advances in understanding of the biology of NETs have resulted in an expansion in treatment options and improved survival for patients. This review focuses on treatment of GEP-NETS and highlights factors that govern the therapeutic approach.

OVERVIEW

Neuroendocrine tumors (NETs) represent a heterogeneous group of neoplasms that arise from cells in the diffuse neuroendocrine system. Although they can occur in multiple organs in the body, they are common in the gastrointestinal (GI) tract and pancreas, where they are thought to originate from enterochromaffin cells of the gut and islets of Langerhans cells in the pancreas.[1] Although relatively rare, the incidence and prevalence of gastroenteropancreatic (GEP)-NETs have been rising in the United States. Classification systems for GEP-NETs that are based on embryologic or anatomic origin, pathologic features, and clinical behavior have been developed and have been utilized to guide therapeutic strategies.

PATHOLOGIC FEATURES

Although once treated as a uniform disease, distinctions have been made in recent years among NETs based on tumor differentiation and grade. In 2010 the World Health Organization (WHO) presented an update to the classification of digestive neuroendocrine neoplasms.[2] The most notable features were the identification of measures to define grading more clearly. A proliferation-based grading system was outlined based on specific Ki-67 proliferation indices and mitotic count cutoffs. This change was made to provide a measurable and more objective system for neuroendocrine cancer definition and, in turn, a useable prognostic indicator for planning of therapy.[2] Since the publication of the 2010 WHO classification, there has been growing recognition that the 2010 WHO-grade categories do not reflect the heterogeneous phenotype of neuroendocrine neoplasms, in particular the prognostic differences between well-differentiated and poorly differentiated grade 3 neuroendocrine neoplasms (Ki-67 >20% or mitotic index >20/10 high-power fields).[3,4] Hence, the recently updated 2019 WHO criteria for GEP-NETs includes categories of well-differentiated grade 1, grade 2, and grade 3 NETs and maintains categories of poorly differentiated grade 3 neuroendocrine carcinomas (**Table 1**).[5] For more on the histologic evaluation of GEP-NETs, see Natalie Patel and colleagues' article, "Neuroendocrine Tumors of the Gastrointestinal Tract and Pancreas," in this issue.

Program in Carcinoid and Neuroendocrine Tumors, Department of Medical Oncology, Dana-Farber Cancer Institute, Harvard Medical School, 450 Brookline Avenue, Boston, MA 02215, USA
* Corresponding author.
E-mail address: Kimberly_perez@dfci.harvard.edu

Surgical Pathology 12 (2019) 1045–1053
https://doi.org/10.1016/j.path.2019.08.011
1875-9181/19/

Table 1
Food and Drug Administration–approved or commonly used therapeutic options for disease control of gastroenteropancreatic neuroendocrine tumors based on primary tumor location

Gastrointestinal Neuroendocrine Tumors (Carcinoid Tumors)	Pancreatic Neuroendocrine Tumors
SSAs	SSA
Everolimus (nonfunctional GI-NET)	Everolimus Sunitinib Alkylating agents • Capecitabine and temozolomide[a] • Streptozocin
^{177}Lu-Dotatate	^{177}Lu-Dotatate

[a] Not FDA approved for this indication.

EMBRYOLOGIC OR ANATOMIC ORIGIN

GEP-NETs have historically been classified according to their site of origin in the embryologic gut and, therefore, divided into foregut, midgut, and hindgut tumors. Foregut tumors develop in the thymus, respiratory tract, esophagus, stomach, duodenum, and pancreas; midgut NETs originate in the appendix, small bowel, cecum, and ascending colon; hindgut NETs begin in remaining large bowel, including rectum.[6] Within this anatomically driven framework, further characterization of NETs has been made based on molecular profiling as well as observations regarding associated clinical and therapeutic phenotypes.

Molecular profiling has uncovered distinctions between poorly differentiated NECs, NETs of the pancreas (pNETs), and those originating from other sites in the GI tract. Poorly differentiated NECs harbor higher incidences of somatic mutations compared with the well-differentiated cohorts, which seem to have a more stable genome.[7] In well-differentiated NETs, when the genome is mutated, variants are most commonly identified in *MEN1*, genes involving the mechanistic (or mammalian) target of rapamycin (mTOR) pathway, *DAXX*, and *ATRX* for pNETs,[8,9] and *CDKN1B* in small bowel NETs.[10] In pNETs, the presence of variants in *DAXX* and *ATRX* not only function as biomolecular markers but also, due to associated chromosomal instability, are correlated with more advanced tumor stage and metastasis, reduced relapse-free survival, and decreased tumor-associated survival.[11]

Survival outcomes seem to vary significantly among NETs of different primary sites. In a recent Surveillance, Epidemiology, and End Results (SEER) database analysis of patients with NETs in the United States, significant differences in survival according to primary tumor location were identified. In this study, 73,782 patients with NETs diagnosed between 1973 and 2014, including those originating in the lung/bronchus, small intestine, rectum, colon, pancreas, and stomach, were analyzed. The median survival duration for the entire cohort was 41 months. Patients diagnosed with NET of the rectum had the best prognosis, followed by small intestine, lung/bronchus, stomach, and colon (Using rectum as a reference: small intestine, HR, 1.660, 95% CI, 1.579 - 1.744; lung/bronchus, HR, 1.786, 95% CI, 1,703 - 1.874; stomach, HR, 1.865, 95% CI, 1.755 - 1.982; and colon, HR, 1.896, 95% CI, 1.799 - 1.999). Patients with pNETs carried the highest risk of mortality (HR 2.034; CI, 1.925).[12] Overall survival (OS) differences depending on primary tumor location also were noted in another analysis using SEER data. In an analysis from this study that controlled for grade and stage of disease, the median survival of patients with distant grade 1 to grade 2 NETs diagnosed between 2000 and 2012 was 103 months for patients with disease originating in the small intestine compared with 60 months for patient with pancreatic primaries.[13]

Therapeutic response has been correlated with anatomic site of origin. Although well-differentiated NETs arising within the digestive system and pancreatic neuroendocrine tumors (pNETs) have similar characteristics on histologic evaluation, the response to anticancer agents is different. Specifically, response rates to cytotoxic agents have been significantly better in pNETs compared with well-differentiated NETs arising elsewhere.[14] In a SEER analysis of patients with NETs conducted between 2000 and 2012, the biggest improvement in survival over the time interval was in pNETs, and this was attributed to the advances in systemic therapies.[13]

FUNCTIONAL STATUS

Neuroendocrine cells and tumor counterparts exhibit physiologic attributes of the neural and endocrine regulatory systems. As a result, NETs are characterized by their ability to secrete peptide hormones that can lead to symptoms related to hormone excess. NETs are classified as functional tumors if patients clinically experience symptoms due to hormone hypersecretion by tumor. The clinical presentation of the syndrome is dependent on the type of hormone produced. The most well-described clinical syndrome is the classical carcinoid syndrome, with manifestations, including diarrhea, flushing, and bronchospasm, related to secretion of serotonin and other vasoactive peptides.[15] Carcinoid syndrome is most common in the setting of disseminated disease, particularly with liver involvement, and a great majority of cases are associated with metastatic tumors originating in the midgut (jejunum, ileum, and cecum). Subtypes of pNETs secreting hormones, including gastrin, insulin, glucagon, vasoactive intestinal peptide, and other peptide hormones, have been identified and are associated with unique clinical manifestations.[16]

SYSTEMIC TREATMENT OF ADVANCED GASTROENTEROPANCREATIC NEUROENDOCRINE TUMORS

Multiple options are available for the management of patients with advanced, metastatic GEP-NETs, including surgical resection, liver-directed therapies for patients with metastases predominantly in the liver, and systemic therapy. Because of the heterogeneity of disease biology and presentation, a multidisciplinary approach to management is critical. The goals of therapy are to improve symptoms related to hormone hypersecretion, slow disease progression, and improve survival. Systemic therapy options include somatostatin analogs (SSAs), radiolabeled SSAs, molecularly targeted agents including everolimus and sunitinib, and cytotoxic chemotherapy (see **Table 1**).

Somatostatin Analogs

Approximately 80% of well-differentiated GEP-NET cells express high levels of somatostatin receptors (SSTRs). Five distinct SSTR subtypes have been identified and characterized. All 5 SSTRs have a G protein coupled to 7 putative membrane-spanning domains.[17] SSAs, including octreotide and lanreotide, bind to SSTRs expressed on NET cells and can result in (1) cell-cycle arrest and/or apoptosis downstream from tumor SSTR activation, (2) inhibition of tumor angiogenesis and the production of growth factors, and (3) decreased secretion of peptide hormones.[18] Through these actions, SSAs have both antisecretory and antiproliferative actions.

The efficacy of SSA for treatment of carcinoid syndrome was first established in a study of 25 patients treated with octreotide, 150 μg subcutaneously, 3 times per day; 88% of patients experienced improvement in flushing and diarrhea, and 72% achieved reduction in serotonin secretion as measured by reduction in urinary levels of its breakdown product 5-hydroxyindolacetic acid (5-HIAA).[19] Utilizing similar mechanisms of action and binding affinities to SSTR subtypes, the long-acting formulation of octreotide and lanreotide, administered every 4 weeks, can also partially or completely improve symptoms of carcinoid syndrome and has eliminated the need for many patients to self-administer injections.[16,20] The efficacy of lanreotide for treatment of carcinoid syndrome was recently evaluated in the ELECT trial, a phase III trial in which patients with carcinoid syndrome were randomized to receive lanreotide, 120 mg, as a deep subcutaneous injection, every 28 days, or placebo. The primary endpoint of this trial was the percentage of days in which short-acting octreotide was used as a rescue medication. The odds ratio of full or partial treatment success (<3 days short-acting octreotide use) was significantly greater with lanreotide compared with placebo (HR 2.4; 95% CI, 1.1–5.3; P = .036).[21] Based on these study results, both octreotide and lanreotide are options for treatment of patients with carcinoid syndrome.

For patients with functional pNETs, variable symptom responses have been described based on peptide produced, with greater benefit described in tumors secreting vasoactive intestinal peptide, glucagon, and somatostatin. More limited therapeutic impact has been described in insulinomas and gastrinomas.[22] In patients with an insulinoma, the clinical benefit of SSAs is limited by 2 factors: (1) only 50% of insulinomas express the SSTR subtype SSTR-2, to which octreotide and lanreotide preferentially bind, and (2) disease-associated hypoglycemia may paradoxically worsen due to inhibition of glucagon secretion caused by SSAs.[23] Therefore, patients with insulinomas need to be closely monitored when initiating therapy with SSA therapy. In patients with a gastrinoma, SSAs can reduce gastrin levels but high-dose proton pump inhibitors have proved more effective in the control of hypergastrinemia-related gastric acid production.[16,24]

In addition to controlling symptoms associated with hormone hypersecretion, SSAs can slow tumor growth. The antiproliferative effects of SSAs were demonstrated in 2 pivotal phase III prospective trials. In the PROMID trial, patients with metastatic well-differentiated (Ki-67 <2%) midgut NETs were randomized to octreotide long-acting repeatable (LAR), 30 mg, every 28 days, or placebo. Treatment with octreotide LAR was associated with an improvement in time to progression of 14.3 months compared with 6 months in the placebo arm (HR 0.34; 95% CI, 0.2–0.59; P = .000072); best response of stable disease was noted in 66.7% of patients compared with 37.2% in the placebo arm.[25,26] In the CLARINET trial, patients with locally advanced or metastatic well-differentiated, low-grade to intermediate-grade (Ki-67 <10%) pNETs or GI-NETs were randomized to lanreotide, 120 mg subcutaneous, every 28 days, or placebo. Median progression-free survival (PFS) was 32.8 months for lanreotide and 18 months for the placebo arm (HR 0.47; 95% CI, 0.30–0.73).[27] Due to their antiproliferative and antisecretory effects, plus ease of administration and tolerability, SSAs generally are considered a first-line therapeutic option in well-differentiated GEP-NETs.

Radiolabeled Somatostatin Analogs

The high rate of SSA expression in NETs provides the rationale for use of peptide receptor radionuclide therapy as a therapeutic strategy. In this form of therapy, SSAs are conjugated with a chelator and a radionuclide to deliver tumoricidal doses of radiation. The most frequently used radionuclides include the β-emitting radionuclide ^{90}yttrium and β-emitting and γ-emitting ^{177}lutetium (^{177}Lu).[28] In the Phase 3 Trial of 177Lu-Dotatate for Midgut Neuroendocrine Tumors (NETTER-1) trial, 229 patients with well-differentiated, metastatic midgut NETs were randomized to receive either ^{177}Lu-Dotatate, at a dose of 7.4 GBq every 8 weeks (4 intravenous infusions plus best supportive care, including octreotide LAR, administered intramuscularly, at a dose of 30 mg), or high-dose octreotide LAR alone, at a dose of 60 mg, every 4 weeks. In the primary analysis, the estimated PFS rate at 20 months was 65.2% in the ^{177}Lu-Dotatate arm compared with 10.8% in the octreotide LAR arm. The median PFS was not reached in the ^{177}Lu-Dotatate group compared with 8.4 months in the control group (HR 0.21; 95% CI, 0.13–0.33). The radiographic response rates were 18% and 3% in the patients receiving ^{177}Lu-Dotatate and high-dose octreotide, respectively; 77% of patients in the ^{177}Lu-Dotatate arm received all 4 infusions. The most common toxicities during treatment included nausea (any grade 59%) and vomiting (any grade 47%) but were attributed to the amino acid infusions infused concurrently for renal protection.[29]

Although the NETTER-1 study was restricted to patients with advanced midgut NETs, retrospective studies have evaluated ^{177}Lu-Dotatate in patients with pNETs and other NETs. In a large retrospective analysis of 443 patients with NETs, including bronchial and GEP-NETs, treated at the Erasmus Medical Center in the Netherlands, the median PFS and median OS durations among all patients were 29 months and 63 months, respectively.[30] Among the 133 patients with pNETs, the radiographic response rate, including complete and partial responses, was 55%; median PFS and OS durations were 30 months and 70 months, respectively. Additional retrospective data from Erasmus from 360 patients with GEP-NET–treated ^{177}Lu-Dotatate demonstrated a radiographic response rate of 16% and median duration of response of 35 months in the responding patients.[31] Based on the results of the NETTER-1 trial and retrospective data from Erasmus, ^{177}Lu-Dotatate is approved in the United States for treatment of SSTR-positive GEP-NETs.

Vascular Endothelial Growth Factor Pathway Inhibitors

NETs are characterized by their hypervascular nature and expression of vascular endothelial growth factor (VEGF), a potent regulator of tumor angiogenesis, and its receptors.[32] Multiple clinical trials have evaluated the role of multitargeted tyrosine kinase inhibitors (TKIs) and monoclonal antibodies that target the VEGF pathway in patients with advanced GEP-NETs. The TKI sunitinib inhibits multiple receptors, including VEGF receptor 1, VEGF receptor 2, and VEGF receptor 3. In a phase II trial with 109 patients with advanced NETs, including pNETs and carcinoid tumors (ie, non-pNETs of various sites), who were treated with sunitinib, 50 mg daily, for 4 weeks of every 6 weeks, the radiographic response rate was higher in patients with pNETs compared with patients with carcinoid tumors, 16.7% versus 2.4%, respectively.[33] In a follow-up phase III study, patients with advanced pNETs were randomized to receive sunitinib, 37.5 mg daily, versus placebo. There was significantly longer median PFS in the sunitinib arm compared with the placebo, 11.4 months compared with 5.5 months, respectively (HR for progression or death, 0.42; 95% CI, 0.26–0.66; $P<.001$).[34] The objective response rate in patients receiving sunitinib was 9.3% versus 0% for patients receiving placebo. Sunitinib is approved by the Food and Drug Administration (FDA) for treatment of patients with advanced pNETs. Other multitargeted TKIs, including pazopanib, lenvantinib, and cabozantinib, have been evaluated in phase II trials and have demonstrated overall response rates of 15% to 20% and median PFS of 14 months to 22 months.[35–37] In the Alliance trial A021202, a randomized phase II trial of patients with progressive carcinoid tumors (non-pancreatic NET), Pazopanib was reported to have an improved PFS compared with placebo with a median PFS of 11.6 and 8.5 months, respectively (HR = 0.53, 1-sided 90% upper confidence limite 0.69, $P = 0.0005$.[38]

The efficacy of bevacizumab, a monoclonal antibody targeting VEGF, in the treatment of NETs has been evaluated in phase II and III trials. Activity of bevacizumab as a single agent in advanced GI-NETs was suggested in a phase II trial demonstrating a relatively high radiographic partial response rate of 18% and significant proportion of patients without disease progression during an 18-week treatment period.[39] These results formed the basis of a phase III trial in which patients with progressive or poor-prognosis advanced GI-NETs and lung NETs were randomized to receive octreotide plus bevacizumab versus octreotide plus interferon.[40] Radiologic responses were more frequent among patients treated with bevacizumab (12% vs 4%), and time to treatment failure was longer in patients treated with bevacizumab (median TTF 9.9 vs 5.6 months; HR 0.72; 95% CI, 0.58–0.90). The primary endpoint of PFS, however, was not significantly different (median PFS 16.6 with bevacizumab vs 15.4 months for placebo; HR, 0.93; 95% CI, 0.73–1.18). Interpretation of these trial results is complicated due to the use of an active control arm; nonetheless, a role for bevacizumab has not been established in patients with advanced GI-NETs.

Mechanistic Target of Rapamycin Inhibitors

mTOR is an intracellular serine/threonine kinase that regulates key cell functions involved in cell survival, proliferation, and metabolism. Signaling through the PI3K phosphatidylinositide 3-kinase/AKT/mTOR pathway leads to increased translation of proteins regulating cell-cycle progression and metabolism.[41] mTOR mediates downstream signaling from several pathways, including VEGF and insulinlike growth factor, that are implicated in NET growth.[42] The activity of the mTOR inhibitor everolimus has been investigated in GEP-NETs in several key phase III randomized trials. In the RAD001 in Advanced Neuroendocrine Tumors (RADIANT)-3 trial, treatment with everolimus was associated with a significant prolongation of PFS in patients with advanced pNETs compared with placebo (11 vs 4.6 months; HR 0.35, 95% CI, 0.27–0.45).[43] The RADIANT-2 trial enrolled patients with low-grade and intermediate-grade NETs with carcinoid syndrome who were randomized to receive octreotide LAR with everolimus versus octreotide LAR with placebo. Although median PFS by central radiology review was longer in patients receiving octreotide and everolimus (16.4 vs 11.3 months; HR 0.77; 95% CI, 0.59–1.00), the result did not meet the predefined level of statistical significance.[44] In the RADIANT-4 trial, patients with advanced nonfunctioning GI-NETs and lung NETs were randomized to receive treatment with everolimus or placebo. Everolimus was associated with an improved median PFS of 11 months compared with 3.9 months for placebo; everolimus was associated with a 52% reduction in the estimated risk of progression or death (HR 0.48; 95% CI, 0.35–0.67).[45] Based on these clinical trial results, everolimus is currently FDA approved for the treatment of patients with advanced pNETs and nonfunctional GI-NETS and lung NETs.

Cytotoxic Chemotherapy

Cytotoxic chemotherapies have been evaluated in advanced well-differentiated GEP-NETs. Activity has been observed with alkylating agents, with more significant responses observed in patients with pNETs compared with GI-NETs. Although streptozocin-based therapy has been a long-standing standard cytotoxic therapeutic option, its use has been limited due to its cumbersome administrative schedule and side-effect profile.[46,47] Temozolomide is an oral alkylating agent with a more favorable administration schedule and toxicity profile. Antitumor activity has been demonstrated with temozolomide-based therapy in both retrospective and prospective trials. Temozolomide has been evaluated prospectively in combination with thalidomide, bevacizumab, and everolimus, with overall response rates of 33% to 45%.[48–50] In a retrospective series of 143 patients who were treated with temozolomide plus capecitabine, the response rate for this combination was 54%.[51] The recently completed Eastern Cooperative Group–American College of Radiology Imaging Network 2211 trial evaluated the activity of the combination of temozolomide plus capecitabine compared with temozolomide alone. In this randomized phase II trial, the median PFS was 22.7 months in patients receiving capecitabine plus temozolomide compared with 14.4 months in those receiving temozolomide alone (HR 0.58; $P = .023$). The radiographic response rate for the combination was higher than for temozolomide monotherapy, 33% versus 28% respectively ($P = .47$).[48] Studies have yielded inconsistent results regarding whether expression of O6-methylguanine DNA methyltransferase (MGMT) or other biomarkers are predictive of response to temozolomide.[52,53] Future evaluation of potential predictors of response will be important to determine whether there are predictors of response or PFS that may allow personalized treatment of patients.

HIGH GRADE NEUROENDOCRINE NEOPLASM

Poorly differentiated, grade 3 neuroendocrine carcinomas are commonly treated with platinum-based chemotherapy regimens using an approach that is similar to treatment of small cell lung carcinoma. There is a subset of patients with NETs that are well differentiated but have Ki-67 proliferation indices greater than 20% that fall into the high-grade range.[4] The most appropriate therapy for this subgroup of patients has not been well established. In a retrospective study of 305 patients with G3 neuroendocrine GEP carcinomas (23% with pancreatic primary site), patients whose disease had a Ki-67 less than 55% had significantly longer median survival compared with patients with higher Ki-67 indices (14 months vs 10 months). Response rates to platinum-based chemotherapy were lower in disease with a Ki-67 less than 55% (15% vs 42%).[54] Because sensitivity to platinum-based chemotherapy seems associated with higher Ki-67 proliferation rates, agents used for low-grade to intermediate-grade NETs, including temozolomide-based therapy, molecularly targeted therapy, or peptide receptor radionuclide therapy (if SSTR positive), may play a role in the treatment of well-differentiated grade 3 NETs. Clinical trials evaluating the optimal treatment of grade 3 neuroendocrine neoplasms are currently ongoing.

Immunotherapy

Immunotherapy-based treatments are currently under investigation in GEP-NETs. Limited activity has been observed with anti-programmed cell death 1 (PD-1) antibody therapy when administered as a single agent. A phase II trial of the anti–PD-1 antibody spartalizumab evaluated in 116 patients with advanced neuroendocrine neoplasms, including 33 with pNETs, 32 with GI-NETs, 30 with thoracic NETs, and 21 with poorly differentiated GEP neuroendocrine carcinomas. Although a response rate of 20% was observed in patients with thoracic NETs, the response rates in 0% and 3% for GI-NETs and pNETs, respectively.[55] The activity of the anti–PD-1 antibody pembrolizumab in patients with well-differentiated or moderately differentiated NETs originating in the lung, GI tract, or pancreas was evaluated in KEYNOTE-158 trial and was noted to be low, with an overall response rate of 3.7%.[56] Trials evaluating checkpoint inhibitors in combination with other immunomodulatory agents are ongoing.

Telotristat

Although SSAs are highly effective in controlling symptoms of carcinoid syndrome, many patients on SSA have suboptimal control or become refractory to SSA over time. In patients in whom SSA efficacy is limited, options include increasing the frequency or dose of SSA, utilizing short-acting SSA breakthrough, and initiating antidiarrheal therapies.[14] Telotristat ethyl is a relatively new option for management of diarrhea in patients with carcinoid syndrome whose symptoms are not well controlled with SSA. Telotristat inhibits the enzyme tryptophase hydroxylase, which mediates the rate-limiting step in the serotonin biosynthesis. In the phase III TELESTAR trial, patients with refractory diarrhea due to carcinoid syndrome, defined by greater than 4 bowel movements per day despite at least standard doses of SSA, were randomized to receive placebo or telotristat, 250 mg or 500 mg orally, 3 times per day. The primary endpoint of the trial was reduction in the mean number of daily bowel movements. In the 3 arms, a total of 44% and 42% of participants who received telotristat, 250 mg and 500 mg, respectively, fulfilled criteria as responders measured by mean reduction of daily bowel activity from baseline to week 12, compared with 20% in the placebo arm. This improvement in mean daily bowel movements also correlated with a drop in urine 5-HIAA.[57] Telotristat has been approved by the FDA in combination with SSA for the treatment diarrhea related to carcinoid syndrome inadequately controlled with SSA alone.

SUMMARY

GEP-NETs are a diverse group of neoplasms whose treatment is based on primary site of disease and clinicopathologic features. In recent years, advances in the understanding of the biology of NETs has resulted in an expansion of treatment options for patients. Given the heterogeneity of disease and clinical presentation in individual patients, a multidisciplinary approach to treatment is critical. For patients with localized disease, surgical resection remains a key to treatment; and for those with liver-predominant metastatic disease, liver-directed therapy can provide symptom and disease control. Systemic treatment options for disease control in GI-NETs include SSAs, everolimus, and radiolabeled SSA therapy with ^{177}Lu-Dotatate; in patients with pNETs, options also include sunitinib and cytotoxic chemotherapy with alkylating agents. Telotristat, an inhibitor of serotonin synthesis, can provide symptom control in patients with carcinoid syndrome not well controlled with SSAs. The role of TKIs, including pazopanib, cabozantinib, and lenvatinib, in non-pNETs remains under investigation with encouraging results seen in phase II trials. With the introduction of new therapeutic options, the challenge ahead is to identify predictors of response and the optimal sequence of therapy. Efforts are under way to better characterize the comparative strengths and weakness of competing therapies, which may allow better personalizing treatment of individual patients.

REFERENCES

1. Modlin IM, Oberg K, Chung D, et al. Gastroenteropancreatic neuroendocrine tumours. Lancet Oncol 2008;9(1):61–72.
2. Rindi G, Petrone G, Inzani F. The 2010 WHO classification of digestive neuroendocrine neoplasms: a critical appraisal four years after its introduction. Endocr Pathol 2014;25(2):186–92.
3. Basturk O, Yang Z, Tang L, et al. The high-grade (WHO G3) pancreatic neuroendocrine tumor category is morphologically and biologically heterogenous and includes both well differentiated and poorly differentiated neoplasms. Am J Surg Pathol 2015;39(5):683–90.
4. Vélayoudom-Céphise FL, Duvillard P, Foucan L, et al. Are G3 ENETS neuroendocrine neoplasms heterogeneous? Endocr Relat Cancer 2013;20(5): 649–57.
5. Klimstra D, Kloppel G, La Rosa S, et al. Introduction to tumours of the digestive system In WHO Classification of Tumours Editorial Board. 5th Edition. Digestive System Tumours. Lyon, France: WHO Press; p.13–20.
6. Kulke MH, Mayer RJ. Carcinoid tumors. N Engl J Med 1999;340(11):858–68.
7. Vijayvergia N, Boland P, Handorf E, et al. Molecular profiling of neuroendocrine malignancies to identify prognostic and therapeutic markers: a Fox Chase Cancer Center Pilot Study. Br J Cancer 2016; 115(5):564–70.
8. Du Y, Ter-Minassian M, Brais L, et al. Genetic associations with neuroendocrine tumor risk: results from a genome-wide association study. Endocr Relat Cancer 2016;23(8):587–94.
9. Scarpa A, Chang D, Nones K, et al. Whole-genome landscape of pancreatic neuroendocrine tumours. Nature 2017;543(7643):65–71.
10. Francis JM, Kiezun A, Ramos A, et al. Somatic mutation of CDKN1B in small intestine neuroendocrine tumors. Nat Genet 2013;45(12):1483–6.
11. Marinoni I, Kurrer A, Vassella E, et al. Loss of DAXX and ATRX are associated with chromosome instability and reduced survival of patients with pancreatic neuroendocrine tumors. Gastroenterology 2014;146(2):453–60.e5.
12. Man D, Wu J, Shen Z, et al. Prognosis of patients with neuroendocrine tumor: a SEER database analysis. Cancer Manag Res 2018;10:5629–38.
13. Dasari A, Shen C, Halperin D, et al. Trends in the Incidence, Prevalence, and Survival Outcomes in Patients With Neuroendocrine Tumors in the United States. JAMA Oncol 2017;3(10):1335–42.
14. Strosberg JR, Halfdanarson R, Belizzi A, et al. The North American Neuroendocrine Tumor Society consensus guidelines for surveillance and medical management of midgut neuroendocrine tumors. Pancreas 2017;46(6):707–14.
15. Maton PN. The carcinoid syndrome. Jama 1988; 260(11):1602–5.
16. Dimitriadis GK, Weickert M, Randeva H, et al. Medical management of secretory syndromes related to gastroenteropancreatic neuroendocrine tumours. Endocr Relat Cancer 2016;23(9):R423–36.
17. Nilsson O, Kolby L, Wangberg B, et al. Comparative studies on the expression of somatostatin receptor subtypes, outcome of octreotide scintigraphy and response to octreotide treatment in patients with carcinoid tumours. Br J Cancer 1998;77(4):632–7.
18. Theodoropoulou M, Stalla GK. Somatostatin receptors: from signaling to clinical practice. Front Neuroendocrinol 2013;34(3):228–52.
19. Kvols LK, Moertel C, O'Connell M, et al. Treatment of the malignant carcinoid syndrome. Evaluation of a long-acting somatostatin analogue. N Engl J Med 1986;315(11):663–6.
20. Rubin J, Ajani J, Schirmer W, et al. Octreotide acetate long-acting formulation versus open-label subcutaneous octreotide acetate in malignant carcinoid syndrome. J Clin Oncol 1999;17(2):600–6.
21. Vinik AI, Wolin E, Liyanage N, et al. Evaluation of lanreotide depot/autogel efficacy and safety as a carcinoid syndrome treatment (elect): a randomized, double-blind, placebo-controlled trial. Endocr Pract 2016;22(9):1068–80.
22. Reubi JC, Kvols K, Waser B, et al. Detection of somatostatin receptors in surgical and percutaneous needle biopsy samples of carcinoids and islet cell carcinomas. Cancer Res 1990;50(18):5969–77.
23. Hirshberg B, Cochran C, Skarulis M, et al. Malignant insulinoma: spectrum of unusual clinical features. Cancer 2005;104(2):264–72.
24. Shojamanesh H, Gibril F, Louie A, et al. Prospective study of the antitumor efficacy of long-term octreotide treatment in patients with progressive metastatic gastrinoma. Cancer 2002;94(2):331–43.
25. Rinke A, Muller H, Schade-Brittinger C, et al. Placebo-controlled, double-blind, prospective, randomized study on the effect of octreotide LAR in the control of tumor growth in patients with metastatic neuroendocrine midgut tumors: a report from the PROMID Study Group. J Clin Oncol 2009;27(28): 4656–63.
26. Rinke A, Wittenberg M, Schade-Brittinger C, et al. Placebo-controlled, double-blind, prospective, randomized study on the effect of octreotide LAR in the control of tumor growth in patients with metastatic neuroendocrine midgut tumors (PROMID): results of long-term survival. Neuroendocrinology 2017; 104(1):26–32.
27. Caplin ME, Pavel M, Cwikla J, et al. Anti-tumour effects of lanreotide for pancreatic and intestinal neuroendocrine tumours: the CLARINET open-label

extension study. Endocr Relat Cancer 2016;23(3): 191–9.
28. Villard L, Romer A, Marincek N, et al. Cohort study of somatostatin-based radiopeptide therapy with [90Y-DOTA]-TOC versus [90Y-DOTA]-TOC plus [177Lu-DOTA]-TOC in neuroendocrine cancers. J Clin Oncol 2012;30(10):1100–6.
29. Strosberg J, El-Haddad G, Wolin E, et al. Phase 3 trial of ^{177}Lu-dotatate for midgut neuroendocrine tumors. N Engl J Med 2017;376(2):125–35.
30. Brabander T, van der Zwan W, Teunissen J, et al. Long-term efficacy, survival, and safety of octreotate in patients with gastroenteropancreatic and bronchial neuroendocrine tumors. Clin Cancer Res 2017;23(16):4617–24.
31. Food and Drug Administration. Summary of basis of approval - Lutathera (lutetium Lu 177 dotatate) injection 2018. Available at: https://www.accessdata.fda.gov/drugsatfda_docs/nda/2018/208700Orig1s000TOC.cfm.
32. Zhang J, Jia Z, Li Q, et al. Elevated expression of vascular endothelial growth factor correlates with increased angiogenesis and decreased progression-free survival among patients with low-grade neuroendocrine tumors. Cancer 2007; 109(8):1478–86.
33. Kulke MH, Lenz H, Meropol N, et al. Activity of sunitinib in patients with advanced neuroendocrine tumors. J Clin Oncol 2008;26(20):3403–10.
34. Raymond E, Dahan L, Raoul J, et al. Sunitinib malate for the treatment of pancreatic neuroendocrine tumors. N Engl J Med 2011;364(6):501–13.
35. Grande E, Capdevila J, Casteliano D, et al. Pazopanib in pretreated advanced neuroendocrine tumors: a phase II, open-label trial of the Spanish Task Force Group for Neuroendocrine Tumors (GETNE). Ann Oncol 2015;26(9):1987–93.
36. Capdevila J, Fazio N, Lopez C, et al. 1307OEfficacy of lenvatinib in patients with advanced pancreatic (panNETs) and gastrointestinal (giNETs) grade 1/2 (G1/G2) neuroendocrine tumors: Results of the international phase II TALENT trial (GETNE 1509). Ann Oncol 2018;29(suppl_8).
37. Chan JA, Faris J, Murphy J, et al. Phase II trial of cabozantinib in patients with carcinoid and pancreatic neuroendocrine tumors (pNET). J Clin Oncol 2017; 35(4_suppl):228.
38. Bergsland E, Mahoney M, Asmis T, et al. Prospective randomized phase II trial of pazopanib versus placebo in patients with progressive carcinoid tumors. JCO 2019;37(15 suppl):4005.
39. Yao JC, Phan A, Hoff P, et al. Targeting vascular endothelial growth factor in advanced carcinoid tumor: a random assignment phase II study of depot octreotide with bevacizumab and pegylated interferon alpha-2b. J Clin Oncol 2008;26(8): 1316–23.
40. Yao JC, Guthrie K, Moran C, et al. Phase III prospective randomized comparison trial of depot octreotide plus interferon alfa-2b versus depot octreotide plus bevacizumab in patients with advanced carcinoid tumors: SWOG S0518. J Clin Oncol 2017;35(15): 1695–703.
41. Ersahin T, Tuncbag N, Cetin-Atalay R. The PI3K/AKT/mTOR interactive pathway. Mol Biosyst 2015; 11(7):1946–54.
42. Zoncu R, Efeyan A, Sabatini DM. mTOR: from growth signal integration to cancer, diabetes and ageing. Nat Rev Mol Cell Biol 2011;12(1): 21–35.
43. Yao JC, Pavel M, Lombard-Bohas C, et al. Everolimus for the treatment of advanced pancreatic neuroendocrine tumors: overall survival and circulating biomarkers from the randomized, phase III RADIANT-3 study. J Clin Oncol 2016;34(32):3906–13.
44. Pavel ME, Baudin E, Oberg K, et al. Efficacy of everolimus plus octreotide LAR in patients with advanced neuroendocrine tumor and carcinoid syndrome: final overall survival from the randomized, placebo-controlled phase 3 RADIANT-2 study. Ann Oncol 2017;28(7):1569–75.
45. Yao JC, Fazio N, Singh S, et al. Everolimus for the treatment of advanced, non-functional neuroendocrine tumours of the lung or gastrointestinal tract (RADIANT-4): a randomised, placebo-controlled, phase 3 study. Lancet 2016;387(10022):968–77.
46. Moertel CG, Lefkopoulo M, Lipsitz S, et al. Streptozocin-doxorubicin, streptozocin-fluorouracil or chlorozotocin in the treatment of advanced islet-cell carcinoma. N Engl J Med 1992;326(8):519–23.
47. Kouvaraki MA, Ajani J, Hoff P, et al. Fluorouracil, doxorubicin, and streptozocin in the treatment of patients with locally advanced and metastatic pancreatic endocrine carcinomas. J Clin Oncol 2004; 22(23):4762–71.
48. Kunz PL, Catalano P, Nimeiri H, et al. A randomized study of temozolomide or temozolomide and capecitabine in patients with advanced pancreatic neuroendocrine tumors: a trial of the ECOG-ACRIN Cancer Research Group (E2211). J Clin Oncol 2018;36(15_suppl):4004.
49. Chan JA, Stuart K, Earle C, et al. Prospective study of bevacizumab plus temozolomide in patients with advanced neuroendocrine tumors. J Clin Oncol 2012;30(24):2963–8.
50. Chan JA, Blaszkowsky L, Stuart K, et al. A prospective, phase 1/2 study of everolimus and temozolomide in patients with advanced pancreatic neuroendocrine tumor. Cancer 2013;119(17): 3212–8.
51. Cives M, Ghayouri M, Morse B, et al. Analysis of potential response predictors to capecitabine/temozolomide in metastatic pancreatic neuroendocrine tumors. Endocr Relat Cancer 2016;23(9):759–67.

52. Kulke MH, Hornick J, Frauenhoffer C, et al. O6-methylguanine DNA methyltransferase deficiency and response to temozolomide-based therapy in patients with neuroendocrine tumors. Clin Cancer Res 2009; 15(1):338–45.
53. Walter T, van Brakel B, Vercherat C, et al. O6-Methylguanine-DNA methyltransferase status in neuroendocrine tumours: prognostic relevance and association with response to alkylating agents. Br J Cancer 2015;112(3):523–31.
54. Sorbye H, Welin S, Langer S, et al. Predictive and prognostic factors for treatment and survival in 305 patients with advanced gastrointestinal neuroendocrine carcinoma (WHO G3): the NORDIC NEC study. Ann Oncol 2013;24(1):152–60.
55. Yao JC, Fazio N, Pavel M, et al. 1308OActivity & safety of spartalizumab (PDR001) in patients (pts) with advanced neuroendocrine tumors (NET) of pancreatic (Pan), gastrointestinal (GI), or thoracic (T) origin, & gastroenteropancreatic neuroendocrine carcinoma (GEP NEC) who have progressed on prior treatment (Tx). Ann Oncol 2018;29(suppl_8).
56. Strosberg JR, Mizuno N, Doi T, et al. Pembrolizumab treatment of advanced neuroendocrine tumors: results from the phase II KEYNOTE-158 study. J Clin Oncol 2019;37(4_suppl):190.
57. Pavel M, Gross D, Benavent M, et al. Telotristat ethyl in carcinoid syndrome: safety and efficacy in the TELECAST phase 3 trial. Endocr Relat Cancer 2018;25(3):309–22.

Neuroendocrine Tumors of the Lung
Updates and Diagnostic Pitfalls

Yin P. Hung, MD, PhD

KEYWORDS

• Typical carcinoid • Atypical carcinoid • Small cell carcinoma • Large cell neuroendocrine carcinoma

Key points

- Primary neuroendocrine tumors of the lung include typical carcinoid, atypical carcinoid, small cell carcinoma, and large cell neuroendocrine carcinoma.
- Classification of pulmonary neuroendocrine tumors is based on mitotic count, necrosis, and cytologic features.
- Immunohistochemistry can help to exclude mimics and confirm neuroendocrine differentiation but should be applied in the context of appropriate histology.
- Although not part of the criteria in classifying pulmonary neuroendocrine tumors, Ki-67 labeling index can be helpful in diagnostic conundrums, including crushed biopsies.
- Pulmonary neuroendocrine tumors are characterized by distinct genetic alterations, although the clinical utility of molecular classification remains to be established.

ABSTRACT

Neuroendocrine tumors of the lung constitute approximately 20% of all primary lung tumors and include typical carcinoid, atypical carcinoid, small cell carcinoma, and large cell neuroendocrine carcinoma. Given their morphologic overlap with diverse mimics, neuroendocrine tumors of the lung can be diagnostically challenging. This review discusses the clinical, histologic, immunophenotypic, and molecular features of pulmonary neuroendocrine tumors, along with common diagnostic pitfalls and strategies for avoidance.

OVERVIEW

Pulmonary neuroendocrine tumors, as encountered routinely in surgical pathology, comprise 4 categories: typical carcinoid (TC), atypical carcinoid (AC), small cell lung carcinoma (SCLC), and large cell neuroendocrine carcinoma (LCNEC).[1] TC, AC, and SCLC/LCNEC are analogous to grades 1, 2, and 3 neuroendocrine tumors in other sites, respectively.[2] This nomenclature, although different from those in other sites and perhaps unfamiliar to nonspecialists, is used in ongoing patient management and research in thoracic oncology. The pathologic diagnosis of pulmonary neuroendocrine tumors is based primarily on histomorphology. Once its neuroendocrine nature is recognized, the tumor is classified into TC, AC, SCLC, or LCNEC based on mitotic activity, the extent of necrosis, and cytologic features (**Table 1**). Mitotic activity is assessed by counting mitoses within the tumor in an area of 2 mm^2, which, depending on the microscope/eyepieces used, translates to 8.3 to 10 high-power fields (at 40× objective).[3]

The diagnosis and classification of pulmonary neuroendocrine tumors can be challenging for

Disclosure Statement: No disclosure.
Department of Pathology, Massachusetts General Hospital, Harvard Medical School, 55 Fruit Street, Boston, MA 02114, USA
E-mail address: yphung@mgh.harvard.edu

Surgical Pathology 12 (2019) 1055–1071
https://doi.org/10.1016/j.path.2019.08.012

Table 1
Overview of pulmonary neuroendocrine tumors

		Typical Carcinoid	Atypical Carcinoid	Small Cell Carcinoma	Large Cell Neuroendocrine Carcinoma
	Grade	**Low**	**Intermediate**	**High**	**High**
Clinical features	Prevalence (% of lung tumors)	1%–2%	~0.2%	10%–15%	2%–3%
	Typical presentation	Solitary nodule	Solitary nodule	Extensive bulky disease	Variable
	Association with smoking	No	No	Yes	Yes
	Overall survival at 5 y	>90%	50%–80%	5%	15%–40%
Histologic criteria	Necrosis	None	Focal or none[a]	Variable (often extensive)	Variable (often extensive)
	Mitoses (per 2 mm^2)	0–1	$\leq$10[a]	$\geq$11	$\geq$11
	Cytologic features	Non–small cell	Non–small cell	Small cell	Non–small cell
IHC	Neuroendocrine marker expression	Diffuse strong	Diffuse strong	Variable	Variable
	Ki-67 LI	<20% (often <5%)	<20%	>50% (often >80%)	$\geq$20% (often approximately 40%–60%)
	Percent of cases with RB1 complete loss	0%	0%	>95%	Approximately 50%
	TTF-1 expression indicative of lung primary	Yes	Yes	No	No
Molecular	Recurrent mutations	*MEN1, ARID1A, PSIP1*		*TP53, RB1*	Variable (subtype-dependent)

[a] AC is defined by having mitoses of 2 to 10 per 2 mm^2 and/or presence of necrosis.

the following reasons. First, their neuroendocrine nature may be difficult to recognize, particularly in small biopsies and intraoperative frozen sections. Second, bona fide mitoses and pyknotic nuclei may look alike, and necrosis may be focal and easily overlooked; thus, tumors that are borderline between categories may be difficult to classify. Third, whether the tumor represents a primary or metastasis may not be apparent clinically. Because these classification criteria are designed specifically for primary neuroendocrine tumors of the lung, it is unclear how these criteria should be applied on metastases in other sites. Not surprisingly, diagnostic disagreements occur among thoracic pathologists in a subset of cases, including distinction between TC and AC[4] and between SCLC and LCNEC.[5–7]

Immunohistochemistry can be helpful in confirming neuroendocrine differentiation. This should be applied, however, in the context of appropriate histology,[8] because each of the commonly used neuroendocrine markers (synaptophysin, chromogranin, and CD56) is not entirely specific for neuroendocrine tumors and can be expressed in up to approximately 30% of lung adenocarcinoma and squamous cell carcinoma[9] as well as other tumors, including metastatic carcinomas from breast, prostate, and other sites. To exclude histologic mimics, immunohistochemistry nonetheless can be valuable.

Unlike neuroendocrine tumors in other sites, Ki-67 labeling index (Ki-67 LI) is not part of the diagnostic criteria for pulmonary neuroendocrine tumors.[2] Ki-67 LI is typically less than 5% in TC, less than 20% in AC, and greater than or equal to 20% in LCNEC/SCLC.[10,11] Ki-67 LI overlaps, however, between TC and AC, between AC and LCNEC, and between LCNEC and SCLC. In TC, compared with those with a Ki-67 LI of less than 5%, those with a Ki-67 LI of greater than or equal to 5% harbor worse prognosis, although both groups remain more indolent than AC.[12] Whether Ki-67 LI imparts additional value to histologic assessment in pulmonary neuroendocrine tumors remains an ongoing debate. Nonetheless, Ki-67 LI can be helpful in certain diagnostic conundrums, such as limited specimens or crushed biopsies, in which mitotic count is practically unfeasible; Ki-67 LI of less than 20% and greater than or equal to 20% favor carcinoid tumors and LCNEC/SCLC, respectively.[10,11]

Next-generation sequencing has increasingly been used to characterize the genetic alterations of pulmonary neuroendocrine tumors, with distinct patterns of mutations found in TC/AC, SCLC, and LCNEC.[13–17] The clinical utility of molecular testing in classifying pulmonary neuroendocrine tumors, however, remains to be established.

TYPICAL CARCINOID

OVERVIEW

Accounting for 1% to 2% of all lung tumors, TC is not associated with smoking history and presents with a wide age range, most commonly in middle-aged patients.[1,18–20] A higher incidence of TC has been reported in those with multiple endocrine neoplasia type 1 (MEN1) syndrome.[21] Some patients present with recurrent pneumonias due to bronchial obstruction, others are asymptomatic, and a small subset (<5%) presents with carcinoid syndrome (in particular those with liver metastases), Cushing syndrome, and other paraneoplastic syndromes.[21] Genetically, a subset of TC harbors recurrent mutations in *MEN1* and other chromatin regulators, such as *ARID1A* and *PSIP1*, whereas mutations in tumor suppressors *RB1* and *TP53* that are common in SCLC/LCNEC are mostly absent.[13,16]

GROSS FEATURES

TC is well circumscribed, round to ovoid or polypoid, and often located near the airways, thus amenable to endobronchial sampling. A small subset of TC is peripheral.

MICROSCOPIC FEATURES

TC is characterized by variably epithelioid-to-spindle cells, generally low-grade nuclei, finely granular chromatin, and inconspicuous nucleoli, although these features can be obscured in crushed biopsies or intraoperative frozen sections (**Fig. 1**A–D). In these instances, its recognition relies on the architecture, with admixture of organoid, solid, trabecular, pseudoglandular, palisading, rosette, or papillary patterns.[22] Scattered cells with characteristic endocrine atypia can be seen focally. Oncocytic morphology has been noted in rare cases.[22,23]

DIAGNOSIS

TC is at least 0.5 cm, exhibits no necrosis, and harbors 0 to 1 mitosis per 2 mm^2. In addition to its neuroendocrine features apparent by light microscopy, TC typically demonstrates strong expression of synaptophysin and chromogranin (**Fig. 1**E). Thyroid transcription factor-1 (TTF-1) expression can be seen in a subset of TC, perhaps more often in peripheral than central tumors.[24] Ki-67 LI is low, often less than 5%, but certainly less than 20% (**Fig. 1**F).[10–12]

DIFFERENTIAL DIAGNOSIS

The chief differential diagnosis of TC is AC, given their shared clinicopathologic features. Unlike

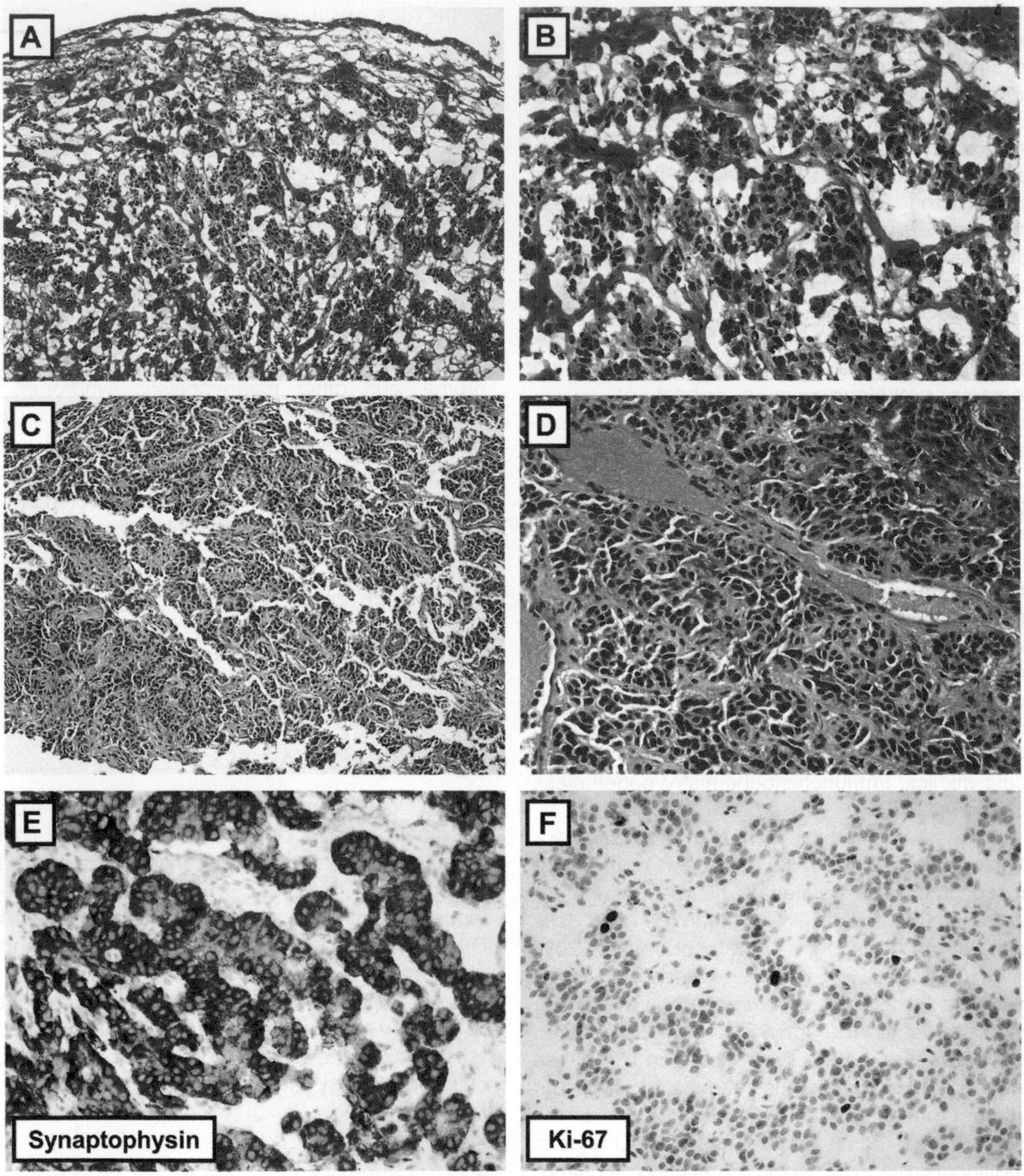

Fig. 1. TC of lung. (*A*) In frozen sections, while the cytologic features can be difficult to assess, diagnostic clues include vague lobulation at low power and frequently a peribronchial location (hematoxylin-eosin, original magnification ×200). (*B*) Tumor cells are generally uniform (hematoxylin-eosin, original magnification ×400). While the findings favor a carcinoid, distinction between TC and AC should be deferred to permanents. (*C*) TC is characterized by neuroendocrine architecture and epithelioid-to-spindle cells (hematoxylin-eosin, original magnification ×200). (*D*) TC shows no necrosis and 0-1 mitosis per 2 mm^2 (hematoxylin-eosin, original magnification ×400). (*E*) Diffuse synaptophysin immunoreactivity is often present (original magnification ×400). (*F*) Ki-67 labeling index in a TC is low, often <5% and universally <20% (original magnification ×400).

TC, AC demonstrates necrosis and/or increased mitoses of 2 to 10 per 2 mm^2. TC should only be diagnosed in a resection, with the tumor entirely submitted for histologic evaluation. A biopsy or frozen section that shows features consistent with TC may represent AC with diagnostic areas not been sampled; the diagnosis in this case should thus be carcinoid tumor, with distinction between TC and AC deferred to resection if available.

TC is at least 0.5 cm, whereas a carcinoid tumorlet is less than 0.5 cm; both invade beyond the basement membrane of the bronchiolar wall, whereas neuroendocrine cell hyperplasia remains confined within the basement membrane. Carcinoid tumorlets and neuroendocrine cell hyperplasia are incidental findings commonly seen in the background lung, including adjacent to approximately 25% of carcinoid tumors.[25] Nonetheless, the presence of multifocal neuroendocrine cell hyperplasia and multiple carcinoid tumorlets suggests diffuse idiopathic neuroendocrine cell hyperplasia (DIPNECH), a condition defined in 1 study as neuroendocrine cell hyperplasia with at least 3 carcinoid tumorlets.[26] In DIPNECH, multiple carcinoid tumors/tumorlets develop synchronously and do not represent intrapulmonary metastases.

Metastases from neuroendocrine tumors of other sites, in particular those that are low-grade, can mimic TC. For low-grade neuroendocrine tumors, transcription factors TTF-1, CDX-2, and PDX-1 are considered site-specific for lung, gastrointestinal, and pancreatic origins, respectively, and can be used for distinction.[27] PAX8 can be useful, because it is expressed in a subset of neuroendocrine tumors from pancreatic, gastrointestinal, and thymic origins but rarely pulmonary carcinoids.[28,29] Given the site-specific behavior and clinical management, distinction between primary pulmonary neuroendocrine tumor and metastasis is important.[2]

Medullary thyroid carcinoma can share histologic and immunophenotypic overlap with pulmonary carcinoids, with TTF-1 expression common in both. Although PAX8 and calcitonin are expressed in most medullary thyroid carcinomas but only rare pulmonary carcinoids,[29,30] distinction between metastatic medullary thyroid carcinoma and a calcitonin-secreting pulmonary carcinoid can be particularly problematic and requires radiologic correlation and additional markers, such as carcinoembryonic antigen (CEA), serotonin, and bombesin.[31]

PROGNOSIS

TC is treated by surgical excision, with a 5-year overall survival of greater than 90%.[3,18,19] A subset (approximately 10%) of patients with TC demonstrates metastases (most commonly nodal),[19,32,33] although their prognosis generally remains favorable. Treatment options for unresectable/metastatic TC include somatostatin analog (octreotide and lantreotide), mTOR inhibitor (everolimus),[34] and peptide receptor radionuclide therapy; there is no consensus to date on the use of chemotherapy.[35]

Key Features of Typical Carcinoid

- Low-grade neuroendocrine tumor of lung with a size of at least 0.5 cm
- Epithelioid-to-spindle cells in an organoid to trabecular or papillary pattern
- Zero to 1 mitosis per 2 mm^2 and no necrosis
- Multifocal to diffuse immunoreactivity for synaptophysin and chromogranin
- Ki-67 LI less than 20% (often <5%)

Pitfalls Diagnosing Typical Carcinoid

! Diagnosis should be made only in resection with the tumor entirely submitted and deferred in biopsies, cytology, and frozen sections (with differentials including AC).

! In intraoperative consultation for a lung mass, beware of carcinoid and do not reflexively diagnose non-small cell lung carcinoma (NSCLC). Although cytologic features may be hard to assess, clues include a vaguely nested architecture and often a peribronchial location. Communicate with the surgeon regarding a possibility of carcinoid tumor as this can alter intraoperative management

! Do not interpret prior biopsy site changes as tumor necrosis.

Differential Diagnosis of Typical Carcinoid

- AC
  - Two to 10 mitoses per 2 mm^2 and/or necrosis (which can be subtle requiring careful search)
- Carcinoid tumorlet
  - Size less than 0.5 cm, with no necrosis
- SCLC
  - Small cell cytomorphology, with nuclear molding and scant cytoplasm
  - Greater than or equal to 11 mitoses per 2 mm^2 with minimal to extensive geographic necrosis

- ○ Synaptophysin and chromogranin immunoreactivity variable and often focal
- ○ Ki-67 LI greater than 50% (particularly useful in crushed specimens)
- • Metastasis from gastrointestinal or pancreatic neuroendocrine tumor
  - ○ Supportive clinical and/or radiographic findings
  - ○ Expresses CDX-2 or PDX-1
  - ○ Lack of TTF-1 immunoreactivity in low-grade tumors
- • Metastatic medullary thyroid carcinoma
  - ○ Supportive clinical and/or radiographic findings
  - ○ Positive for TTF-1, PAX8, calcitonin, and CEA
  - ○ Negative for serotonin and bombesin

ATYPICAL CARCINOID

OVERVIEW

AC is approximately 10-fold less common than TC and comprises approximately 0.2% of all lung tumors. Similar to TC, AC shows a predilection for middle-aged patients, with no established association with smoking.[1,18–20] Patients present incidentally or with signs of bronchial obstruction, rarely with carcinoid syndrome in the setting of liver metastases or other paraneoplastic syndromes.[21] Genomic studies have identified recurrent mutations in epigenetic regulators *MEN1*, *PSIP1*, and *ARID1A* in a subset of AC, whereas mutations in tumor suppressors, including *RB1* and *TP53*, are largely absent.[13,16]

GROSS FEATURES

Typically well-circumscribed, AC is located centrally near the airways or peripherally. Even if present microscopically, necrosis is often not apparent grossly.

MICROSCOPIC FEATURES

AC is characterized by variably epithelioid-to-spindle cells with a neuroendocrine architecture, with organoid, solid, trabecular, pseudoglandular, palisading, and/or papillary patterns, similar to those seen in TC (**Fig. 2**A). Occasional nucleoli may be prominent. If present, necrosis can be patchy and subtle (**Fig. 2**B).

DIAGNOSIS

AC exhibits 2 to 10 mitoses per 2 mm^2 and/or necrosis.[1,3] By immunohistochemistry, AC is typically positive for synaptophysin and chromogranin, with TTF-1 expression noted in a subset of cases.[24] Although not a formal diagnostic criterion, Ki-67 LI is less than 20%.[10–12]

DIFFERENTIAL DIAGNOSIS

Morphologic mimics of AC include other pulmonary neuroendocrine tumors (TC, carcinoid-like LCNEC, and SCLC) as well as metastasis and other rare tumors.

AC is histologically akin to TC, albeit with increased mitoses and/or necrosis (see **Table 1**). Necrosis can be focal and easily missed, requiring thorough sampling and careful search. LCNEC can rarely show a carcinoid-like morphology, mimicking AC[36]; however, its mitotic count of greater than or equal to 11 per 2 mm^2 would by

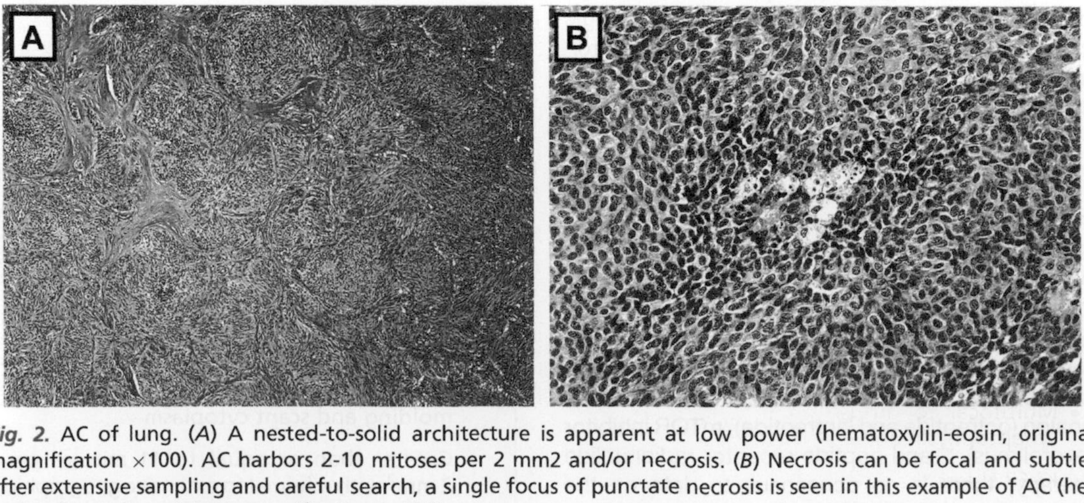

Fig. 2. AC of lung. (*A*) A nested-to-solid architecture is apparent at low power (hematoxylin-eosin, original magnification ×100). AC harbors 2-10 mitoses per 2 mm2 and/or necrosis. (*B*) Necrosis can be focal and subtle; after extensive sampling and careful search, a single focus of punctate necrosis is seen in this example of AC (hematoxylin-eosin, original magnification ×400).

definition exclude AC. Albeit rare, carcinoid tumors with crush artifact can be mistaken for SCLC. Ki-67 LI of less than 20% and greater than 50% is noted in carcinoid tumors and SCLC, respectively.[10,11]

Metastases from gastrointestinal or pancreatic neuroendocrine tumors can mimic AC. Correlation with radiologic findings as well as a panel of immunohistochemical stains, including TTF-1, CDX-2, and PDX-1,[27] can aid the distinction and primary site determination. Furthermore, synaptophysin, chromogranin, and CD56 are not entirely specific; each can be expressed in diverse tumors, including metastatic carcinoma from breast (**Fig. 3**) or prostate, melanoma, and rare cases of Ewing sarcoma, all of which may be misdiagnosed as AC.[37,38]

Finally, the diagnosis of metastatic AC in other sites, such as liver, can be difficult. With entrapped bile ductules, the tumor may simulate the appearance of a metastatic adenocarcinoma. Also, how the classification criteria (based on mitotic count and necrosis) should be applied to metastases remains unclear; a metastasis with mitoses slightly greater than or equal to 11 per 2 mm^2 may originate from AC, rendering its distinction from LCNEC challenging based on these metastasis specimens alone.[39]

PROGNOSIS

AC has a 5-year overall survival of 50% to 80%, with distant metastases in up to 50% of AC.[3,18,19,32,33] The adverse outcome compared with TC highlights the importance of distinguishing AC from TC. AC is treated by surgical excision, whereas treatment options for unresectable or metastatic AC include somatostatin analog (octreotide and lantreotide), mTOR inhibitor everolimus,[34] peptide receptor radionuclide therapy, and chemotherapy.[35]

Key Features of Atypical Carcinoid

- Intermediate-grade neuroendocrine tumor of lung, with some clinicopathologic similarities to TC
- Epithelioid-to-spindle cells in an organoid to trabecular or papillary pattern
- Two to 10 mitoses per 2 mm^2 and/or necrosis
- Multifocal to diffuse immunoreactivity for synaptophysin and chromogranin
- Ki-67 LI less than 20%

Pitfalls Diagnosing Atypical Carcinoid

! Necrosis can be focal and subtle, requiring thorough sampling and careful search to distinguish AC from TC.

! Metastatic pulmonary carcinoid tumor in other sites, such as liver, can entrap adjacent bile ductules and be mistaken for metastatic adenocarcinoma.

! Synaptophysin and chromogranin are not specific for AC and are expressed in metastatic neuroendocrine tumors of other sites, metastatic carcinoma (see **Fig. 3**), melanoma, rare Ewing sarcoma, and others. Recognition requires select immunohistochemical stains, correlation with radiologic findings, and a high index of suspicion.

Differential Diagnosis of Atypical Carcinoid

- TC
  - Zero to 1 mitosis per 2 mm^2 and lack of necrosis
- SCLC
  - Small cell cytomorphology, with nuclear molding and scant cytoplasm
  - Greater than or equal to 11 mitoses per 2 mm^2 with minimal to extensive geographic necrosis
  - Synaptophysin and chromogranin immunoreactivity variable and often focal
  - Ki-67 LI greater than 50% (particularly useful in crushed specimens)
- LCNEC
  - High-grade NSCLC with neuroendocrine histology and evidence of neuroendocrine differentiation (by ultrastructural and/or immunohistochemical studies)
  - Greater than or equal to 11 mitoses per 2 mm^2
- Metastasis from gastrointestinal or pancreatic neuroendocrine tumor
  - Supportive clinical and/or radiographic findings
  - Expresses CDX-2 (gastrointestinal) or PDX-1 (pancreatic)
  - Lack of TTF-1 immunoreactivity in low-grade tumors

- Metastatic medullary thyroid carcinoma
  - Supportive clinical and/or radiographic findings
  - Positive for TTF-1, PAX8, calcitonin, and CEA
  - Negative for serotonin and bombesin
- Metastatic carcinoma from breast or prostate
  - Supportive clinical and/or radiographic findings
  - Expresses mammaglobin/GATA3 (breast) or PSA/PSAP/NKX3.1 (prostate)
  - Lack of TTF-1 immunoreactivity
- Metastatic melanoma
  - Supportive clinical and/or radiographic findings
  - Expresses S-100, SOX10, HMB45, and/or other melanocytic markers
  - Lack of TTF-1 or keratin immunoreactivity
- Ewing sarcoma
  - Small round blue cell tumor with generally uniform nuclei
  - Expresses CD99 in a diffuse fashion and NKX2.2
  - Harbors *EWSR1* or *FUS* gene rearrangement

SMALL CELL CARCINOMA

OVERVIEW

SCLC constitutes 10% to 15% of all lung cancers and affects primarily heavy smokers,[40] with less than 2% of patients being nonsmokers.[41] SCLC is highly aggressive; most patients present with extensive disease, with bulky mediastinal involvement and metastases to liver, bone, brain, and/or other sites.[42] A subset of patients presents with paraneoplastic syndromes, such as syndrome of inappropriate antidiuretic hormone secretion and other paraneoplastic syndromes.[21] Localized solitary SCLC has been described in a small subset of patients.[43]

Genetically, SCLC is characterized in nearly all cases by biallelic inactivation of *TP53* and *RB1*.[14,44–47] Diverse copy-number alterations, including amplification of *MYC* family genes, are seen in a subset of tumors.[14] SCLC most commonly arises de novo but can arise as part of the resistance mechanism in a subset of patients with *EGFR*-mutant lung adenocarcinoma treated with tyrosine kinase inhibitor.[48,49]

GROSS FEATURES

Although seldom resected, SCLC is fleshy, with poorly marginated to infiltrative borders and prominent necrosis.

MICROSCOPIC FEATURES

The prototypical appearance of SCLC is sheets of blue cells with scant cytoplasm and nuclear molding,[50] often with crush artifact, prominent geographic necrosis, and focal desmoplastic stroma. In noncrushed areas, multiple mitoses can be seen in each high-power field. Nonetheless, tumor cells in SCLC may appear larger in resections[43] or frozen sections (**Fig. 4**), precluding their recognition by those unfamiliar with this histologic pattern.

DIAGNOSIS

Although diagnosis of SCLC can be rendered in cases with prototypical histology, immunohistochemistry has been shown to improve concordance among pathologists[7] and can be helpful for diagnostic confirmation, particularly in cases of unusual clinical history (eg, never smoker) or suboptimal (limited or crushed) specimens. SCLC shows variable expression of TTF-1, synaptophysin, chromogranin (**Fig. 5**A–C), and CD56; nonetheless, absence of neuroendocrine marker expression does not exclude SCLC and is noted in up to approximately 25% of cases.[51] Keratin staining is variable and may be dotlike when present. Napsin A and p40 are generally negative (**Fig. 5**D). Ki-67 LI is greater than 50%, typically greater than 80 to 90% (**Fig. 5**E).[10,11] Loss of RB1 expression is seen in nearly all SCLC, with intact nuclear staining in the control stromal cells (**Fig. 5**F).[52]

DIFFERENTIAL DIAGNOSIS

SCLC can be confused with diverse mimics: basaloid squamous cell carcinoma (including NUT carcinoma), poorly differentiated adenocarcinoma, other pulmonary neuroendocrine tumors (carcinoid tumors and LCNEC), and other small round blue cell tumors (melanoma, lymphoma, Merkel cell carcinoma, Ewing sarcoma, poorly differentiated synovial sarcoma, and desmoplastic small round cell tumor).

Distinction between SCLC and NSCLC (LCNEC, adenocarcinoma, and squamous cell carcinoma) is usually straightforward, based on the gestalt assessment of cytologic and architectural features. On low power, SCLC appears blue, whereas most NSCLCs (aside from basaloid squamous cell carcinoma) look pink. Features that favor SCLC include nuclear molding, scant cytoplasm, and inconspicuous nucleoli, whereas features that favor

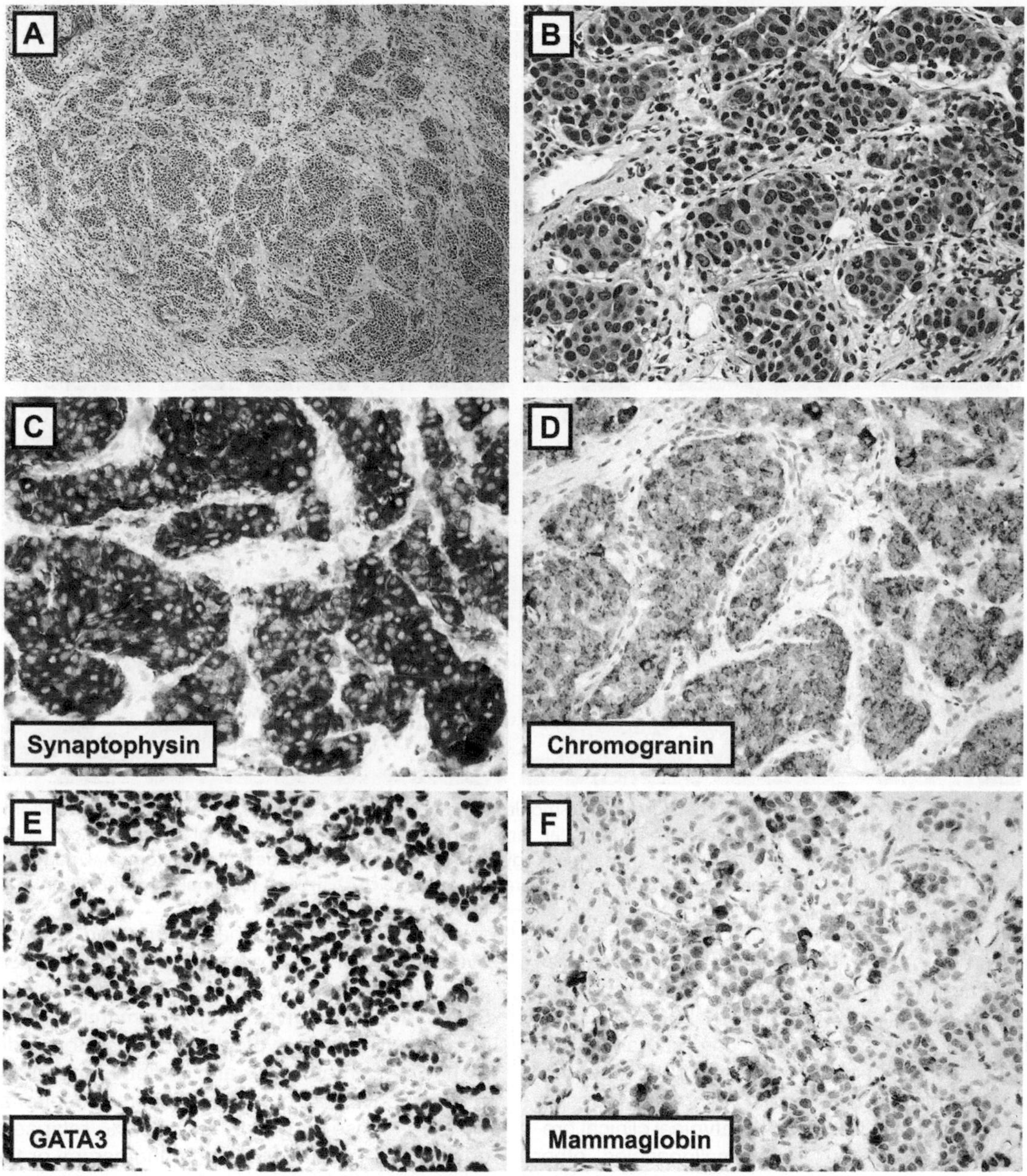

Fig. 3. Metastatic breast carcinoma mimicking a pulmonary neuroendocrine tumor. (*A*) This lung nodule is characterized by a lobular architecture, reminiscent of a carcinoid tumor (hematoxylin-eosin, original magnification ×100). (*B*) Tumor cells are arranged in small nests, with occasional hyperchromatic nuclei and variably conspicuous nucleoli (hematoxylin-eosin, original magnification ×400). (*C*) This tumor shows diffuse synaptophysin expression (original magnification ×400). (*D*) Diffuse cytoplasmic granular chromogranin immunoreactivity is present (original magnification ×400). However, the presence of (*E*) diffuse nuclear GATA3 (original magnification ×400) and (*F*) focal mammaglobin expression (original magnification ×400), along with the clinical history (breast cancer), confirms the diagnosis of metastatic breast carcinoma.

NSCLC include nuclear palisading, abundant eosinophilic cytoplasm, and conspicuous nucleoli. Nevertheless, some tumors lie in a morphologic continuum between SCLC and LCNEC with significant interobserver variability in their classification.[6,7,53] Despite its resemblance to SCLC, basaloid squamous cell carcinoma is negative for neuroendocrine markers and is instead positive for p40, p63, and CK5/6. In approximately 25% of SCLCs, an associated NSCLC component is present; these tumors are classified as combined SCLC.[18,43]

In suboptimal specimens with limited quantity and/or distorted by significant crush artifact, a diagnosis of SCLC should be rendered particularly

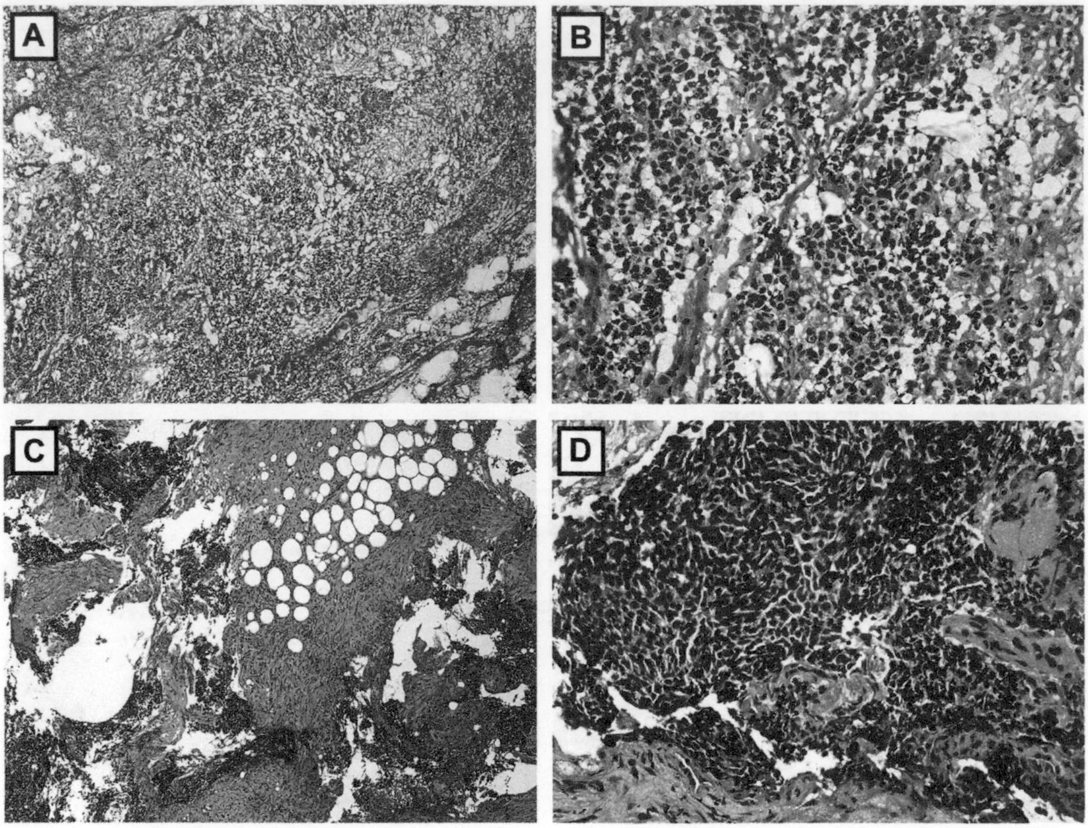

Fig. 4. SCLC. (*A*) In frozen sections, background desmoplasia may be seen but can be variable and subtle (original magnification ×100). (*B*) The nuclei of SCLC appear larger and relatively intact (original magnification ×400). (*C*) Permanents of the same case show prototypical histology, with prominent stromal desmoplasia (original magnification ×100), along with (*D*) nuclear molding, scant cytoplasm, and variable crush artifact (original magnification ×400).

with caution, because similar histologic appearance may be seen in carcinoid tumors[10] or even collections of lymphocytes. Immunohistochemical studies, including Ki-67 LI, are helpful for distinction. Also, synaptophysin, chromogranin, and CD56 each can be expressed in a subset of other small round blue cell tumors, which can represent a diagnostic pitfall. In cases of atypical clinical presentation or history of prior malignancies, other immunohistochemical markers and molecular testing may be considered to exclude melanoma (S-100, SOX10, and HMB45), lymphoma (CD45, CD3, and CD20), Merkel cell carcinoma (CK20), Ewing sarcoma (CD99, NKX2.2, *EWSR1* and *FUS* gene rearrangements), poorly differentiated synovial sarcoma (TLE1 and *SS18* gene rearrangement), and desmoplastic small round cell tumor (*EWSR1* gene rearrangement).[7,54]

PROGNOSIS

SCLC can be staged as limited (with disease confined to a radiation port) or extensive.[42] The prognosis of SCLC is dismal, with a median overall survival of less than 1 year and a 5-year overall survival of approximately 5% with extensive disease.[3,18] Localized SCLC has a higher 5-year overall survival of approximately 35%.[18] Treatment regimen typically includes etoposide/platinum chemotherapy and radiotherapy, along with prophylactic cranial radiation. Despite an initial response of greater than 50%, relapse is common. Clinical trials on immunotherapy or targeting poly (ADP-ribose) polymerase in SCLC are ongoing.[55,56]

Key Features of Small Cell Carcinoma

- High-grade neuroendocrine carcinoma, nearly all with biallelic inactivation of *TP53* and *RB1*
- Predilection for smokers, often with bulky disease and metastases at presentation
- Sheets of blue tumor cells with scant cytoplasm, nuclear molding, and frequent crush artifact

- Greater than or equal to 11 mitoses per 2 mm^2 with minimal to extensive geographic necrosis
- Synaptophysin, chromogranin, and CD56 staining variable and often focal; keratin staining variable and sometimes dotlike; complete loss of RB1 expression in most cases
- Ki-67 LI greater than 50% (often >80%–90%)

Pitfalls in Diagnosing Small Cell Carcinoma

! A nonspecific diagnosis of high-grade neuroendocrine carcinoma often is insufficient in thoracic oncology, because treatments of SCLC and LCNEC differ.

! Diagnose SCLC with caution, particularly in crushed specimens where mitoses and cytologic details are difficult to assess. Immunohistochemistry including Ki-67 LI can help to exclude a crushed carcinoid tumor.

! In frozen sections and resections, tumor cells in SCLC may appear larger with no apparent nuclear molding.

! Staining of neuroendocrine markers, in particular chromogranin, can be focal and requires evaluation at high power.

! TTF-1 expression is not indicative of lung primary for high-grade neuroendocrine tumors, including SCLC. SCLCs originating at other sites, such as prostate and cervix, often express TTF-1.

Differential Diagnosis of Small Cell Carcinoma

- Basaloid squamous cell carcinoma
  - Expresses p40, p63, and CK5/6
  - Lack of synaptophysin or chromogranin expression in most cases
- NUT carcinoma
  - Aggressive variant of poorly differentiated squamous cell carcinoma
  - Monomorphic primitive-appearing cells; abrupt keratinization may be present
  - Nuclear NUT expression, with variable expression of keratin, p40, p63, TTF-1, CD34, and CD99
  - Harbors *NUT* gene rearrangement, with fusion to *BRD4* in most cases
- Poorly differentiated lung adenocarcinoma
  - Diverse histologic patterns, including solid and cribriform
  - Expresses napsin A in a subset of cases
  - Mucicarmine stain may highlight focal mucin consistent with glandular differentiation.
- Carcinoid tumors
  - Necrosis at most focal and generally not extensive
  - Zero to 10 mitoses per 2 mm^2
  - Show diffuse strong staining for synaptophysin and chromogranin in most cases
  - Ki-67 LI less than 20%
- LCNEC
  - High-grade tumor with neuroendocrine histology and evidence of neuroendocrine differentiation
  - Non–small cell cytomorphology, with nuclear palisading, abundant eosinophilic cytoplasm, and conspicuous nucleoli
  - Intact RB1 expression in approximately 50% of cases
- Melanoma
  - Supportive clinical and/or radiographic findings
  - Expresses S-100, SOX10, HMB45, and/or other melanocytic markers
  - Lack of TTF-1 or keratin immunoreactivity
- Lymphoma
  - Sheets of discohesive tumor cells
  - Expresses lymphoid markers and lacks immunoreactivity for TTF-1 or keratins
- Ewing sarcoma
  - Small round blue cell tumor with generally uniform nuclei
  - Expresses CD99 in a diffuse fashion and NKX2.2
  - Harbors *EWSR1* or *FUS* gene rearrangement
- Desmoplastic small round cell tumor
  - Typically presents in young patients with extensive peritoneal disease
  - Nests and trabeculae of crushed small blue cells admixed with prominent desmoplastic stroma
  - Polyphenotypic, with variable expression of keratins, desmin, neuron-specific enolase (NSE), synaptophysin, and chromogranin
  - Harbors *EWSR1* gene rearrangement

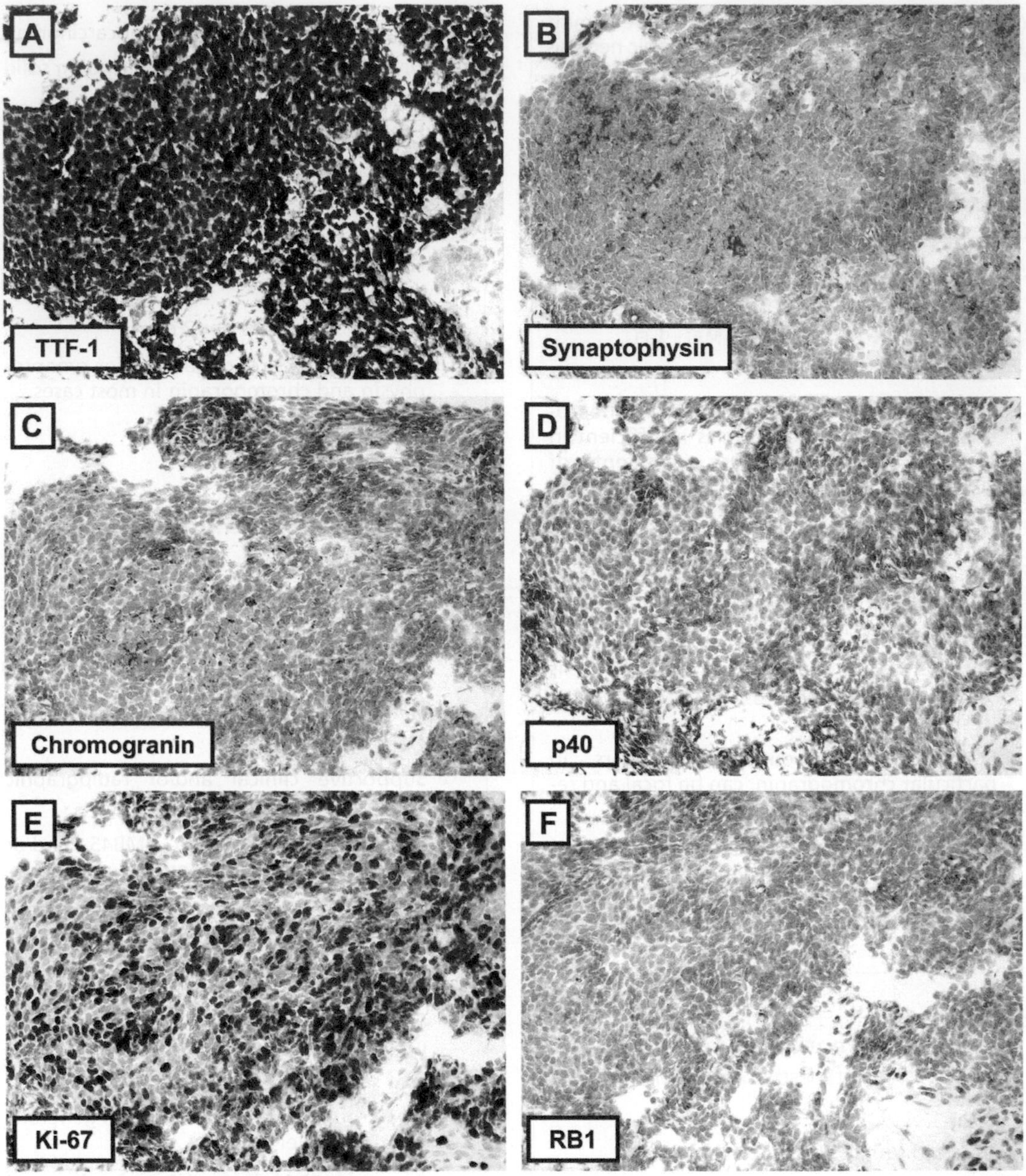

Fig. 5. Immunohistochemistry for SCLC. (*A*) TTF-1 expression is variable and, when present, accentuates the appearance of nuclear molding (original magnification ×400). (*B–C*) Synaptophysin immunoreactivity (original magnification ×400) and chromogranin immunoreactivity (original magnification ×400) can be variable and focal, requiring evaluation at high power. (*D*) p40 is negative (original magnification ×400). (*E*) Ki-67 labeling index is useful and typically >50% in SCLC (original magnification ×400). (*F*) Complete loss of RB1 expression is seen in nearly all cases (original magnification ×400).

LARGE CELL NEUROENDOCRINE CARCINOMA

OVERVIEW

LCNEC is a highly aggressive non–small cell lung tumor showing neuroendocrine features histologically with evidence of neuroendocrine differentiation.[1,22] Accounting for 1% to 3% of all lung tumors, LCNEC has a predilection for the elderly, men, and smokers.[57,58] Mutations in *TP53*, *RB1*, and *STK11/KEAP1* are overall present in approximately 80% to 90%, 40% to 50%, and 20% to 30% of LCNEC, respectively.[15,17,59] Nonetheless, LCNEC comprises multiple distinct molecular subgroups: SCLC-like (with recurrent biallelic inactivating mutations in *TP53* and *RB1*), NSCLC-like (with recurrent mutations in *KRAS*, *STK11*, and *KEAP1*), and carcinoid-like (with recurrent *MEN1* mutations).[15,17]

GROSS FEATURES

LCNEC can be solitary or multiple, with poor margination, fleshy cut surface, and necrosis.

MICROSCOPIC FEATURES

LCNEC is histologically characterized by an organoid, solid, lobular to trabecular architecture; tumor cells typically show moderate eosinophilic cytoplasm, coarse chromatin, variably prominent nucleoli, with variable pleomorphism. Geographic necrosis and conspicuous mitoses are apparent (**Fig. 6**A, B).

DIAGNOSIS

A diagnosis of LCNEC requires the fulfillment of all 4 criteria: (1) the presence of neuroendocrine features by light microscopy; (2) the presence of neuroendocrine differentiation, as confirmed by electron microscopy (detection of dense-core granules) and/or immunohistochemistry (expression of synaptophysin, chromogranin, and/or CD56 [**Fig. 6**C, D]); (3) greater than or equal to 11 mitoses per 2 mm^2; and (4) non–small cell cytomorphology, with low nuclear-to-cytoplasmic ratio, eosinophilic cytoplasm, and prominent nucleoli.[1,22] By immunohistochemistry, LCNEC is positive for chromogranin and CD56 in greater than 80% of cases, and synaptophysin and TTF-1 in approximately 40 to 50% of cases.[1,22]

Although a definitive diagnosis of LCNEC can be rendered in resections, it can be challenging in biopsies or cytology specimens; final classification in this instance should be deferred to resection if available, and a diagnosis of NSCLC with neuroendocrine morphology and positive neuroendocrine markers, possible LCNEC is sufficient.[60] Nonetheless, LCNEC may be suspected in biopsies when the tumor shows high-grade neuroendocrine features with no overt squamous or glandular differentiation and expresses more than one neuroendocrine marker (synaptophysin, chromogranin, and/or CD56).[9]

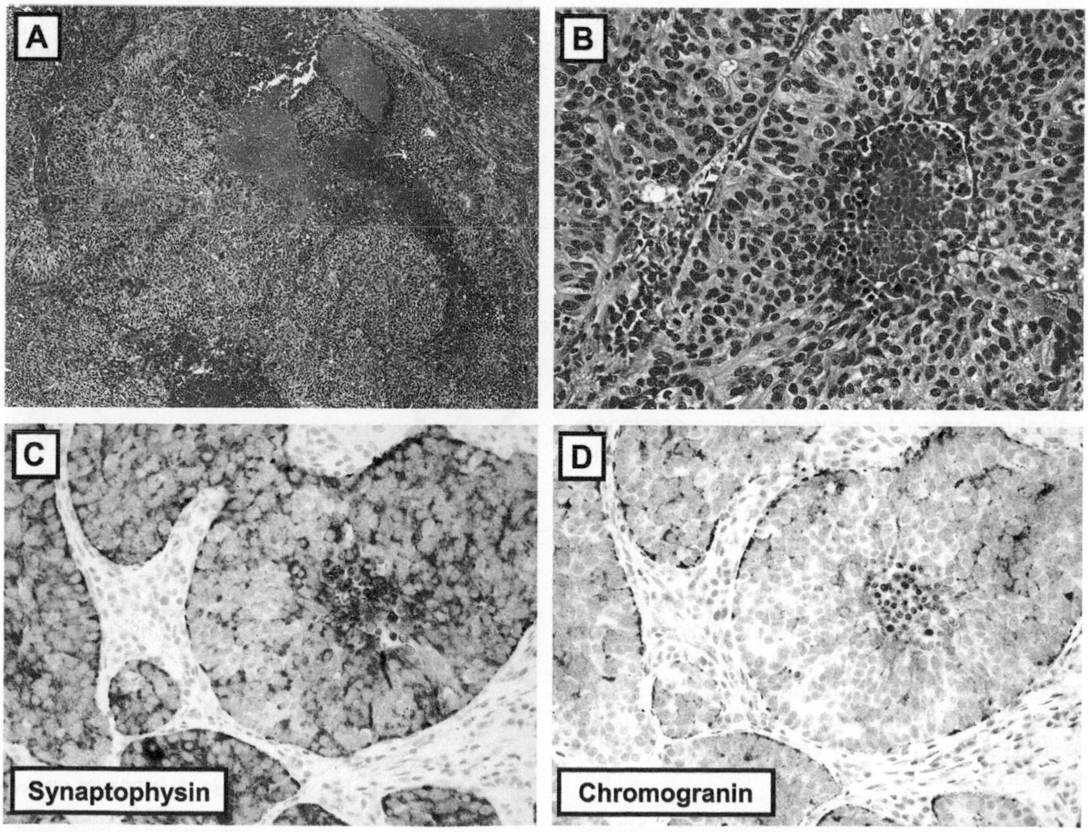

Fig. 6. LCNEC of lung. (*A*) Histologically, an organoid to trabecular architecture is apparent (hematoxylin-eosin, original magnification ×100). (*B*) Tumor cells show moderate eosinophilic cytoplasm, coarse chromatin, variably prominent nucleoli (hematoxylin-eosin, original magnification ×400). In addition to the neuroendocrine morphology, the presence of neuroendocrine differentiation is confirmed by immunohistochemistry for (*C*) synaptophysin (original magnification ×400) and (*D*) chromogranin (original magnification ×400) in this example.

DIFFERENTIAL DIAGNOSIS

Among pulmonary neuroendocrine tumors, the diagnosis of LCNEC may be the most challenging, given its wide morphologic spectrum and tremendous overlap with SCLC, poorly differentiated adenocarcinoma/squamous cell carcinoma, carcinoid tumors, and metastasis.

For a subset of LCNECs, distinction from SCLC or combined SCLC-LCNEC can be problematic, with considerable nuclear size overlap[53,61] and interobserver variability.[6,7] Both LCNEC and SCLC are high-grade tumors with overlapping expression of neuroendocrine markers, TTF-1, and Ki-67 LI. Because complete loss of RB1 expression is found in greater than 95% of SCLCs and approximately 50% of LCNECs,[7,15,52,59] intact RB1 expression in equivocal cases may favor LCNECs over SCLCs.

A subset of LCNECs morphologically resembles poorly differentiated lung adenocarcinoma (in particular, the cribriform/solid variant) and squamous cell carcinoma.[62] Up to 30% of lung adenocarcinoma and squamous cell carcinoma can be positive for a neuroendocrine marker (synaptophysin, chromogranin, or CD56).[9] Neuroendocrine marker expression alone is thus not sufficient for the diagnosis of LCNEC without supportive neuroendocrine histomorphology.[8] Conversely, napsin A can be focally seen in LCNEC (in particular those with NSCLC-like genomic features), although not in a diffuse fashion typical of most lung adenocarcinomas.[63]

A small subset of LCNECs appears carcinoid-like[36] and may correspond to cases with carcinoid-like genomic features[15]; by definition, a mitotic count of greater than or equal to 11 per 2 mm^2 would exclude carcinoid tumors.

LCNEC may be confused with metastasis, such as from breast or prostatic carcinoma, or gastrointestinal or pancreatic neuroendocrine carcinoma. Diagnostic clues that favor metastasis include history of prior malignancy, lack of smoking history, and small circumscribed peripheral tumor(s). In high-grade neuroendocrine carcinomas, including LCNEC and SCLC, TTF-1 expression is not specific for lung origin and not useful for primary site determination. Correlation with clinical history and radiologic findings as well as select immunohistochemical stains (mammaglobin for breast and PSA and PSAP for prostatic primary) may aid the distinction between pulmonary LCNEC and metastasis.

PROGNOSIS

LCNEC has a 5-year overall survival of approximately 15% to 40%, with frequent metastases to liver, brain, and/or bone.[3,18,22,58] Resectable LCNEC is treated by surgical excision. For unresectable LCNEC, treatment options include chemotherapy and/or radiotherapy. Optimal systemic treatment of LCNEC has not been established, however; patients may be treated with SCLC-regimen (etoposide/platinum) or NSCLC-regimen, although LCNEC appears overall more aggressive than most NSCLC and less responsive to SCLC-regimen.[57,58] Recent data suggest *RB1* status as a potential biomarker in selecting LCNEC patients for SCLC-regimen versus NSCLC-regimen, with LCNEC carrying wild-type *RB1* or showing intact RB1 expression to be more responsive to NSCLC-regimen.[59]

Key Features of Large Cell Neuroendocrine Carcinoma

- High-grade NSCLC with neuroendocrine histology and evidence of neuroendocrine differentiation (by ultrastructural and/or immunohistochemical studies)
- Greater than or equal to 11 mitoses per 2 mm^2 with minimal to extensive geographic necrosis
- Predilection for smokers
- Genetically heterogeneous with distinct molecular subgroups: SCLC-like, NSCLC-like, and carcinoid-like

Pitfalls in Diagnosing Large Cell Neuroendocrine Carcinoma

! Without supportive neuroendocrine histomorphology, neuroendocrine marker expression alone is not sufficient for the diagnosis of LCNEC.

! Metastases (from breast or prostatic carcinoma, or gastrointestinal or pancreatic neuroendocrine carcinoma) can be close mimics. Clues that favor metastases include history of prior malignancy, lack of smoking history, and small circumscribed peripheral tumor(s). Select immunohistochemical stains (mammaglobin for breast and PSA/PSAP for prostate) aid distinction.

! TTF-1 is expressed in some high-grade neuroendocrine carcinomas of other sites and is not specific for lung primary.

ΔΔ *Differential Diagnosis* of Large Cell Neuroendocrine Carcinoma

- SCLC
  - Small cell cytomorphology, with nuclear molding, scant cytoplasm, and inconspicuous nucleoli
- Poorly differentiated lung adenocarcinoma
  - Diverse histologic patterns, including solid and cribriform
  - Expresses napsin A in a subset of cases; diffuse napsin A staining favors adenocarcinoma over LCNEC
  - Mucicarmine stain may highlight focal mucin consistent with glandular differentiation.
- Squamous cell carcinoma
  - Expresses p40, p63, and CK5/6
  - Lack of synaptophysin or chromogranin expression in most cases
- Carcinoid tumors
  - Necrosis at most focal and generally not extensive
  - 0 to 10 mitoses per 2 mm^2
  - Show diffuse strong staining for synaptophysin and chromogranin in most cases
  - Ki-67 LI less than 20%
- Metastasis from gastrointestinal or pancreatic neuroendocrine tumor
  - Supportive clinical and/or radiographic findings
  - TTF-1 expression not specific
- Metastatic carcinoma from breast or prostate
  - Supportive clinical and/or radiographic findings
  - Expresses mammaglobin (breast) or PSA/PSAP (prostate)
  - Lack of TTF-1 immunoreactivity

REFERENCES

1. Travis WD, Brambilla E, Burke A, et al. Pathology and genetics of tumors of the lung, pleura, thymus, and heart. 4th edition. Lyon (France): IARC Press; 2015.
2. Rindi G, Klimstra DS, Abedi-Ardekani B, et al. A common classification framework for neuroendocrine neoplasms: an International Agency for Research on Cancer (IARC) and World Health Organization (WHO) expert consensus proposal. Mod Pathol 2018;31(12):1770–86.
3. Travis WD, Rush W, Flieder DB, et al. Survival analysis of 200 pulmonary neuroendocrine tumors with clarification of criteria for atypical carcinoid and its separation from typical carcinoid. Am J Surg Pathol 1998;22(8):934–44.
4. Swarts DR, van Suylen RJ, den Bakker MA, et al. Interobserver variability for the WHO classification of pulmonary carcinoids. Am J Surg Pathol 2014; 38(10):1429–36.
5. Travis WD, Gal AA, Colby TV, et al. Reproducibility of neuroendocrine lung tumor classification. Hum Pathol 1998;29(3):272–9.
6. den Bakker MA, Willemsen S, Grunberg K, et al. Small cell carcinoma of the lung and large cell neuroendocrine carcinoma interobserver variability. Histopathology 2010;56(3):356–63.
7. Thunnissen E, Borczuk AC, Flieder DB, et al. The use of immunohistochemistry improves the diagnosis of small cell lung cancer and its differential diagnosis. An international reproducibility study in a demanding set of cases. J Thorac Oncol 2017; 12(2):334–46.
8. Travis WD, Brambilla E, Nicholson AG. Testing for neuroendocrine immunohistochemical markers should not be performed in poorly differentiated NSCCs in the absence of neuroendocrine morphologic features according to the 2015 WHO classification. J Thorac Oncol 2016;11(2):e26–7.
9. Derks JL, Dingemans AC, van Suylen RJ, et al. Is the sum of positive neuroendocrine immunohistochemical stains useful for diagnosis of large cell neuroendocrine carcinoma (LCNEC) on biopsy specimens? Histopathology 2019;74(4):555–66.
10. Pelosi G, Rodriguez J, Viale G, et al. Typical and atypical pulmonary carcinoid tumor overdiagnosed

as small-cell carcinoma on biopsy specimens: a major pitfall in the management of lung cancer patients. Am J Surg Pathol 2005;29(2):179–87.

11. Fabbri A, Cossa M, Sonzogni A, et al. Ki-67 labeling index of neuroendocrine tumors of the lung has a high level of correspondence between biopsy samples and surgical specimens when strict counting guidelines are applied. Virchows Arch 2017;470(2): 153–64.
12. Marchevsky AM, Hendifar A, Walts AE. The use of Ki-67 labeling index to grade pulmonary well-differentiated neuroendocrine neoplasms: current best evidence. Mod Pathol 2018;31(10):1523–31.
13. Fernandez-Cuesta L, Peifer M, Lu X, et al. Frequent mutations in chromatin-remodelling genes in pulmonary carcinoids. Nat Commun 2014;5:3518.
14. George J, Lim JS, Jang SJ, et al. Comprehensive genomic profiles of small cell lung cancer. Nature 2015;524(7563):47–53.
15. Rekhtman N, Pietanza MC, Hellmann MD, et al. Next-generation sequencing of pulmonary large cell neuroendocrine carcinoma reveals small cell carcinoma-like and non-small cell carcinoma-like subsets. Clin Cancer Res 2016;22(14):3618–29.
16. Simbolo M, Mafficini A, Sikora KO, et al. Lung neuroendocrine tumours: deep sequencing of the four World Health Organization histotypes reveals chromatin-remodelling genes as major players and a prognostic role for TERT, RB1, MEN1 and KMT2D. J Pathol 2017;241(4):488–500.
17. George J, Walter V, Peifer M, et al. Integrative genomic profiling of large-cell neuroendocrine carcinomas reveals distinct subtypes of high-grade neuroendocrine lung tumors. Nat Commun 2018;9(1):1048.
18. Asamura H, Kameya T, Matsuno Y, et al. Neuroendocrine neoplasms of the lung: a prognostic spectrum. J Clin Oncol 2006;24(1):70–6.
19. Ferolla P, Daddi N, Urbani M, et al. Tumorlets, multicentric carcinoids, lymph-nodal metastases, and long-term behavior in bronchial carcinoids. J Thorac Oncol 2009;4(3):383–7.
20. Rugge M, Fassan M, Clemente R, et al. Bronchopulmonary carcinoid: phenotype and long-term outcome in a single-institution series of Italian patients. Clin Cancer Res 2008;14(1):149–54.
21. Kaltsas G, Androulakis II, de Herder WW, et al. Paraneoplastic syndromes secondary to neuroendocrine tumours. Endocr Relat Cancer 2010;17(3):R173–93.
22. Travis WD, Linnoila RI, Tsokos MG, et al. Neuroendocrine tumors of the lung with proposed criteria for large-cell neuroendocrine carcinoma. An ultrastructural, immunohistochemical, and flow cytometric study of 35 cases. Am J Surg Pathol 1991;15(6):529–53.
23. Tsuta K, Kalhor N, Raso MG, et al. Oncocytic neuroendocrine tumors of the lung: histopathologic spectrum and immunohistochemical analysis of 15 cases. Hum Pathol 2011;42(4):578–85.
24. Du EZ, Goldstraw P, Zacharias J, et al. TTF-1 expression is specific for lung primary in typical and atypical carcinoids: TTF-1-positive carcinoids are predominantly in peripheral location. Hum Pathol 2004;35(7):825–31.
25. Miller RR, Muller NL. Neuroendocrine cell hyperplasia and obliterative bronchiolitis in patients with peripheral carcinoid tumors. Am J Surg Pathol 1995; 19(6):653–8.
26. Marchevsky AM, Wirtschafter E, Walts AE. The spectrum of changes in adults with multifocal pulmonary neuroendocrine proliferations: what is the minimum set of pathologic criteria to diagnose DIPNECH? Hum Pathol 2015;46(2):176–81.
27. Srivastava A, Hornick JL. Immunohistochemical staining for CDX-2, PDX-1, NESP-55, and TTF-1 can help distinguish gastrointestinal carcinoid tumors from pancreatic endocrine and pulmonary carcinoid tumors. Am J Surg Pathol 2009;33(4):626–32.
28. Long KB, Srivastava A, Hirsch MS, et al. PAX8 Expression in well-differentiated pancreatic endocrine tumors: correlation with clinicopathologic features and comparison with gastrointestinal and pulmonary carcinoid tumors. Am J Surg Pathol 2010;34(5):723–9.
29. Weissferdt A, Tang X, Wistuba II, et al. Comparative immunohistochemical analysis of pulmonary and thymic neuroendocrine carcinomas using PAX8 and TTF-1. Mod Pathol 2013;26(12):1554–60.
30. Vahidi S, Stewart J, Amin K, et al. Metastatic medullary thyroid carcinoma or calcitonin-secreting carcinoid tumor of lung? A diagnostic dilemma in a patient with lung mass and thyroid nodule. Diagn Cytopathol 2018;46(4):345–8.
31. Duan K, Mete O. Algorithmic approach to neuroendocrine tumors in targeted biopsies: practical applications of immunohistochemical markers. Cancer Cytopathol 2016;124(12):871–84.
32. Chong CR, Wirth LJ, Nishino M, et al. Chemotherapy for locally advanced and metastatic pulmonary carcinoid tumors. Lung Cancer 2014;86(2):241–6.
33. Caplin ME, Baudin E, Ferolla P, et al. Pulmonary neuroendocrine (carcinoid) tumors: European Neuroendocrine Tumor Society expert consensus and recommendations for best practice for typical and atypical pulmonary carcinoids. Ann Oncol 2015;26(8):1604–20.
34. Yao JC, Fazio N, Singh S, et al. Everolimus for the treatment of advanced, non-functional neuroendocrine tumours of the lung or gastrointestinal tract (RADIANT-4): a randomised, placebo-controlled, phase 3 study. Lancet 2016;387(10022):968–77.
35. Hendifar AE, Marchevsky AM, Tuli R. Neuroendocrine tumors of the lung: Current challenges and advances in the diagnosis and management of well-differentiated disease. J Thorac Oncol 2017;12(3): 425–36.

36. Quinn AM, Chaturvedi A, Nonaka D. High-grade neuroendocrine carcinoma of the lung with carcinoid morphology: a study of 12 cases. Am J Surg Pathol 2017;41(2):263–70.
37. Gupta R, Dastane A, McKenna RJ Jr, et al. What can we learn from the errors in the frozen section diagnosis of pulmonary carcinoid tumors? An evidence-based approach. Hum Pathol 2009;40(1):1–9.
38. Doyle LA, Wong KK, Bueno R, et al. Ewing sarcoma mimicking atypical carcinoid tumor: detection of unexpected genomic alterations demonstrates the use of next generation sequencing as a diagnostic tool. Cancer Genet 2014;207(7–8):335–9.
39. Derks JL, Speel EJ, Thunnissen E, et al. Neuroendocrine cancer of the lung: a diagnostic puzzle. J Thorac Oncol 2016;11(3):e35–8.
40. Govindan R, Page N, Morgensztern D, et al. Changing epidemiology of small-cell lung cancer in the United States over the last 30 years: analysis of the surveillance, epidemiologic, and end results database. J Clin Oncol 2006;24(28):4539–44.
41. Varghese AM, Zakowski MF, Yu HA, et al. Small-cell lung cancers in patients who never smoked cigarettes. J Thorac Oncol 2014;9(6):892–6.
42. Micke P, Faldum A, Metz T, et al. Staging small cell lung cancer: Veterans Administration Lung Study Group versus International Association for the Study of Lung Cancer–what limits limited disease? Lung Cancer 2002;37(3):271–6.
43. Nicholson SA, Beasley MB, Brambilla E, et al. Small cell lung carcinoma (SCLC): a clinicopathologic study of 100 cases with surgical specimens. Am J Surg Pathol 2002;26(9):1184–97.
44. Harbour JW, Lai SL, Whang-Peng J, et al. Abnormalities in structure and expression of the human retinoblastoma gene in SCLC. Science 1988;241(4863):353–7.
45. Takahashi T, Nau MM, Chiba I, et al. p53: a frequent target for genetic abnormalities in lung cancer. Science 1989;246(4929):491–4.
46. Peifer M, Fernandez-Cuesta L, Sos ML, et al. Integrative genome analyses identify key somatic driver mutations of small-cell lung cancer. Nat Genet 2012; 44(10):1104–10.
47. Rudin CM, Durinck S, Stawiski EW, et al. Comprehensive genomic analysis identifies SOX2 as a frequently amplified gene in small-cell lung cancer. Nat Genet 2012;44(10):1111–6.
48. Niederst MJ, Sequist LV, Poirier JT, et al. RB loss in resistant EGFR mutant lung adenocarcinomas that transform to small-cell lung cancer. Nat Commun 2015;6:6377.
49. Lee JK, Lee J, Kim S, et al. Clonal history and genetic predictors of transformation into small-cell carcinomas from lung adenocarcinomas. J Clin Oncol 2017;35(26):3065–74.
50. Azzopardi JG. Oat-cell carcinoma of the bronchus. J Pathol Bacteriol 1959;78:513–9.
51. Guinee DG Jr, Fishback NF, Koss MN, et al. The spectrum of immunohistochemical staining of small-cell lung carcinoma in specimens from transbronchial and open-lung biopsies. Am J Clin Pathol 1994;102(4):406–14.
52. Igarashi T, Jiang SX, Kameya T, et al. Divergent cyclin B1 expression and Rb/p16/cyclin D1 pathway aberrations among pulmonary neuroendocrine tumors. Mod Pathol 2004;17(10):1259–67.
53. Marchevsky AM, Gal AA, Shah S, et al. Morphometry confirms the presence of considerable nuclear size overlap between "small cells" and "large cells" in high-grade pulmonary neuroendocrine neoplasms. Am J Clin Pathol 2001;116(4):466–72.
54. Hung YP, Fletcher CD, Hornick JL. Evaluation of NKX2-2 expression in round cell sarcomas and other tumors with EWSR1 rearrangement: imperfect specificity for Ewing sarcoma. Mod Pathol 2016;29(4):370–80.
55. Lok BH, Gardner EE, Schneeberger VE, et al. PARP inhibitor activity correlates with SLFN11 expression and demonstrates synergy with temozolomide in small cell lung cancer. Clin Cancer Res 2017;23(2):523–35.
56. Sabari JK, Lok BH, Laird JH, et al. Unravelling the biology of SCLC: implications for therapy. Nat Rev Clin Oncol 2017;14(9):549–61.
57. Fasano M, Della Corte CM, Papaccio F, et al. Pulmonary large-cell neuroendocrine carcinoma: From epidemiology to therapy. J Thorac Oncol 2015; 10(8):1133–41.
58. Naidoo J, Santos-Zabala ML, Iyriboz T, et al. Large cell neuroendocrine carcinoma of the lung: Clinico-pathologic features, treatment, and outcomes. Clin Lung Cancer 2016;17(5):e121–9.
59. Derks JL, Leblay N, Thunnissen E, et al. Molecular subtypes of pulmonary large-cell neuroendocrine carcinoma predict chemotherapy treatment outcome. Clin Cancer Res 2018;24(1):33–42.
60. Travis WD, Brambilla E, Noguchi M, et al. Diagnosis of lung cancer in small biopsies and cytology: implications of the 2011 International Association for the Study of Lung Cancer/American Thoracic Society/ European Respiratory Society classification. Arch Pathol Lab Med 2013;137(5):668–84.
61. Hiroshima K, Iyoda A, Shida T, et al. Distinction of pulmonary large cell neuroendocrine carcinoma from small cell lung carcinoma: a morphological, immunohistochemical, and molecular analysis. Mod Pathol 2006;19(10):1358–68.
62. Jiang SX, Kameya T, Shoji M, et al. Large cell neuroendocrine carcinoma of the lung: a histologic and immunohistochemical study of 22 cases. Am J Surg Pathol 1998;22(5):526–37.
63. Rekhtman N, Pietanza CM, Sabari J, et al. Pulmonary large cell neuroendocrine carcinoma with adenocarcinoma-like features: Napsin A expression and genomic alterations. Mod Pathol 2018;31(1): 111–21.

UNITED STATES POSTAL SERVICE®

Statement of Ownership, Management, and Circulation (All Periodicals Publications Except Requester Publications)

1. Publication Title	2. Publication Number	3. Filing Date
SURGICAL PATHOLOGY CLINICS	025 – 478	9/18/2019
4. Issue Frequency	5. Number of Issues Published Annually	6. Annual Subscription Price
MAR, JUN, SEP, DEC	4	$213.00

7. Complete Mailing Address of Known Office of Publication (Not printer) (Street, city, county, state, and ZIP+4®)
ELSEVIER INC.
230 Park Avenue, Suite 800
New York, NY 10169

Contact Person: STEPHEN R. BUSHING
Telephone (Include area code): 215-239-3688

8. Complete Mailing Address of Headquarters or General Business Office of Publisher (Not printer)
ELSEVIER INC.
230 Park Avenue, Suite 800
New York, NY 10169

9. Full Names and Complete Mailing Addresses of Publisher, Editor, and Managing Editor (Do not leave blank)

Publisher (Name and complete mailing address)
TAYLOR BALL, ELSEVIER INC.
1600 JOHN F KENNEDY BLVD. SUITE 1800
PHILADELPHIA, PA 19103-2899

Editor (Name and complete mailing address)
KATERINA HEIDHAUSEN, ELSEVIER INC.
1600 JOHN F KENNEDY BLVD. SUITE 1800
PHILADELPHIA, PA 19103-2899

Managing Editor (Name and complete mailing address)
PATRICK MANLEY, ELSEVIER INC.
1600 JOHN F KENNEDY BLVD. SUITE 1800
PHILADELPHIA, PA 19103-2899

10. Owner (*Do not leave blank. If the publication is owned by a corporation, give the name and address of the corporation immediately followed by the names and addresses of all stockholders owning or holding 1 percent or more of the total amount of stock. If not owned by a corporation, give the names and addresses of the individual owners. If owned by a partnership or other unincorporated firm, give its name and address as well as those of each individual owner. If the publication is published by a nonprofit organization, give its name and address.*)

Full Name	Complete Mailing Address
WHOLLY OWNED SUBSIDIARY OF REED/ELSEVIER, US HOLDINGS	1600 JOHN F KENNEDY BLVD. SUITE 1800 PHILADELPHIA, PA 19103-2899

11. Known Bondholders, Mortgagees, and Other Security Holders Owning or Holding 1 Percent or More of Total Amount of Bonds, Mortgages, or Other Securities. If none, check box → ☐ None

Full Name	Complete Mailing Address
N/A	

12. Tax Status (*For completion by nonprofit organizations authorized to mail at nonprofit rates*) (*Check one*)
The purpose, function, and nonprofit status of this organization and the exempt status for federal income tax purposes:
☒ Has Not Changed During Preceding 12 Months
☐ Has Changed During Preceding 12 Months (*Publisher must submit explanation of change with this statement*)

13. Publication Title: SURGICAL PATHOLOGY CLINICS
14. Issue Date for Circulation Data Below: JUNE 2019

15. Extent and Nature of Circulation			Average No. Copies Each Issue During Preceding 12 Months	No. Copies of Single Issue Published Nearest to Filing Date
a. Total Number of Copies (*Net press run*)			265	309
b. Paid Circulation (By Mail and Outside the Mail)	(1)	Mailed Outside-County Paid Subscriptions Stated on PS Form 3541 (include paid distribution above nominal rate, advertiser's proof copies, and exchange copies)	186	236
	(2)	Mailed In-County Paid Subscriptions Stated on PS Form 3541 (*Include paid distribution above nominal rate, advertiser's proof copies, and exchange copies*)	0	0
	(3)	Paid Distribution Outside the Mails Including Sales Through Dealers and Carriers, Street Vendors, Counter Sales, and Other Paid Distribution Outside USPS®	45	68
	(4)	Paid Distribution by Other Classes of Mail Through the USPS (e.g., First-Class Mail®)	0	0
c. Total Paid Distribution [*Sum of 15b (1), (2), (3), and (4)*]			231	304
d. Free or Nominal Rate Distribution (By Mail and Outside the Mail)	(1)	Free or Nominal Rate Outside-County Copies included on PS Form 3541	34	5
	(2)	Free or Nominal Rate In-County Copies Included on PS Form 3541	0	0
	(3)	Free or Nominal Rate Copies Mailed at Other Classes Through the USPS (e.g., First-Class Mail)	0	0
	(4)	Free or Nominal Rate Distribution Outside the Mail (*Carriers or other means*)	0	0
e. Total Free or Nominal Rate Distribution (*Sum of 15d (1), (2), (3) and (4)*)			34	5
f. Total Distribution (*Sum of 15c and 15e*)			265	309
g. Copies not Distributed (*See Instructions to Publishers #4 (page #3)*)			0	0
h. Total (*Sum of 15f and g*)			265	309
i. Percent Paid (*15c divided by 15f times 100*)			87.17%	98.38%

* If you are claiming electronic copies, go to line 16 on page 3. If you are not claiming electronic copies, skip to line 17 on page 3.

16. Electronic Copy Circulation	Average No. Copies Each Issue During Preceding 12 Months	No. Copies of Single Issue Published Nearest to Filing Date
a. Paid Electronic Copies		
b. Total Paid Print Copies (Line 15c) + Paid Electronic Copies (Line 16a)		
c. Total Print Distribution (Line 15f) + Paid Electronic Copies (Line 16a)		
d. Percent Paid (Both Print & Electronic Copies) (16b divided by 16c × 100)		

☒ **I certify that 50% of all my distributed copies (electronic and print) are paid above a nominal price.**

17. Publication of Statement of Ownership
☒ If the publication is a general publication, publication of this statement is required. Will be printed in the DECEMBER 2019 issue of this publication. ☐ Publication not required.

18. Signature and Title of Editor, Publisher, Business Manager, or Owner
Stephen R. Bushing
STEPHEN R. BUSHING - INVENTORY DISTRIBUTION CONTROL MANAGER
Date: 9/18/2019

I certify that all information furnished on this form is true and complete. I understand that anyone who furnishes false or misleading information on this form or who omits material or information requested on the form may be subject to criminal sanctions (including fines and imprisonment) and/or civil sanctions (including civil penalties).

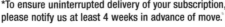

Printed and bound by CPI Group (UK) Ltd, Croydon, CR0 4YY
03/10/2024
01041527-0001

Printed and bound by CPI Group (UK) Ltd, Croydon, CR0 4YY
03/10/2024
01040307-0001